CORONARY STENOSIS MORPHOLOGY:
ANALYSIS AND IMPLICATION

Developments in Cardiovascular Medicine

M.LeWinter. H. Suga and M.W. Watkins (eds.): *Cardiac Energetics: From Emax to Pressure-volume Area*. 1995   ISBN 0-7923-3721-2
R.J. Siegel (ed.): *Ultrasound Angioplasty*. 1995 ISBN 0-7923-3722-0
D.M. Yellon and G.J. Gross (eds.): *Myocardial Protection and the Katp Channel*. 1995   ISBN 0-7923-3791-3
A.V.G. Bruschke. J.H.C. Reiber. K.I. Lie and H.J.J. Wellens (eds.): *Lipid Lowering Therapy and Progression of Coronary Atherosclerosis*. 1996
                ISBN 0-7923-3807-3
A.S.A. Abd-Elfattah and A.S. Wechsler (eds.): *Purines and Myocardial Protection*. 1995   ISBN 0-7923-3831-6
M. Morad, S. Ebashi, W. Trautwein and Y. Kurachi (eds.): *Molecular Physiology and Pharmacology of Cardiac Ion Channels and Transporters*. 1996
                ISBN 0-7923-3913-4
A.M. Oto (ed.): *Practice and Progress in Cardiac Pacing and Electrophysiology*. 1996   ISBN 0-7923-3950-9
W.H. Birkenhager (ed.): *Practical Management of Hypertension. Second Edition*. 1996   ISBN 0-7923-3952-5
J.C. Chatham, J.R. Forder and J.H. McNeill(eds.):*The Heart In Diabetes*. 1996   ISBN 0-7923-4052-3
M. Kroll, M. Lehmann (eds.): *Implantable Cardioverter Defibrillator Therapy: The Engineering-Clinical Interface* 1996   ISBN 0-7923-4300-X
Lloyd Klein (ed.): *Coronary Stenosis Morphology: Analysis and Implication* 1996   ISBN 0-7923-9867-X
Julio E. Perez, Roberto M. Lang, (eds.): *Echocardiography and Cardiovascular Function: Tools for the Next Decade* 1996   ISBN 0-7923-9884-X

CORONARY STENOSIS MORPHOLOGY:
ANALYSIS AND IMPLICATION

edited by

Lloyd W. Klein, M.D.
Department of Cardiology
Rush-Presbyterian-St. Luke's Medical Center
Rush Medical School
Chicago, IL

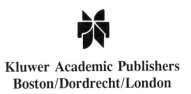

Kluwer Academic Publishers
Boston/Dordrecht/London

DISTRIBUTORS

For North America:

Kluwer Academic Publishers
101 Philip Drive
Norwell, Massachusetts 02061 USA

For all other countries:

Kluwer Academic Publishers Group
Distribution Centre
Post Office Box 322
3300 AH Dordrecht, THE NETHERLANDS

Library of Congress Cataloging-in-Publication Data

Coronary stenosis morphology: analysis and implication/edited by Lloyd W. Klein.
       p. cm. -- (Developments in cardiovascular medicine)
                  Includes index.
    ISBN 0-7923-9867-X (alk. paper)
    1. Coronary artery stenosis. I.. Klein, Lloyd W. II. Series.
    [DNLM: 1. Coronary Disease--diagnosis. 2. Coronary Disease--physiopathology.
    3. Coronary Disease--therapy. WG 300 C82564 1997]
    RC685.C58C676   1997
    616.1'23075--dc21
    DNLM/DLC   for Library of Congress   96-53049
                                             CIP

Copyright 1997 by Kluwer Academic Publishers

Printed on acid-free paper.

Printed in the United States of America

Contents

List of Contributors

Introduction: Clinical Analysis and Utilization of Coronary Stenosis Morphology
Lloyd W. Klein, M.D.

Section One: Assessment of Stenosis Morphology

1. Morphologic analysis of coronary stenoses by coronary
    angiography: Subjective variability and accuracy
    Nasser M. Lakkis and Neil Kleiman   1

2. Intravascular ultrasound: Equipment, technique and
    applications in clinical practice and research
    Steven Nissen and Lloyd W. Klein   31

3. Quantitative analysis of lesion morphology by
    computerized techniques
    G. B. John Mancini and Gilles Hudon   53

4. Intravascular angioscopy in the analysis of stenosis
    morphologic and composition: Therapeutic implications
    Steve Feld and Richard Smalling   83

5. Computerized three-dimension intravascular
    reconstruction
    Richard R. Heuser, T Laas, B Prebil, and DB Reid   103

Section Two: Implications of Stenosis Morphology on Pathogenesis

6. Coronary stenosis morphology: The importance of lesion
    length, stenosis eccentricity, severity, and coronary blood
    flow in clinical decision making
    Morton Kern, Thomas J. Donohue and Richard G. Bach   121

7. Angiographic stenosis and acute coronary syndromes:
    Progression of stenoses to myocardial infarction
    William Little and Robert J. Applegate   161

8. Unstable angina and non-Q wave myocardial infarction:
    Pathogenetic mechanisms and morphology of the unstable
    plaque
    Lloyd W. Klein   177

9. Defining coronary pathology and clinical syndromes by
    coronary angioscopy
    James Forrester, Frank Litvack, Neal Eigler and
    Robert J. Siegel   211

10. Usefulness of intravascular ultrasound for detecting
    atherosclerosis progression or regression
    Mun K. Hong, Martin B. Leon and Gary Mintz   239

**Section Three: Selection of Treatment Options Guided by
Morphologic Assessment**

11. Stenosis morphology and risk assessment in balloon
    angioplasty
    Steven Ellis and Koon-Hou Mak   251

12. Intravascular ultrasound -guided selection of new
    coronary devices in coronary intervention
    Stuart Higano and David R. Holmes   281

13. Lesion morphology and composition: Risk of restenosis
    following coronary interventions
    Bradley Strauss and Madhu K. Natarajan   311

14. Pitfalls and practical approach to the use of
     imaging techniques in developing clinical
     strategies
     Terry R. Bowers, Barry M. Kaplan and
     William W. O'Neill   343

Index   383

List of contributors

Lloyd W. Klein
Associate Professor of Medicine
Director, Interventional Cardiology
Co-Director, Cardiac Catheterization Laboratories
Section of Cardiology
Rush-Presbyterian-St. Luke's Medical Center
Chicago, Illinois

Neil Kleiman
Associate Professor of Medicine
Assistant Director of Cardiac Catheterization Laboratories
Section of Cardiology
Baylor College of Medicine
Houston, TX

Nasser M Lakkis
Section of Cardiology
Baylor College of Medicine
Houston, TX

James Forrester
Professor of Medicine
Buirns and Allen Chair in Cardiology
Director, Division of Cardiology
Cedars-Sinai Med Center
Los Angeles, CA

Frank Litvack
Associate Director of Medicine
Co-Director, Division of Cardiology
Cedars-Sinai Med Center
Los Angeles, CA

Neal Eigler
Co-Director, Cardiovascular Intervention Center
Division of Cardiology
Associate Professor of Medicine
UCLA School of Medicine
Cedars-Sinai Med Center
Los Angeles, CA

Robert J. Siegel
Division of Cardiology
Cedars-Sinai Med Center
Los Angeles, CA

Stephen G. Ellis
Director, Sones Cardiac Catheterization Laboratories
Department of Cardiology
Cleveland Clinic foundation
Cleveland, OH 44106

Koon-Hou Mak, M.B.B.S.
Cardiology Interventional Fellow
Interventional Cardiology
Cleveland ClinicFfoundation
Cleveland, OH 44106

Steven Nissen
Vice Chairman of Cardiology
Director, Clinical Cardiology
Cleveland Clinic Foundation
Cleveland, OH

Gary Mintz
Direrctor, Intravascular Ultrasound Program
Section of Cardiology
Washington Hospital Center
Washington, DC

Mun K. Hong
Director, Experimental Physiology and Pharmacology
Section of Cardiology
Washington Hospital Center
Washington, DC

Martin B. Leon
Director, Cardiovascular Research
Section of Cardiology
Washington Hospital Center
Washington, DC

G. B. Mancini
Eric W. Hamber Professor and Head
Department of Internal Medicine
University of B.C. and Vancouver Hospital
Vancouver, B.C., Canada

Giles Hudon, M.D.
Head, Department of Radiology
Montreal Heart Institute
Associate Professor, Radiology
University of Montreal
Montreal, CA

Richard Smalling
Professor of Medicine
Co-Director, Division of Cardiology
University of Texas Health Science Center
Houston, TX

Steven Feld
Cardiology Interventional Fellow
Shaare Zedek Hospital
Jerusalem, Israel

Richard Heuser
Arizona Heart Institue
Phoenix, AZ

Terry Laas
Quinton Imaging Division
Sunnyvale, CA
Brian Prebil
Research and Education
Arizona Heart Institue
Phoenix, AZ

Donald B. Reid, M.D.
Arizona Heart Institue
Phoenix, AZ

Morton J. Kern
Director, Cardiac Catheterization Laboratories
Dept. of Internal Medicine
St. Louis University
St. Louis, Mo

Thomas J. Donohue
Assistant Professor of Medicine
Co-Director, J.G. Mudd Cardiac Cath Laboratory
St. Louis University
St. Louis, MO

Richard G. Bach
Assistant Professor of Medicine
J.G. Mudd Cardiac Cath Laboratory
St. Louis University
St. Louis, MO

William Little
Professor of Medicine
Chief, Division of Cardiology
Bowman Grey School of Medicine
Winston-Salem, NC

Robert J. Applegate
Associate Professor, Internal Medicine
Section of Cardiology
Bowman Gray School of Medicine
Wake Forest University
Winston-Salem, NC

Lloyd W. Klein
Director, Interventional Cardiology
Co-Director, Cardiac Catheterization Laboratories
Associate Professor of Medicine
Rush Medical College and
Rush-Pres.-St. Luke's Medical Center
Chicago, IL

Stuart Higano
Assistant Professor of Medicine
Division of Cardiovascular Diseases
Mayo Clinic
Rochester, MN

David Holmes
Director, Adult Cardiac Catheterization Laboratories
Professor of Medicine
Mayo Clinic
Rochester, MN

Bradley Strauss
Staff Physician, Division of Cardiology
Assistant Professor of Medicine
St. Michael's Hospital
Toronto, Ontario

Madhu K. Natarajan
Clinical Research Fellow
Division of Cardiology
St. Michael's Hospital
Toronto, Ontario

William O'Neill
Division of Cardiology
William Beaumont Hospital
Royal Oak, MI

Terry R. Bowers
Division of Cardiology
William Beaumont Hospital
Royal Oak, MI

Barry M. Kaplan
Division of Cardiology
William Beaumont Hospital
Royal Oak, MI

1.

MORPHOLOGIC ANALYSIS OF CORONARY STENOSES BY CORONARY ANGIOGRAPHY: SUBJECTIVE VARIABILITY AND ACCURACY

Nasser M. Lakkis, M. D.
Neal S. Kleiman, M. D.
The Methodist Hospital-Baylor College of Medicine
Cardiology Section, Houston, Texas

Introduction

Coronary angiography remains the standard technique to evaluate the significance of coronary arterial lesions. It allows identification of severe stenoses that cause ischemia, helps to determine prognosis, to define optimal therapy and the feasibility of angioplasty or bypass surgery. Early studies of coronary angiography demonstrated a link between the number of vessels with severe narrowings and the likelihood of long-term survival (1,2). Concomitantly, a series of experiments, typified by the classic studies of Gould et al (3,4) and Gregg (5) established the relationship between coronary stenosis and the limitation of flow. These findings, coupled historically with the ability of non-invasive testing to detect arterial stenoses, and the advent of coronary artery bypass surgery, further tied interpretations of coronary arteriograms to estimating the severity of stenoses and counting the number of trunks with severe disease. The ultimate impact of these important developments was to increase the appreciation of the relationship between the extent of disease and clinical prognosis, however, an unfortunate result was to obscure other important information about lesion morphology and its pathophysiologic implications.

A series of three developments within the past decade has led to the use of coronary arteriography to study the morphologic characteristics of atherosclerotic lesions: the recognition of plaque rupture as the central pathophysiologic feature of acute ischemic syndromes; the development of percutaneous revascularization techniques such as percutaneous transluminal coronary angioplasty (PTCA), atherectomy, and stenting; as well as refinement of the optical equipment used to obtain and process cineangiograms. However the description of coronary lesions has been complicated by a great deal of subjective variability which is explained on the basis of three broad categories: those related to the performance of angiography, the angiographic equipment, and the observer's expertise.

As is seen with most other surgical procedures, obtaining angiograms adequate to define coronary arterial lesion morphology is operator-dependent. It requires adequate injection of contrast, adequate duration of filming runs, and most importantly, careful selection of projection angles which can isolate the lesion in question without foreshortening or overlap with other structures. Additionally, appropriate interpretation of angiograms also requires considerable diligence and attention to detail. Multiple views are usually necessary since in one view a lesion may look smooth while complex features are seen only in other projections. While the use of orthogonal projections to delineate the stenosis in question is often recommended, obtaining truly orthogonal views (opposed by 90 degrees) is often not feasible for technical reasons, and one of the two paired views may be inadequate due to overlap or foreshortening. Moreover, the best angiographic analysis is often obtained by combining both stop-frame and in-motion views, since images are more easily integrated while they are in motion.

Histologic and Biochemical Correlates of Complex Lesions:

In general, lesions that are not totally occlusive are divided into two types: simple and complex. The angiographic features of 'complicated' plaques were first described by Levin and Fallon (6) who performed post-mortem angiography on the coronary arteries of 39 patients who had died following acute myocardial infarction or coronary artery bypass grafting. A strong relationship was found between complex stenosis as determined angiographically and histologic features of plaque rupture, hemorrhage or thrombi. These pathologic features corresponded to a distinctive angiographic appearance characterized by eccentric, irregular, and shaggy borders with intraluminal haziness. The sensitivity of post mortem angiography was 88% and the specificity was 79% for detecting 'complicated' lesions.

Recently biochemical correlating markers of thrombus formation with complex coronary lesion morphology have been reported. Fibrinopeptide A (FPA), a peptide which is released by thrombin during the formation of fibrin, and which is used as an indicator of thrombin activity, is one of the first coagulation markers measured in patients with complex angiographic coronary lesion morphology. Eisenberg et al (7) correlated the angiographic findings in 29 patients presenting with unstable angina with their FPA levels in an attempt to identify a subgroup of patients with ongoing thrombosis. Seven of 11 (64%) patients with type II eccentric lesions (Ambrose classification, see text later) were found to have increased FPA levels

The expression of tissue factor within atherosclerotic plaque may also play an important role in the thrombotic events associated with plaque disruption. The excision and retrieval of atherosclerotic plaque during coronary atherectomy (DCA) affords an excellent opportunity to study the expression of tissue factor in patients with unstable coronary syndromes. Using a monoclonal anti-tissue factor antibody Marmur et al (8) have identified tissue factor antigen within human atherectomy samples in 8 of 24 (33%) lesions obtained from 24 patients treated with DCA. Lesions in which tissue factor was detected had a higher incidence of complex angiographic morphology (ulceration, irregular borders, or filling defects) compared with lesions in which tissue factor was not detected (6/8 versus 4/16, p=0.03). Lucore et al (9) measured the tissue factor procoagulant activity in human atherosclerotic plaques recovered from patients with unstable coronary syndromes. Nine of 11 plaques (82%) with increased procoagulant activity were obtained from patients with Ambrose type II lesions compared with only 2 plaques obtained from patients with type I eccentric and concentric lesions. These preliminary data suggest that variability of tissue factor expression may help explain the variable thrombotic tendency of different lesions. The association of tissue factor antigen with complex angiographic lesions supports a role of tissue factor in the increased frequency of thrombotic events which occur at these lesions.

There is no study to date correlating markers of platelet activation such as thromboxane metabolites or other markers of platelet activation such as IIb/IIIa receptor or P-selectin with specific lesion morphologies in patients with unstable angina.

In clinical practice, most of the characteristics which describe complex lesions are applied in an arbitrary fashion and reflect what

4

seem to be primarily qualitative features. With careful attention to detail, the analysis of symmetry and irregularity can be reproducible. Some investigators have reported inter and intra-observer consistency of up to 90% (10). However the lack of a common standard between different operators and laboratories, and the absence of uniformly accepted system to grade lesions quantitatively and thus detect subtle changes in response to therapy has led to the development of a variety of different systems for grading morphologic abnormalities. In this context, quantitative measures refer to the assignment of a numeric parameter to substitute for an otherwise descriptive characteristic of a narrowed area. The first attempt to quantify the morphologic features of coronary lesions was published by Mancini et al (11) who described an automated computer program that analyzed digitized angiograms and extracted quantitative morphometric parameters using standard mathematical formulas based on vector and fractal analysis used to describe shapes in engineering applications. This method was originally validated by substituting various mathematical functions for the arterial borders. It allows all lesion characteristics to be described in a continuous fashion and thus avoids the problem of assigning a lesion to a particular predetermined category. The major advantage of this analysis is that it avoids subjective visual inspection. However, the clinical application of this system did not gain widespread usage, and for the most part morphologic characteristics of coronary arterial lesions continue to be either qualitative or semi-quantitative methods.

Morphologic Characteristics of Arterial Lesions:

What follows is a comprehensive review of the commonly described characteristics which are generally regarded as indicators of plaque complexity.

Eccentricity:

Pathologically the vast majority of atheromatous lesions are eccentric. However, this finding is seen less common angiographically since the latter represents the artery in a 2-dimensional view. An eccentric lesion is characterized by a lumen lying in the outer quadrant of the main lumen diameter of the coronary artery (12), leaving a variable arc of normal or nearly normal wall. It can be either smooth or associated with abrupt or overhanging edges, or with steep inflow angles (formed by the main axis of the vessel and a line from the proximal border of the lesion to its maximal narrowing). The latter type of lesion is often seen in patients with acute coronary syndromes (10,13).

The determination of axis symmetry requires knowledge of the location of the vessel lumen with respect to the location of the vessel wall. When the coronary arteries are particularly tortuous this makes the localization of the normal vessel wall very difficult and therefore appropriate views must be selected. It is particularly important in the determination of eccentricity that multiple views be obtained since a lesion may appear concentric in one view but eccentric when viewed from another angiographic. Accordingly any single arbitrary angle of view may significantly misrepresent the eccentric nature of lesions. Theoretically, 2 orthogonal angiograms should accurately reflect the eccentricity of many lesions, but orthogonal views may be unobtainable due to overlapping side branches, disease at bifurcation sites or radiographic foreshortening, and even if all these limitations are overcome, the orthogonal views chosen may still not transect the lesion in its most eccentric plane.

The first attempt to measure the degree of eccentricity in coronary arterial lesions was reported by Fischell et al (14) who defined lumen eccentricity by comparing the ratio of the difference of the lengths between the centerline of the lesion and the estimated vessel wall (a) and the length of the centerline and normal wall at the adjacent segment (b) (Figure 1). This ratio was less than 0.5 in eccentric lesions.

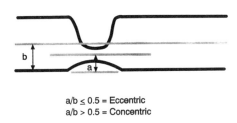

a/b ≤ 0.5 = Eccentric
a/b > 0.5 = Concentric

Figure 1: Eccentricity index as defined by the ratio of difference of centerline of lesion and estimated normal edge and centerline of adjacent segment and normal wall as defined by Fischell et al (14).

Ambrose et al (15) studied lesion morphology in 63 patients with unstable angina and 47 patients with stable angina. Based on angiographic findings, he subclassified eccentric lesions qualitatively into 2 types (Figure 2) : _Type I_ _lesions_ characterized by asymmetric narrowings in the form of convex intraluminal obstructions with smooth borders and a wide neck, or any asymmetric narrowing with smooth borders, _Type II_ _lesions_ are those with eccentric stenoses in the form of convex intraluminal obstructions with a narrow neck due to one or more overlapping edges or irregular and scalloped borders or both. Type II lesions are characterized by rough and irregular edges that appear as small perturbations in the vessel lumen edges within a coronary lesion.

Under this classification, 54% of lesions in patients with unstable angina were type II eccentric compared with 7% of lesions in patients with stable angina (table 1).

ECCENTRIC LESIONS

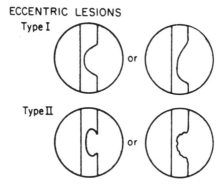

Figure 2: Schematic representation of eccentric lesion morphology used by Ambrose et al (15) in evaluating cineangiograms in patients with coronary syndromes.

Similar findings have been reported by Williams et al (16) demonstrating a strong association between unstable angina and the presence of plaques with eccentric angiographic morphology. The classification of eccentric lesions into 2 types has not found its way into routine clinical use, since its clinical utility (i.e. predicting a response to pharmacologic or mechanical management) has not yet been established.

Table I: Lesion Morphology in Patients with Stable
Angina Versus Patients with Unstable Angina

	SA (47pts)	USA (63 pts)	p-value
Concentric	47%	26%	p=0.01
Type I eccentric	35%	17%	p<0.05
Type II eccentric	7%	54%	p<0.001

SA = Stable Angina
USA = Unstable Angina

Ulceration

Ulcerations are contrast-opacified craters within or adjacent to a stenotic lesion, which resemble ulcers seen on barium studies of the gastrointestinal tract. Ulcerated lesions are frequently seen in patients with rest angina and those recovering from acute myocardial infarction. It is believed that they result from plaque rupture (12,17). They are usually of different shapes (round, ovoid or club shaped) and sizes. The TIMI 4 study investigators (18) developed a qualitative ulceration grading system to assess the severity of ulcerated lesions and found that it predicted the occurrence of early reocclusion after thrombolysis. Grade 0 = no angiographic evidence of ulceration; grade1= lesion contains a neck with contrast material dissecting under the plaque either proximally or distally; grade 2= distinct extravasation of contrast material. Reocclusion occurred in 3% of patients with grade 0 ulceration and 10.7% in patients with grades 1 or 2 (p=0.009).

In an attempt to characterize ulcerations objectively, Wilson et al (13), studied coronary angiograms from 15 patients with recent myocardial infarction (4-13 days), unstable angina (10 patients) or stable angina (15 patients). Coronary stenoses were measured by serial coronary artery diameter determination throughout the length of the stenosis. An index of ulceration was determined and defined as the ratio of the diameter of the least severe narrowing within the non-ulcerated lesion to the maximum intra-lesion diameter (presumed to be the maximal diameter of the "ulcerated" portion of the vessel). This index was inversely related to the extent of the angiographic ulceration and independent of the severity of the stenosis. It was found to be significantly different in lesions responsible for myocardial infarction (0.61 ± 0.05) and unstable angina (0.61 ± 0.03) compared to lesions in stable angina ($0.96\pm0.01, p<0.05$), or from indexes of lesions in the non-infarct related artery (0.90 ± 0.02, $p<0.05$).

Later, Davies et al (19) modified this index, as the ratio of the maximal to the minimal intralesional diameter and used it successfully as a predictor of clinical instability following thrombolytic therapy. The median plaque ulceration index of the infarct related lesion was 6.7 (95% confidence limits 6.3,10) in the 15 patients with an unstable course versus 3.3 (95% confidence limits 2,4.4) in those with stable course ($p<0.001$) (Figure 3). This indices continue to have a limited use by investigators as well as practicing cardiologists for at least 2 reasons: first, these indices are not part of the curriculum in most cardiology programs and trainees are unaware of them; second, the impact of these findings on the clinical outcome of patients has not been validated in large clinical studies.

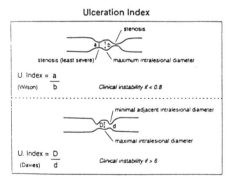

Figure 3: Quantitative morphologic analysis of an ulceration index method as developed by Wilson et al (top) and later modified by Davies et al (bottom). The indices derived are useful to identify patients with unstable angina.

Filling Defects (thrombi)

Filling defects are intracoronary ovoid or polypoid lucencies that are either partially or totally occlusive (20). They are usually globular in shape and are surrounded by contrast on three or more sides. They are usually attached to an underlying plaque and can occur proximal, within, or distal to a coronary stenosis (Figure 4a and 4b). When smooth and well delineated by the contrast media, filling defects are virtually pathognomonic of intraluminal thrombi. However, dense calcific deposits within the rim of an eccentric stenosis can occasionally mimic the appearance of an intravascular filling defect. Older, laminated thrombi usually do not protrude into the vascular lumen and often do not appear as filling defects.

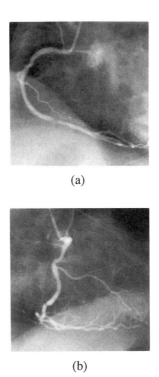

(a)

(b)

Figure 4: Right coronary angiogram obtained from a patient admitted with unstable angina. Figure 4a demonstrates a filling defect that is localized at the site of stenosis as shown in 4b suggesting the presence of an intracoronary thrombus.

Occlusive thrombi are often characterized by a rectangular or a convex (vertex facing upstream) termination, creating a "stump". As intravascular thrombi age, endogenous thrombolytic mechanisms result in partial resolution of the thrombus and often lead to partial restoration of the vascular lumen. These thrombi can assume the appearance of adherent intraluminal masses with irregular borders creating eccentric lumina and are often difficult to distinguish from the underlying atheroma. Thrombi which remain occlusive cause stasis of blood in the proximal portion of the artery and ultimately undergo extension proximally. This process usually progresses until the occluded segment of vessel reaches a large side branch which has brisk flow. The "runoff" provided by such a branch usually causes the process to stop at this point. Thus, a useful characteristic for distinguishing acute from chronic thrombotic occlusion is that chronic obstructions usually end at a terminal side branch while acute occlusions may be seen in the middle of a segment with gaps of one or more centimeters between the end of the column of contrast and the last large side branch.

The TIMI IIIA (21) investigators devised a semi-quantitative thrombus grading system in patients with unstable angina: *grade 0=* no cineangiographic characteristics of thrombus present; *grade 1=* possible thrombus present (angiography demonstrates characteristics, such as reduced contrast density, haziness, irregular lesion contour or a smooth convex meniscus at the site of total occlusion suggestive but not diagnostic of a thrombus); *grade 2=* small thrombus present (definite thrombus with greatest dimensions < 50% of the vessel diameter); *grade 3 =* moderate thrombus present (definite thrombus present but with greatest linear dimension> 50% but less than 2 vessel diameters); *grade 4=*large thrombus present (as in grade 3 but with largest diameter > 2 vessel diameters). Thrombus grades 2 to 4 were combined to determine the incidence of angiographically apparent thrombus and they predicted the angiographic response to an infusion of t-PA.

Angiographically visible thrombus is more frequently found in patients with unstable angina compared to patients with stable angina (table 2) and it has been correlated with a high risk of ischemic events in patients with unstable angina as well as post PTCA.

Williams et al (16) reported that cardiac events occurred in 73 % of patients with angiographic evidence of intracoronary thrombi compared to 17% of patients without thrombi. Similar results were found by Freeman et al (20) who reported adverse cardiac events in

23 of 32 (73%) patients with unstable angina with angiographic coronary thrombi. Mabin et al (25) reported that complete occlusion complicated PTCA in 11 of 15 cases with an intracoronary clot compared to 18 out of 223 patients with no thrombus. This finding was also confirmed by Myler et al (26) who reported that in a series of 1000 lesions in 533 consecutive patients treated by PTCA the presence of an intracoronary thrombus was the only independent predictor of complications post PTCA by univariate (p<0.003) and multivariate analysis (p<0.006).

TABLE 2: Incidence of Thrombus in Patients
with Stable vs. Unstable Angina

AUTHOR	PATIENTS (N)	INCIDENCE
Bresnahan 85 (22)	67 USA 201 SA	35% vs. 2.5%
Capone et al 85 (23)	119 USA 35 SA	37 vs. 0%
Cowley et al 89 (24)	69 USA 20 SA	58% vs. 5%

SA = Stable Angina
USA = Unstable Angina

With the advent of intracoronary angioscopy, the sensitivity of coronary angiography for detecting coronary thrombi has come into question. Teirstein et al (27) compared the accuracy of angiography and angioscopy in determination of the presence of intracoronary thrombi in 75 patients undergoing interventional procedures. Thrombus was defined angiographically as non-calcified filling defect outlined on at least 3 sides by contrast media. The angioscopic presence of thrombus was defined as red material protruding into the lumen or adherent to the luminal wall. Thrombus was detected in 12% of episodes by angiography compared with 41% by angioscopy (p<0.05). In 28% of the angiographically determined filling defects, angioscopy found no evidence of thrombus and provided an alternative explanation for the filling defect (tissue flaps or plaque fragments). When angioscopy was used as a reference standard, the sensitivity of angiography to detect thrombus was 20.8% and the specificity was 94.2%. The sensitivity of angiography to detect intraluminal thrombus alone was 100% compared to 10% for intramural thrombi in the same study.

de Feyter et al (28) assessed the characteristics of the ischemia-related lesions with coronary angiography, intracoronary angioscopy and intravascular ultrasound in 44 patients with unstable angina and 23 patients with stable angina. The angiographic images were classified as either stable (smooth surfaces) or complex (irregular borders, thrombi). Angioscopic images were classified as either stable or thrombotic (red thrombus). The ultrasound characteristics of lesions were classified as poorly echo-reflective, highly echoreflective with shadowing or highly echo reflective without shadowing. Fifty five percent of angiographically complex lesions were seen in patients with unstable angina while 61% of patients with stable angina had simple lesions. Comparatively, an angioscopic thrombotic lesion was concordant with unstable angina in 68% of the cases and stable lesions were concordant in 83% of patients with stable angina. The ultrasound obtained composition of the plaque was similar in patients with stable versus unstable angina. Recently, White et al (29) reported the results of percutaneous coronary angioscopy performed on 122 patients undergoing PTCA. In this study, angioscopy identified coronary thrombi in 61% of the lesions and angiography in only 20% (p<0.001).

By depicting both color and texture, angioscopy can readily distinguish white or yellow plaque fragments protruding into the vessel lumen from red thrombus. However, angioscopy is limited by its inability to distinguish between white thrombi from tissue elements such as tissue flaps or plaque fragments that may be present in the vessel lumen. In addition, the validity of this new modality has not been established yet. One of the early attempts to devise a classification system for coronary angioscopic observations was undertaken by the European Working Group on Coronary Angioscopy (30). Using the "Ermenonville" classification the Kappa values for chance corrected intra-observer agreement were 0.51-0.67. However, the mean Kappa values for interobserver variability were very low 0.13-0.29. Therefore angioscopic diagnosis should, at least currently, be made with caution until a standard system is found.

Contrast Streaming

Streaming of contrast medium is the result of non-uniform mixing of blood with the contrast medium when contrast is injected into the coronary artery. Consequently, mobile areas of radiolucency can often be seen within the column of contrast. This phenomenon is frequently the result of an inadequate contrast volume being injected during the cine run. However, pathophysiologic conditions can also lead to streaming, as stagnation of contrast medium can occur proximal to a clot. Therefore, streaming despite an adequate contrast injection can often be used as a clue that a thrombus is present. Such pathophysiologic streaming can be distinguished from an artifact of injection since its location remains relatively constant within the artery and is usually located distal to an area of stenosis or irregularity, in contrast to artifactually induced streaming which appears to move through the various portions of the proximal artery during different portions of a cineangiographic run (Figure 5).

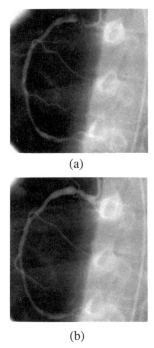

(a)

(b)

Figure 5 (a and b): Angiogram of the right coronary artery from a 50 year old post heart transplant patient demonstrating contrast streaming in the proximal segment of the vessel (5a), that disappear during a second injection of dye (5b) suggesting inadequate contrast volume injected during the initial cine run.

14

Irregularities and lesion roughness

Irregular lesions have coarse and rough edges that lack definition because of hazy margins (17). They may represent partially resolved thrombi, healed ulcerations, or remodeled plaques. Angiographically, they appear as variations in the vessel wall that invaginate into the lumen of the vessel. Multiple irregularities may exist in the same vessel simultaneously. (Figure 6). A technique which has been used to assess roughness of coronary lesions is to determine the angle that the lesion creates with the presumed axis of blood flow into and out of the lesion. Steep inflow and outflow angles have been reported to predict future sites of myocardial infarction (31).

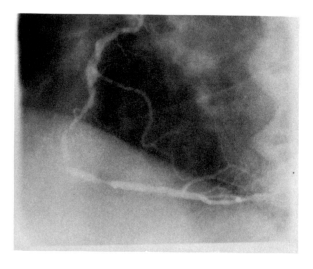

Figure 6: Multiple irregularities and diffuse narrowing of the right coronary artery obtained from a patient with unstable angina.

Ambrose et al (15) defined *multiple irregularities* as three or more serial and severe (>70%) closely spaced obstructions in a coronary artery. This classification included coronary arteries with severe diffuse irregularities or arteries in which a segment of a coronary artery lying between two severe obstructions also exhibited significant diffuse luminal irregularities. Using this classification, the intra and inter-observer reproducibility has been 95 and 88 % respectively. Little et al (32) and Ellis et al (17) reported that irregularities of the coronary wall predicted the site of future myocardial infarction and coronary obstruction.

The roughness of a vessel can be determined quantitatively by comparing the local variation of a vessel edge from a smooth line with the average variation over a longer segment of the vessel. Shape may be quantitatively measured by dividing the vessel edge into small segments. The radius of the curves generated by the small segments can be determined by a process called curvature analysis[a] (33). The major advantages of this method include the ease and rapidity with which analysis can be performed and that it lacks reliance on expert users.

a: In curvature analysis, each point along a vessel edge line is considered to lie on the edge of a circle and the radius of the circle at that point is determined. By determining the inverse of the radius of the circle for all points along a vessel edge line, a "curvature" signature can be derived. Using this method a straight line has a curvature signature line of zero. The more irregular a vessel wall the more it deviates from zero. Four quantitative parameters were based on the curvature signature of the vessel edge line. The parameters included the numbers of the peaks of the curve per centimeter, the sum of the maximum curve or deviation in curvature, the integrated error per centimeter and the number of features per centimeter as defined by a characteristic triplet shape of the curvature signature.

16

Lesion length:

Traditionally, lesion length is determined by measuring the length of a segment with>50% lumen encroachment (Figure 7).

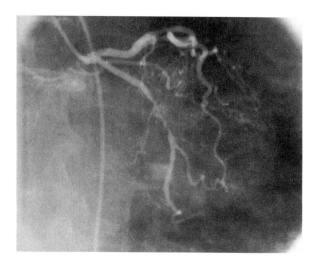

Figure 7: Angiogram of the left coronary system obtained from a 65 year old male with unstable angina demonstrating a long atherosclerotic stenotic lesion of the left circumflex artery.

The length of a coronary lesion varies significantly among different vessels in the same patient or different vessels in different patients. Baroldi (34) examined angiographically the length of 565 severe coronary stenoses and found it less than 5 mm in 13%, 5-20 mm in 38%, and greater than 20 mm in 49%.

The length of a coronary lesion is an important factor in determining blood flow, particularly at high levels of blood viscosity[b] , and a powerful predictor of abrupt closure and of restenosis following percutaneous interventions. The length of a lesion may be defined as the area between the apparent shoulders of the lesion, or in terms of the length of the region whose lumenal narrowing exceeding 30%, 50%, or 70% of the coronary arterial diameter (35). Unfortunately, of all the morphologic characteristics, determination of lesion length suffers from the greatest degree of intra-and inter-observer variability. Although lesion length lends itself readily to quantitative measurements, deciding where a lesion begins and ends is sometimes difficult; as lesion length increases, such determinations become increasingly imprecise . Kleiman et al (36) reported a 66% agreement on lesion length when 2 experienced angiographers reviewed 150 angiograms of patients undergoing balloon angioplasty. Since it is a lumenographic technique, coronary angiography routinely underestimates the extent of atherosclerosis within a tubular structure such as an artery and thus cannot identify precisely the ends of a tapered atherosclerotic deposit. Consequently, the length of a lesion is often severely underestimated by coronary angiography compared with pathologic findings. Wilson et al (13) found that lesions in the infarct related artery were 44% longer than those in patients with stable angina, and 81% longer than lesions in the non-infarct-related vessel. In addition, lesions associated with unstable angina were marginally longer than those associated with stable angina.

[b]: *Basic considerations of fluid mechanics indicate that the pressure drop across a stenosis varies directly with the length of the stenosis and inversely with fourth power of the radius (Poiseuille equation* $\Delta p = 8\mu LQ)/\Pi R^4$

18

Calcified lesions:

Calcific deposits are commonly observed histologically in coronary arterial segments. Calcium is deposited early in the formation of the atherosclerotic plaque, and calcification therefore can be used as an early clue of the atherosclerotic process (Figure 8). Calcified lesions are defined angiographically as radiolucencies within the vessel wall noted with flouroscopy or cineangiography. Often, vessel calcification is seen more easily using flouroscopy than cineangiography.

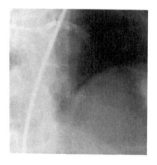

Figure 8: Flouroscopy of the left anterior descending artery showing the presence of severe calcification of the proximal portion of the vessel (8a).

Calcium deposition may occur in aging coronary arteries as part of a degenerative process involving the intima and rarely the media (Monckeberg medial sclerosis) (37). In the latter type calcification is confined to the media and does not encroach on the vessel wall. Therefore as patients age increases, the ability of calcification to predict obstructive atheromatous disease decreases (38).

Intracoronary ultrasound studies have demonstrated that calcification is systematically underestimated by angiography as calcium is easily detected by ultrasonography because of its intense echoreflective characteristics. Recently ultra fast CT has been used to detect CAD based on the amount of coronary calcium and the number of calcified vessels, and is reported to have a high sensitivity to detect CAD. However, correlations of ultrafast CT with angiography were weak, and the sensitivity of this test differs in different age groups. Kosling et al (39) studied the angiographic findings of 24 patients with coronary artery disease and compared them with the qualitative and quantitative detection of coronary calcification by ultrafast computerized tomography. There was a one third false positive and a one third false negative results with the latter technique compared to angiography. What remains to be determined is intraobserver and the interobserver variability in interpreting these studies.

Since calcification is believed to begin at the endothelial surface, angiographically visible coronary arterial calcification is an important clue to assess the severity of luminal narrowing by defining the original coronary lumen(a). Because the density of calcium is similar to that of the contrast medium, the absence of non-calcified plaques between a large calcific deposit and an adjacent column of contrast can lead to overestimation of luminal patency.

Angiographic Assessment of Coronary Arterial Flow and its Relation to Lesion Morphology

The assessment of coronary flow has taken an increased importance since reperfusion therapy has become the treatment of choice for patients with acute myocardial infarction. Rentrop (40) and later the investigators of the Western Washington Studies (41) distinguished complete and partial restoration of blood flow after thrombolysis. Subsequently, the quality of flow has been characterized further by the TIMI I investigators (42). Although originally devised to characterize the response to intravenous thrombolysis, this system is also commonly used to describe flow in the non infarct related arteries and flow after coronary angioplasty. TIMI *grade 0* flow represents the absence of penetration by contrast material beyond the proximal aspect of the thrombus. TIMI *grade 1*, describes penetration of the blood clot by dye but without complete opacification of the distal artery. TIMI *grade 2* represents faint and delayed opacification of the distal vessel but contrast clears more slowly than in non infarct related vessels. In TIMI *grade 3* flow, the distal vessel is completely opacified by contrast. Flow grading should be interpreted with several caveats because of its subjective nature. The assessment of antegrade flow is generally a subjective determination. Hackworthy et al (43) reported a 25% interobserver variability in the distinction between TIMI grade 2 and grade 3 flow. Although this degree of variability might be predicted, discordance between grade 0 or grade 1 versus 2 or 3 also occurred in 5% of the 1615 angiographic readings. Even among vessels in which it is universally agreed that grade 3 flow is present, there are likely to be differences in the degree to which perfusion is restored to the myocardium. Ito et al (44) performed myocardial contrast echocardiography before and immediately after successful reperfusion (either primary PTCA or intracoronary urokinase) with intracoronary injection of sonicated Ioxoglate. Immediately after reflow, 30 of 39 patients showed significant contrast enhancement within the risk area which correlated with greater improvement in global and regional left ventricular function. However, 9 patients with angiographic grade 3 flow had poor contrast perfusion to the myocardium, and had less improvement of wall motion in the infarct distribution. The authors concluded that angiographically successful reflow cannot be used as an indicator of successful reperfusion. Recent studies with an intracoronary Doppler tipped flow wire have confirmed significant variability in coronary flow reserve among patients with TIMI grade 3 flow. Recognizing that TIMI flow grading is limited by its subjective and categorical nature, Gibson et al (45) adopted a method that relies on corrected TIMI frame count (CTFC) to analyze coronary flow. The method involves counting the number of cine frames required for contrast to first reach standardized distal coronary landmarks in the infarct related artery. The first frame used for TIMI counting is the first frame in which radiographic contrast material fully enters the artery as determined by the following criteria: first, a column of nearly full or full concentrated dye must extend across the entire width of the origin of the artery. Second, contrast must touch both borders of the origin of the artery; third, there must be antegrade flow. The last frame is counted or included as one of the frames and occurs when dye first enters the distal landmark branch. This method revealed total overlap in the distribution of the CTFC for TIMI 2 versus TIMI 3 flow and they were not distinct populations with slow or fast flow. This method was also reproducible and independent of the number of injections, catheter sizes, hemodynamic parameters or coronary collaterals. Further prospective studies are however required to validate the relationship of this technique with clinical outcome.

LESION MORPHOLOGY AND PERCUTANEOUS TRANSLUMINAL CORONARY ANGIOPLASTY:

The final reason behind efforts to characterize angiographic lesions according to their morphologic characteristics has been the need to select patients for percutaneous revascularization procedures as well as to match revascularization technologies with specific arterial characteristics. The association between various angiographic characteristics and both the risk of important procedural complications as well as the likelihood of procedural success has been recognized since the advent of coronary angioplasty. These characteristics were initially categorized in reports from the first National Heart Lung and Blood Institute Registry of Coronary Angioplasty (46) which indicated that stenosis >90%, multiple discrete or diffuse lesion morphology ,thrombus and total occlusion were predictors of complications after PTCA. In 1988, a Subcommittee Report on PTCA of the AHA/ACC Task Force (47) proposed a lesion specific classification of angiographic patterns (Table 3). This classification was devised in an attempt to predict the likelihood of a successful PTCA as well as the likelihood of developing abrupt closure after PTCA. Although evolution of the process of coronary angioplasty has led to modification of the predicted outcome, and of the classification itself, this classification is still used as a benchmark to predict the outcome of a variety of percutaneous interventions and to select patients for revascularization procedures. *Type A* lesions have characteristics that allow an anticipated success rate of >85% and have a low risk of abrupt closure. *Type B* lesions have those characteristics that result in lower than optimal success rate ranging from 60-85% , a moderate risk of abrupt closure or both. *Type C* lesions have those characteristics that result in an unacceptable low success rate (<60%) or that have a high risk of closure or both.

Subsequently, Ellis et al (48) distinguished 2 gradations of type B lesions: B1(indicating the presence of only one type B characteristic) and B2 (a combination of 2 or more type B characteristic). Subsequent procedural complications occurred in 4 and 10% in patients with type B1 and B2 lesions respectively, compared to 2 and 21% in patients types A and C lesions respectively. In a series of 97 patients with 328 lesions, Moushmoush et al (49) reported found no clinically significant difference in success rate between patients with Type A lesions (84%) versus those with type B lesions (89%). However, there was a significant difference in the success rate between type A and B versus the success rate for type C (P< 0.0001). Based on these findings, the authors reported that the angiographic characteristics of diffuse disease (> 20 mm in length), tortuous segment, extremely angulated segments and chronic total occlusions were particularly predictive of adverse procedure outcome. Since less subjective judgment is required to determine these characteristics than some of the other elements incorporated within the ACC/AHA classification (eccentricity or irregularity, for example), these authors felt that restricting the characteristics described to those mentioned above might be simpler and more relevant for clinical use.

Table 3: Characteristics of Type A, Type B, and Type C Lesions Influencing Successful PTCA:

Type A lesions (high success, >85%; low risk)	
Discrete (<10 mm length)	Little or no calcification
Concentric	Less than totally occlusive
Readily accessible	Not ostial in location
Nonangulated segment <45°	No major branch involvement
Smooth contour	Absence of thrombus
Type B Lesions (moderate success, 60-80%; moderate risk)	
Tubular (10-20mm long)	Moderate to heavy calcification
Eccentric	
Moderator tortousity of proximal segment	Total occlusion <3 months old
Moderately angulated segment (>45 but <90°)	Ostial location
Irregular contour	Bifurcation lesions requiring double guide wires
	Some thrombus present
Type C lesions (low success, <60%; high risk)	
Diffuse (>20mm length)	Total occlusion >3 months old. Inability to protect major side branches.
Excessive tortousity of proximal segment	
Extremely angulated segment >90 °	Degenerated Vein grafts with friable lesions

Since the elements of each of the ACC/AHA classification consist of subjectively determined morphological characteristics, it is logical that when the characteristics are combined the inter and intra observer variability increases. In a study of 150 cineangiograms obtained prior to angioplasty, two angioplasty operators who had worked together over a period of 4 years agreed on the lesion classification in only 61% of angiograms. Total agreement on all individual ACC/AHA characteristics was achieved in only 12% of angiograms (36). Similar results were reported by Klein et al (49), with eccentricity and irregularity representing the main points of disagreement. Although this classification is still very useful to predict the outcome of interventional procedures, this degree of variability makes it very difficult to compare success rates between operators or between technologies when lesions are graded according to the ACC/AHA scale.

Conclusion

Coronary angiography has been traditionally used to assess the severity and eccentricity of coronary atherosclerotic lesions. However, the morphologic characteristics of coronary lesions have been underutilized despite the available literature which showed that the analysis of coronary morphology helps to uncover important pathologic mechanisms that are critical to the understanding of the clinical findings in our patients. The use of quantitative measures of morphology provides a means of standardization of the morphological features and enables clinicians and researchers to improve reproducibility of studies of coronary artery disease. A key question is whether the angiographic correlates of risk can be used to ascertain which patients would benefit from preventive pharmacologic or mechanical therapies.

Acknowledgment

We would like to thank Ms. Martha Gary for her valuable technical assistance in preparing this manuscript.

References:

1. Bruschke AV, Proudfit WL, Sones FM Jr: Progress study of 590 consecutive non-surgical cases of coronary followed 5.9 years with arteriographic correlations. Circulation. 1973; 47:1147-1153.

2. Humphries JO, Kuller L, Ross RS, Freisinger GC, Page EE: Natural history of ischemic heart disease in relation to arteriographic findings. A twelve year-study of 224 patients. Circulation. 1974;49:489-497.

3. Gould KL, Lipscomb K: Effects of coronary stenoses on coronary flow reserve and resistance. Am J Cardiol. 1974;34:48-55.

4. Gould KL, Lipscomb K: Physiologic basis for assessing critical coronary stenosis. Instantaneous flow response and regional distribution during coronary hyperemia as measures of coronary flow reserve. Am J Cardiol 1974;33: 87-94.

5. Gregg D: The George E. Brown memorial lecture: Physiology of the coronary circulation. Circulation 1963;28:1128-1137.

6. Levin DC, Fallon JT. Significance of the angiographic morphology of localized coronary stenoses. Histopathologic correlations. Circulation 1982;66:316-320.

7. Eisenberg PR, Kenzone JL, Sobel be, Ludbrook PA, Jaffe AS. Relation between ST segment shifts during ischemia and thrombin activity in patients with unstable angina. J Am Coll Cardiol 1991;18: 898-903.

8. Marmur JD, Fyle B, Sharma SK, Ambrose JA, Habert M, Eisenberg S, Torre SR, Nemerson Y, Taubman M. Immunohistochemical detection of tissue factor in human coronary atheroma. J Am Coll Cardiol 1994; (suppl):64A.

9. Lucore CL, Winters KJ, Eisenberg PR. Procoagulant activity of coronary atherosclerotic plaques (abstract). Circulation 1992;86:1-20.

10. Ambrose JA, Winters SL, Arora RR, Haft JI, Goldstein J, Rentrop KP, et al. Coronary angiographic morphology in myocardial infarction: a link between the pathogenesis of unstable angina and myocardial infarction. J Am Coll Cardiol 1985;6:1233-1238.

11. Mancini GB, Deboe SF, Anselmo E, Simon SB, LeFree MT, Vogel RA. Quantitative regional curvature analysis: an application of shape determination for the assessment of segmental left ventricular function in man. Am Heart J 1987;113:326-334.

12. Ambrose JA, Tannenbaum MA, Alexopoulos D, Hjemdahl-Monsen CE, Leary J, Weiss M, et al: Angiographic progression of coronary artery disease and the development of myocardial infarction . J Am Coll Cardiol 1988;12:56-62.

13. Wilson RF, Holida MD, White CW: Quantitative angiographic morphology of coronary stenoses leading to myocardial infarction or unstable angina: Circulation 1986;73:286-293.

26

14. Fischell TA, Bausback KN. Effects of luminal eccentricity on spontaneous coronary vasoconstriction after successful PTCA. Am J Cardiol 1991;68:530-534.

15. Ambrose JA, Winters SL, Stern A, Teichholz LE, Gorlin J, et al. Angiographic morphology and the pathogenesis of unstable angina pectoris. J Am Coll Cardiol 1985;5:609-616.

16. Williams AE, Freeman MR, Chisolm RJ, Patt NL, Armstrong PW. Angiographic morphology in unstable angina pectoris. Am J Cardiol 1988;62:1024-1027.

17. Ellis S, Alderman EL, Cain K, Wright A, Bourassa M, Fisher L, et al and the participants of the Coronary Artery Surgery Study (CASS). Morphology of the left anterior descending coronary territory lesions as a predictor of anterior myocardial infarction: a CASS registry study. J Am Coll Cardiol 1988;13:1481-1491.

18. Gibson CM, Cannon CP, Piana RN, Breall JA, Sharaf B, et al: Angiographic predictors of reocclusion after thrombolysis: Results from the Thrombolysis in Myocardial Infarction (TIMI) 4 Trial. J Am Coll Cardiol 1995;25:582-589.

19. Davies SW, Marchant B, Lyons JP, Rothman MT, Layton CA, et al. Irregular coronary lesion morphology after thrombolysis predicts clinical instability. J Am Coll Cardiol 1991; 18: 669-674.

20. Freeman MR, Williams AE, Chisolm RJ, Armstrong PW. Intracoronary thrombus and complex morphology in unstable angina. Relation to timing of angiography and in-hospital cardiac events. Circulation 1989;80:17-23.

21. The TIMI IIIA Investigators. Early effects of tissue-type plasminogen activators added to conventional therapy on the culprit coronary lesions in patients presenting with ischemic cardiac pain at rest. Results of The Thrombolysis in Myocardial Ischemia (TIMI IIIA) trial. Circulation 1993;87:38-52.

22. Bresnahan DR, Davis JL, Holmes DR Jr, Smith HC. Angiographic occurrence and clinical correlates of intraluminal coronary artery thrombosis: role of unstable angina: J Am Coll Cardiol 1985;6:285-289.

23. Capone G, Wolf NM, Meyer B, Meister SG. Frequency of intracoronary filling defects by angiography in angina pectoris at rest. Am J Cardiol 1985;56:403-406.

24. Cowley MJ, Disciascio G, Rehr RB, Vetrovec GW. Angiographic observations and clinical relevance of coronary thrombus in unstable angina pectoris: Am J Cardiol 1989;63:108E-13E.

25. Mabin TA, Holmes DR Jr, Smith HC, Vliestran RE, Bore AA, Reeder GS, et al: Intracoronary thrombus: role in coronary occlusion complicating percutaneous transluminal coronary angioplasty: J Am Coll Cardiol 1985;5:198-202.

26.   Myler RK, Shaw RE, Streider SH, Hecht HS, Ryan C, Rosenblum J, et al: Lesion morphology and coronary angioplasty, current experience and analysis: J Am Coll Cardiol 1992;19:1641-1652.

27.   Teirstein PS, Schatz RA, De Nardo SJ, Jensen EE, Johnson AD. Angioscopic versus angiographic detection of thrombus during coronary interventional procedures. Am J Cardiol 1995;75:1083-1095.

28.   de Feyter PJ, Ozuki Y, Baptista J, Escaned J, Di Mario C, et al. Ischemia related lesion characteristics in patients with stable or unstable angina. A study with intracoronary angioscopy and ultrasound. Circulation 1995;92:1408-1413.

29.   White C, Ramee S, Collins T, Escobar A, Karsan A, et al: Coronary thrombi increase PTCA risk: Angioscopy as a clinical tool. Circulation 1996;93:259-265.

30.   The Ermenonville classification of observations at coronary angioscopy-evaluation of intra and inter observer agreement , European Working Group on Coronary Angioscopy. Eur Heart J 1994;15:815-822.

31.   Taeymans Y, Theroux P, Lesperance J, Waters D: Quantitative angiographic morphology of the coronary artery lesions at risk for thrombotic occlusion: Circulation 1992;85:78-85.

32.   Little WC, Constantinescu M, Applegate RJ, Kutcher MA, Burrows MT, Kahl FR, et al: Can coronary angiography predict the site of a subsequent myocardial infarction in patients with mild to moderate coronary artery disease?   Circulation 1988;78:1157-1166.

33.   Kalbfleisch J, McGillen MJ, Simon SB et al. Automated quantitation of indexes of coronary lesion complexity: comparison between patients with stable and unstable angina. Circulation 1988;82:439-447.

34.   Baroldi G.   Disease of the coronary arteries.   In Cardiovascular Pathology. VI I. Churchill Livingstone , New York 1983;317-391.

35.   Ellis, SG, Roubin GS, King SB, et al.   Angiographic and clinical predictors of acute closure after native coronary angioplasty. Circulation 1988;77:372-379.

36.   Kleiman NS, Rodriguez AR, Raizner AE. Interobserver variability in the grading of coronary arterial narrowings using the ACC/AHA grading criteria. Am J Cardiol 1992;69:13-415.

37.   Mockenberg GJ: Uber die reine media verkalkung der extremitat enartenen und ihr verhalten zur arteriosklerose. Virchows Archiv 1903; 171: 14-30.

38.   Shirani J, Yousefi J, Roberts WC.   Major cardiac findings at necropsy in 366 American octogenarians. Am J Cardiol 1995; 75: 151-156.

39.   Kosling S, Hoffman V, Leiberenz S, Rather T, Weber P, et al.   First experience with electron beam computed tomography of the heart: comparison with heart catheterization and echocardiographic findings (German) ROFO 1995;163:111-118.

40. Rentrop P, Blanke H, Karsch KR, Kaiser H, Kostring H, et al. Selective intracoronary thrombolysis in acute myocardial infarction and unstable angina pectoris. Circulation 1981; 63: 307-315.

41. Kennedy JW, Richie JL, Davis KB, Stadius ML, Maynard C, et al. The Western Washington randomized trial of intracoronary streptokinase in acute myocardial infarction: a 12 month follow up report. N Engl J Med 1985;312:1073-1078.

42. TIMI Study Group. Thrombolysis in myocardial infarction: N Engl J Med 1985;312:932-936.

43. Hackworthy RA, Sorensen SG, Fitzpatrick PG, Barry WH, Menlove RL, et al. Dependence of assessment of coronary artery reperfusion during acute myocardial infarction on angiographic criteria and interobserver variability. Am J Cardiol 1988; 62:538-542.

44. Ito H, Tomooka T, Sahai N, Yu H, Fuji K, et al. Lack of myocardial perfusion immediately after successful thrombolysis. A predictor of poor recovery of left ventricular function in anterior myocardial infarction. Circulation 1992;85:1699-1705.

45. Gibson MC, Cannon CP, Daley WL, Dodge JT, Alexander B, for the TIMI 4 Study Group. The TIMI Frame Count: a quantitative method of assessing coronary artery flow. Circulation 1996;93:879-888.

46. Kelsey SF, Miller DP, Holubkov R, Lu AS, Cowley MJ, et al. Comparison of complication during percutaneous transluminal coronary angioplasty from 1977 to 1981 and from 1985 to 1986: The National Heart, Lung and Blood Institute percutaneous transluminal coronary angioplasty registry. J Am Coll Cardiol 1988;12:1149-1155.

47. ACC/AHA Task Force Report: Guidelines for percutaneous transluminal coronary angioplasty: J Am Coll Cardiol 1988;12:529-545.

48. Sutton JM, Ellis SG, Roubin GS et al for the Gianturco-Roubin intracoronary Stent Investigator Group: Major clinical events after coronary stenting: The multicenter registry of acute and elective Gianturco-Roubin stent placement. Circulation 1994;89:1126-1137.

49. Mashmoush B, Kramer B, Hsieh AM, Klein LW. Does the AHA/ACC task force grading system predict outcome in mulivessel coronary angioplasty? Cath and Cardiovas Diag 1992;27:97-105.

Neal S. Kleiman, M.D.
Associate Professor of Medicine
Section of Cardiology
Baylor College of Medicine

Assistant Director
Cardiac Catheterization Laboratories
The Methodist Hospital
Houston, Texas

Nasser M. Lakkis, M.D.
Cardiology Fellow
Baylor College of Medicine
Houston, Texas

2.

INTRAVASCULAR ULTRASOUND: EQUIPMENT, TECHNIQUE
AND APPLICATIONS IN CLINICAL PRACTICE AND RESEARCH

Steven Nissen, M.D., Cleveland Clinic Foundation, Cleveland, Ohio

Lloyd W. Klein, M.D., Rush-Presbyterian-St. Luke's Medical Center and
The Rush Heart Institute, Chicago, Illinois

INTRODUCTION
Morphological and quantitative assessment of coronary artery
disease *in vivo* represents an important, although difficult, challenge in
cardiovascular research and clinical practice. Until recently,
atherosclerotic coronary lesions could not be visualized directly by any
available imaging modality. Accordingly, detection of coronary
obstructions has relied principally upon indirect methods that either
depict the vessel lumen (angiography) or expose the ischemic effect of
coronary narrows (nuclear or stress echocardiography). However, both
methods are insensitive to the early, minimally obstructive disease
associated with the dramatic and often lethal consequences of coronary
atherosclerosis - acute coronary syndromes.
In the absence of a direct method for visualizing atherosclerotic
plaques, angiography, following its introduction by Sones et al in 1958,
has constituted the principal modality used by clinicians and investigators
to determine the anatomic severity of coronary artery disease. Since
that discovery, coronary angiography has represented the "gold
standard" for diagnosis of coronary disease, growing in frequency to
more than 1 million procedures annually in the United States. The
diagnostic preeminence of coronary angiography remained unchallenged
during the development in the 1980's of balloon angioplasty and other
percutaneous coronary revascularization techniques. This practice has
resulted in a particularly singled-minded, non-critical acceptance by
clinicians of the "luminogram" as the principal determinant of the
indications and success of coronary interventions.[1]
Now, in the 1990's, for the first time, an alternative imaging
modality, intravascular ultrasound, is challenging the dominance of

coronary angiography in diagnosis and therapy of coronary disease. Catheter-based ultrasound represents a radically different approach to the imaging of vascular anatomy. The incremental value of coronary ultrasound originates principally from two key features - the cross-sectional, tomographic perspective of the images and the ability to directly image atheromata. Whereas angiography depicts the complex cross-sectional anatomy of a human coronary as a planar silhouette, ultrasound *directly* examines the anatomy within the vessel wall, allowing the operator to measure precisely atheroma size, distribution, and composition (Figure 1). Accordingly, coronary ultrasound is yielding important insights into diverse phenomena, ranging from the pathophysiology of coronary syndromes to the mechanical effects of interventional devices.

Limitations of Coronary Angiography

The rationale for intracoronary ultrasound arises from well-established limitations of coronary angiography. In the 1960's and 70's, investigators first began questioning the accuracy and reproducibility of the coronary angiogram.[2,3] Studies established that visual interpretation of angiograms exhibit significant observer variability.[2] Other investigations reported major discrepancies between the apparent lesion severity and post-mortem examination.[3] More recently, investigators have documented major differences between the apparent severity of lesions and measurements of the physiologic effects of stenoses.[4] Although quantitative coronary angiography has improved the reproducibility of coronary luminal measurements, this technique is limited by magnification errors, inability to detect disease at the reference segment and the limited number of the projections available.[1]

In the setting of percutaneous intervention, the theoretical limitations of angiography are particularly relevant. Radiographic imaging depicts complex coronary cross-sectional anatomy from a planar silhouette of the contrast-filled lumen. Most mechanical interventions exaggerate the extent of luminal eccentricity by fracturing or dissecting the atheroma.[5] This disruption of the atherosclerotic plaque permits extravasation of contrast media into (or beneath) the atheroma. The silhouette (angiographic appearance) of the complex post-intervention vessel often consists of an enlarged, although frequently "hazy" lumen. In the setting of extensive plaque fracture, the hazy, broadened angiographic silhouette may overestimate the vessel cross-section and misrepresent the actual gain in lumen size.

Angiography represents an indirect and relative measure of luminal narrowing. The traditional methods for characterizing lesion severity by angiography depend upon visual or computer measurements of the percent stenosis. This process requires comparison of minimum luminal dimensions within both the coronary lesion and an adjacent uninvolved "normal" reference segment. However, post-mortem studies have consistently demonstrated that coronary atherosclerosis is typically a diffuse, rather than focal, process. Accordingly, no truly normal reference segment exists from which to calculate percent. In this setting, the calculated percent diameter stenosis will underestimate the true lesion severity by comparing the lesion diameter to a narrowed reference segment. Atherosclerotic involvement of the reference segment also has important implications for interventional practice, because reference segment disease will affect assessment of the target vessel, influencing device selection, sizing, and assessment of results.

Theoretical Advantages

Atherosclerotic plaque morphology constitutes a critical determinant of the prognosis and natural history of coronary disease. Intravascular ultrasound represents the first and only diagnostic technique that provides direct visualization of atherosclerotic coronary plaques *in vivo*. The tomographic orientation of ultrasound enables visualization of the full 360 degree circumference of the vessel wall, not merely a silhouette of the lumen. This capability permits direct measurements of lumen dimensions, including minimum and maximum diameter and cross-sectional area. The constant velocity of sound in soft tissue permits ultrasound scanners to overlay a highly accurate, electronically-generated distance scale within the image. This capability obviates the need to correct for radiographic magnification, a troublesome requisite of angiographic methods.[1]

TECHNIQUES AND EQUIPMENT

Approaches to Catheter Design

The equipment required for intracoronary ultrasound examination consists of two major components, a catheter incorporating a miniaturized transducer and an console containing the necessary electronics to reconstruct an ultrasound image. The current generation of catheters range in size from 2.9 to 3.5 French (0.96 to 1.17 mm.) The basic principles underlying the development of intravascular ultrasound imaging catheters are relatively simple. As the frequency of the ultrasound transmission increases, structural resolution increases proportionately. However, this increasing resolution occurs at the expense of decreasing penetration. Standard 2.25 - 3.50 MHz transthoracic ultrasound transducers have a two-point structural resolution of 5-10 mm with an imaging penetration up to 30 cm. At the frequency emitted by intravascular ultrasound transducers increases to the range of 20 - 40 MHz, the two-point structural resolution becomes <0.1 mm, but the depth of penetration is limited to 3 - 10 mm. The most advanced devices yield remarkably high image quality, primarily as a consequence of the high operating frequency and close proximity to the target. Axial resolution typically approaches 80 μm, while lateral resolution is depth dependent averaging about 200 μm.

There are two approaches to the design of intracoronary ultrasound devices - mechanical transducers and multi-element electronic designs. Mechanical devices employ an external motor drive to rotate a single piezoelectric transducer mounted near the distal end of the catheter. Mechanical transducers typically operate at 1800 revolutions per minute to yield 30 frames per second. Rotating mechanical devices provide greater acoustic power than multi-element systems, because acoustic energy is directed to a single ultrasound element. The higher power yields greater dynamic range and tissue penetration than electronic probes resulting in better image quality, although this gap appears to be narrowing.

Some recent catheter designs employ a different approach in which sheath-type covering is advanced distally into the vessel, the guidewire removed, and the ultrasound transducer is passed freely within the sheath to image the vessel. Recent sheath-type devices incorporate a distal lumen that is shared by the transducer and guidewire, a feature that allows maximum transducer size with minimum sheath size. The electronic approach to ultrasound catheter design employs 32 elements mounted in an annular array near the distal catheter tip.[6] Precise, sequential timing of various groups of these elements results in a sweep of the ultrasound signal through the 360° vessel arc. The main advantages of this approach include excellent shaft flexibility, and optimal guidewire tracking. However, an image quality disadvantage stems from a lower frequency (20 MHz), reduced acoustic power, and a smaller aperture, which limits lateral resolution.

A unique version of the multi-element catheter recently approved by the FDA, the Oracle-Micro™ (Endosonics Corp.), employs an imaging transducer mounted a few millimeters proximal to a standard angioplasty balloon. This device allows examination of the vessel before and after angioplasty without requiring a catheter exchange.

Laboratory Technique

Catheter handling procedures are similar to standard interventional techniques The operator subselective cannulates the vessel using a steerable guidewire and interrogates the vessel by carefully advancing or retracting the imaging catheter over the wire.[7] As the transducer is moved to various points along the vessel, the operator examines the vessel in real time, recording images on videotape for subsequent quantitative analysis. Although currently available ultrasound devices are quite flexible and allow atraumatic coronary examination, these probes have handling characteristics distinctly inferior to modern angioplasty balloons. While typical ultrasound catheters are small and flexible enough for routine imaging, interrogation of heavily diseased or distally located coronary segments remains challenging. Monorail designs facilitate rapid catheter exchanges and allow a guidewire to remain safely in position well beyond critical coronary stenoses.

CLINICAL IMAGING

Safety of Coronary Ultrasound

Although intravascular imaging requires intracoronary instrumentation, studies have demonstrated few serious untoward effects. Transient coronary spasm occurs in about 5% of patients, but usually responds rapidly to administration of intracoronary nitroglycerin. The imaging transducer may temporarily obstruct or severely reduce coronary flow when advanced into tight stenoses or small distal vessels, but patients generally do not experience chest pain if the catheter is promptly withdrawn. In both the diagnostic and interventional catheterization, most experienced practitioners administer heparin (5,000 to 10,000 units) prior to intracoronary imaging.

Despite, the relative safety of coronary ultrasound, any intracoronary instrumentation carries the potential risk of intimal injury or vessel dissection. Although, many centers employ ultrasound during diagnostic catheterization, most laboratories limit credentialing for intravascular imaging procedures to personnel with interventional training. In the unlikely event of intimal disruption, this safety measure ensures that the necessary personnel and equipment are immediately available to initiate appropriate corrective action. Particular prudence is warranted when imaging intracoronary stents with short monorail catheter systems. The potential exists for "snagging" the stent during imaging with catastrophic consequences.

Artifacts and Limitations

Current intravascular ultrasound imaging devices generate artifacts that may adversely affect image quality. Mechanical transducers may exhibit cyclical oscillations in rotational speed, *non-uniform rotational distortion* (NURD), which arises from mechanical drag on the catheter drive-shaft producing visible distortion NURD is most evident when the drive-shaft is bent into a small radius of curvature by a tortuous vessel and is recognized as circumferential "stretching" of a portion of the image with compression of the contralateral vessel wall. An additional artifact, *transducer ring-down*, appears in virtually all medical ultrasound devices. This artifact arises from acoustic oscillations in the piezoelectric transducer material resulting in high-amplitude signals that obscure the near-field imaging. The resultant inability to image structures immediately adjacent to the transducer yields a device with an "acoustic" size larger than its physical size.

An additional limitation of all intravascular imaging systems originates from vulnerability to geometric distortion produced by oblique catheter orientation. When the ultrasound beam interrogates an imaging plane not orthogonal to the vessel walls, a circular lumen appears elliptical in shape. The nature of ultrasound imaging results other important limitations. All ultrasonography relies upon differences in the acoustic impedance of tissues to reconstruct an image. As a result, two very different structures may exhibit similar acoustic properties when examined by ultrasound. It is therefore important to recognize that intravascular ultrasound can delineate the thickness and echogenicity of vessel wall structures, but does not provide actual histology.

INTERPRETATION OF MORPHOLOGY

Normal Anatomy

A series of investigations have characterized the appearance of normal coronary anatomy by intravascular ultrasound.[8-10] At higher frequencies (25 MHz and above), the vessel lumen is characterized by faint, finely textured, specular echoes that move and swirl during active blood flow. The echogenicity within the lumen presumably arises the reflection of acoustic energy by circulating blood elements. In many situations, blood "speckle" assists image interpretation by providing a means to confirm the communication between tissue planes and the lumen.

Morphology in normal arteries consists of two basic patterns - a trilaminar appearance with three discrete layers or monolayered vessel wall. (Figure 2) Although there is still some controversy regarding the genesis of the three ultrasonic layers in normal subjects, most authorities agree that the innermost band represents reflections from the internal elastic lamina, while the middle sonolucent layer is principally composed of the vessel media. In normal segments without a trilaminar appearance, the internal elastic lamina is thin and reflects the ultrasound signal poorly, resulting in a monolayered appearance. In normals, the intimal thickness averages 0.15 ± 0.07 mm with many investigators using 0.25 to 0.30 mm as an upper limit (2 standard deviations > normal). The deepest layer of the arterial wall represents the adventitia and peri-adventitial tissues, exhibiting a characteristic "onionskin" pattern.

Abnormal Morphology

Arteries with coronary atherosclerosis exhibit a diversity of abnormal features which reflect the distribution, severity and composition of the atheroma.[8,11] Sites with minimal disease show generalized or focal thickening of the intimal leading-edge, while advanced lesions appear as large echogenic masses encroaching upon the lumen. Most classification schemes differentiate coronary atheromata into one of three categories (soft, fibrous or calcified) according to plaque echogenicity. (Figure 3-5) Plaques are termed "soft" if they are less echogenic than the adventitia because *in vitro* studies demonstrate a high lipid content. Plaques with an echodensity similar to the adventitia are described as "fibrous" because studies demonstrate that increasing echogenicity correlates with increasing fibrous tissue content. "Calcified" lesions are recognized as highly echogenic plaques that attenuate transmission of the ultrasound signal thereby obscuring deeper layers.

Caution is warranted in interpretation of intravascular ultrasound images. Methods do not yet exist for automated classification of atheromatous lesions. Although currently available devices produce remarkably detailed views of the vessel wall, interpretation employs visual inspection of acoustic reflections to determine morphology. The echogenicity and texture of different histological features may exhibit comparable acoustic properties and therefore appear quite similar by intravascular ultrasound. For example, sonolucent plaque may represent intracoronary thrombus, while another nearly identical atheroma may result from a plaque with a high lipid content. Thus, intravascular ultrasound can delineate the thickness and echogenicity of vessel wall structures, but does not provide actual histology.

Despite these limitations, the general classification of coronary plaques into the categories of soft, fibrous, or calcified has significant clinical implications for the interventional practitioner. Initial experience suggests that the three different categories often respond differently to interventional devices. For example, densely fibrotic or calcified plaques resist removal with the current generation of directional atherectomy devices. Armed with this information, the prudent practitioner may choose an alternative revascularization device such as rotational atherectomy, for such lesions.

DIAGNOSTIC APPLICATIONS

Angiographically Silent Disease

Coronary ultrasound commonly detects atherosclerotic abnormalities at sites containing no apparent lesion by angiography.[9,12] There are four principle mechanisms by which angiography may underestimate the amount of atherosclerosis or completely fail to diagnose coronary disease. First, angiography relies upon comparison one segment of the vessel to another to detect disease, whereas atherosclerosis is typically a diffuse process. A diffusely diseased vessel may be reduced in caliber along its entire length and contain no truly normal segment for comparison. (Figure 6) In the absence of a focal stenosis, the angiographer could erroneously conclude that the vessel is simply "small in caliber".

Eccentric lesions, plaques that occupy only a portion of the vessel circumference, represent a second important source of false negative angiography. There exist major limitations to obtaining optimal angiographic projections. For example, at certain angles overlapping structures such as adjacent vessels often obscure segments of the coronary, while limits in mechanical positioning of the x-ray gantry may preclude other potentially useful views. Therefore, an eccentric lesion may not be visualized by angiography because the operator could not obtain an appropriate projection angle tangential to the lesion.

A third important mechanism underlying false-negative angiography results from the phenomenon of coronary remodeling.[13] At atherosclerotic sites, compensatory enlargement ("remodeling") of the vessel wall overlying the plaque often preserves lumen diameter resulting in an angiographic lumen size identical to adjacent, uninvolved segments. Finally, vessel foreshortening can conceal short "napkin-ring" lesions (usually less than 1-2mm).

For each of these mechanism of false negative angiography, ultrasound can readily confirm the presence and estimate the severity of the lesion. There are important clinical implications for the higher sensitivity of intravascular ultrasound in detecting coronary atherosclerosis. Patients who present with symptoms suggestive of coronary disease, but who have "normal" angiograms represent a common and perplexing group. In our experience, ultrasound will demonstrate coronary atherosclerosis in the majority of such patients, a finding that impacts on the choice of therapy. Indeed, by the time angiography detects the first luminal irregularity, nearly all of the coronary system will have abnormal intimal thickening by ultrasound.

Ambiguous Coronary Lesions

Despite thorough radiographic examination using multiple projections, angiographers commonly encounter lesions which elude accurate characterization. Lesions of uncertain severity often include ostial lesions and moderate stenoses (angiographic severity ranging from 40 to 75%) in patients whose symptomatic status is difficult to evaluate. For these ambiguous lesions, ultrasound provides a precise tomographic measurements, enabling quantitation of the stenosis independent of the radiographic projection.[14] Bifurcation lesions are particularly difficult to assess by angiography. Examination of bifurcation lesions by ultrasound involves specialized techniques, requiring subselective placement of the transducer in the main trunk and each of the daughter branches.

We compared angiographic and ultrasound dimensions in patient subgroups stratified by the extent of eccentricity determined by ultrasound.[8] In these normal subjects demonstrating a nearly circular lumen, the correlation between angiographic and ultrasound derived diameter was close, r = 0.92, demonstrating concordance between planar and tomographic measurement. In approximately two thirds of atherosclerotic vessels, the lumen was concentric in shape and the correlation between ultrasound and angiography was also close, r = 0.93. However, in the subgroup of patients with an eccentric lumen shape regression analysis demonstrated significant disagreement between angiographic and ultrasonic diameters, r = 0.78. This reduced correlation is likely results from the irregular, non-circular cross-sectional profile of atherosclerotic arteries. These data demonstrate the potential superiority of a tomographic technique, such as intravascular ultrasound, in measurement of coronary dimensions for the complex, eccentric vessels commonly encountered in patients with atherosclerosis.

Identification of atherosclerotic lesions in cardiac allograft recipients represents a particularly important and challenging task for diagnostic intravascular ultrasound.[15] These patients may have diffuse vessel involvement which, for reasons already enumerated, conceals the atherosclerosis from the angiographer. Many centers now routinely perform intravascular ultrasound at the time of annual catheterization in all cardiac transplant recipients. Recent studies in our laboratory have revealed dual pathways to transplant atherosclerosis, with some patients receiving atherosclerotic plaques from the donor heart, while others develop immune-mediated vasculopathy.

Risk Stratification of Atherosclerotic Lesions.

In the early 1980's, Little et al confirmed that plaques of minimal to moderate angiographic severity were the most likely to rupture and cause acute myocardial infarction. When intracoronary ultrasound interrogates lesions associated with acute coronary syndromes, the most of these plaques contain a relatively echolucent material, consistent with a high lipid content. If a fibrous cap is present, this thick layer is most often ruptured and overlies a large, echolucent, lipid-laden area. Recent research indicates that lipids are the most thrombogenic component of atherosclerotic plaque. The ability of intravascular ultrasound to differentiate predominantly fibrous or calcified plaques from atheromata with a high lipid content offers the potential to determine which plaques are most susceptible to progression to acute coronary syndromes.

INTERVENTIONAL APPLICATIONS

Quantitative Luminal Measurements

In interventional practice, the precise measurement of vascular dimensions from a tomographic perspective constitutes an important application of intravascular ultrasound. Most investigators report a relatively poor correlation between ultrasonic and angiographic dimensions following intervention. This discrepancy reflects the inability of angiography to accurately portray the complex, irregular cross-sectional profiles of atherosclerotic vessels following mechanical intervention. Careful comparisons of ultrasound and angiographic findings following balloon angioplasty have confirmed that angiography often overestimates the actual gain in luminal cross sectional area.[16]

Two factors influence the overly optimistic tendency of angiographic imaging. At the reference site, angiography tends to underestimate the true vessel diameter because of the frequent presence of unrecognized atherosclerosis. At the target site, angiography tends to overestimate the actual gain in luminal diameter, because contrast material penetrates into complex cracks and fissures produced by the balloon, giving the appearance of a more enlarged lumen. To calculate a post-procedure percent diameter stenosis, the diameter at the target site (an overestimate) is divided by the reference diameter (an underestimate), resulting in a more favorable impression of the actual gain in luminal dimensions. Accordingly, when quantitative angiography reports a residual stenosis of 10-15%, ultrasound not uncommonly reports that 60-80% of the vessel is still occupied by plaque.

Characterization of Restenosis

It seems likely that the morphology of the vessel wall following interventions will provide valuable insights into phenomena such as elastic recoil, pathologic dissection, abrupt occlusion, and restenosis. The relatively poor correlation between angiographic and ultrasonic dimensions following-angioplasty raises provocative clinical and scientific issues. In certain patients, does "restenosis" represent a failure to adequately augment luminal area, rather than the subsequent over-exuberant proliferation of cellular elements? Can ultrasound assessment of the residual lumen predict acute post-interventional complications or identify patients with a high likelihood of poor long-term results? Several multicenter clinical trials, currently underway, are examining whether ultrasound can reliably predict restenosis following intervention. These include several multi-center trials in which the interventional practitioner is blinded to the ultrasound findings.

Preliminary unpublished observations obtained by serial intravascular ultrasound studies have challenged the prevailing assumptions about the genesis of the restenotic lesion. These initial investigations report that 50 to 80% of the loss in lumen size following balloon angioplasty is derived from "remodeling", a process characterized by "shrinkage" in the adventitia rather than neointimal proliferation. If confirmed, these insights would explain much of the benefit of intracoronary stenting and suggest other innovative approaches to the prevention of restenosis.

Post-Angioplasty Analysis

Necropsy studies in patients who have died shortly after balloon angioplasty describe plaque fracturing or disruption as the most common mechanism of successful balloon dilatation.[5] Ultrasound studies have confirmed that plaque fissuring is the most common mechanism of luminal enlargement, occurring in 40% to 80% of patients. Ultrasound often shows other mechanisms of luminal enlargement after balloon angioplasty that cannot be discerned in *post mortem* analyses.[7] Careful pre- and post-PTCA imaging reveals that stretching of the vessel wall occurs in at least 20% of patients, while apparent "compression" of the atheromatous material occurs in at least 10%. More recent studies using automatic pullback devices (which withdraws the ultrasound catheter at a constant rate through the target site) have shown that "compression" may represents redistribution of plaque along the long axis of the vessel.Guidance of Directional Atherectomy.

Intravascular ultrasound has proven particularly valuable in guiding directional coronary atherectomy.[17,18] By determining both the location and composition of the target atheroma, ultrasound enables optimal pre-procedural planning and improved intraprocedural decision-making. Lesions that appear concentric by angiography are often eccentric by ultrasound and conversely, angiographically eccentric lesions are often concentric by ultrasound. The spatial improved perspective provided by ultrasound can assist in the proper orientation of atherectomy cuts. However, successful application of this approach requires experience, patience, and careful planning because precise orientation of the intravascular image remains a difficult challenge. Experienced operators will carefully examine the target vessel prior to atherectomy to locate anatomic landmarks, especially side branches, and will use these landmarks to orient the ultrasound image. With this information, the operator can then direct atherectomy cuts toward the appropriate side of the vessel. Some operators use repeat ultrasound examinations between passes of the atherectomy device to determine the extent of plaque removal and assess the need for additional cuts.

With currently available directional atherectomy devices, the presence and extent of vessel calcification can dramatically affect the efficiency of plaque removal. In detection of calcification, ultrasound is more sensitive than angiography, permitting identification of extensively calcified atheromata despite the absence of any apparent calcification on fluoroscopy.[19] In our experience, calcification at the luminal surface usually precludes successful tissue removal. However, ultrasound can determine not only the presence of calcification, but also its depth in relation to the lumen. Ultrasound studies have demonstrated that target lesions with extensive calcification deep within the atheroma can undergo successful atherectomy.

In striking contrast to balloon angioplasty, ultrasound studies before and after directional atherectomy confirm that plaque removal is the primary mechanism of luminal enlargement. Nevertheless, ultrasound also reveals that despite a successful angiographic result (<15% residual stenosis), 40-60% or more of the target site is still occupied by plaque.[18] Some investigators have proposed that a larger lumen after atherectomy would result in a lower restenosis rate (compared to balloon angioplasty). However, it remains untested whether a larger post-procedure lumen can be achieved using angiographic guidance without an concomitant increase in dissection, perforation, or other complications. In our experience, more aggressive plaque removal is most safely accomplished with the use of ultrasound guidance. Development of a combined atherectomy-ultrasound device represents a major focus of current commercial ventures.

Guidance of Rotational Atherectomy.

Rotational ablation (Rotablator™, Heart Technology, Bellevue, WA) employs a high speed diamond-coated burr to debulk atheromata within coronary stenoses. This approach has been proven particularly effective at removing superficial calcium from stenotic vessels. Interestingly, this morphological subset represents precisely the type of vessel least suitable for directional atherectomy. As previously discussed, there is a poor correlation between ultrasound and fluoroscopy in assessment of the presence and amount of calcification.[19] Accordingly, in our laboratory, practitioners not uncommonly abandon an intended directional atherectomy in favor of rotational ablation because pre-interventional ultrasound revealed extensive calcification.

Vessels revascularized using rotational ablation are frequently diffusely diseased and the "normal" dimension can be difficult to determine angiographically. Ultrasound-guided vessel sizing can facilitate the selection of the largest burr. Observational ultrasound studies to date have confirmed that ablation of plaque constitutes the primary mechanism of rotational atherectomy, particularly the more fibrotic or calcified components of the lesion.[20] The residual lumen is usually round or ellipsoid, and may result in a lumen with a15-20% greater area than the largest burr used, presumably due to lateral movement of the burr during the procedure. In certain lesions, rotational atherectomy may be the only device capable of removing a hard, superficial layer of calcium, yet even after this layer is removed, a large volume of plaque may remain. Post-Rotablator™ ultrasound can quantitate the size of the neo-lumen, characterizes the morphology of the remaining plaque, and guide the technique and size of device used for further luminal enlargement. (Figure 7) In other target vessels, ultrasound may document restoration of luminal size, obviating the need for an adjunctive device.

Coronary Stent Deployment

Recent studies demonstrating a reduced restenosis rate have stimulated renewed interest in coronary stenting. However, the requirement for vigorous post-deployment anticoagulation have limited more widespread application of this technique. Ultrasound studies have demonstrated that angiography is often inadequate to guide stent deployment. Some stents may appear successfully deployed by angiography, but are actually incompletely apposed to the vessel wall (Figure 8). In such cases, angiographic contrast presumably penetrates the porous stent, giving the false appearance of a large lumen. In other cases, although the stent is well-apposed to the wall, the lumen cross sectional area is considerably reduced in comparison to a proximal or distal reference site.

Ultrasound examination can easily diagnose both of these circumstances. The metallic structure of current coronary stents produces a distinct appearance. Individual struts appear as echodense objects with acoustic shadowing similar to vessel wall calcification. A single-center, retrospective analysis has documented that the level of systemic anticoagulation may be safely reduced if ultrasound confirms both adequate stent apposition and restoration of near-normal lumen dimensions, defined as 60% or more of the area of the lumen in a normal or near-normal adjacent segment.[21] However, prospective trials will be required before any widespread application of the practice of reduced anticoagulation

Intravascular ultrasound is occasionally useful in determining the true longitudinal extent of a dissection before placement of a stent for vessel salvage. Thus, intracoronary imaging is more sensitive in detecting the presence of a dissection, and more accurate in determining the true length of a dissection. In questionable cases, ultrasound examination before stenting can define the limits of the dissection determine where (and how many) stents should be placed. Although ultrasound is unquestionably useful of following stenting, there remain questions of safety in passing any monorail-type catheter through a fine-wire, coil design, such as the Gianturco-Roubin™ (Cook) stent. It is theoretically possible to dislodge the stent by "snagging" a loop of the struts between the monorail catheter and the guidewire..

Future Directions of Intravascular Ultrasound

During the next several years technological advances in intravascular imaging will undoubtedly expand the utility of this procedure. Industry engineers anticipate further reductions in the size of imaging catheters and animal testing of a guidewire-sized device (<0.025 inches) has already begun. This guidewire-sized ultrasound probe will improve the ease and safety of the examination and may also enable simultaneous imaging during the revascularization procedure. Very small devices would also enable imaging of virtually any coronary stenosis prior to treatment. Combination devices will likely undergo refinement, permitting on-line guidance during revascularization procedures. An angioplasty balloon with an ultrasound transducer (Endosonics - Oracle™) is FDA approved, and a transducer combined with an atherectomy device is also under development.

SUMMARY

Recent advances in microelectronic and piezoelectric technology have permitted development of miniaturized ultrasound devices capable of real-time tomographic intravascular imaging. Initial studies have successfully employed intravascular ultrasound to augment angiography in both diagnostic and therapeutic catheterization. The cross-sectional perspective of intravascular ultrasound appears ideally suited for precision measurements of luminal diameter and cross-sectional area. In addition, ultrasound improves assessment of problem lesions such as ostial stenoses or disease at bifurcations. Intravascular imaging provides unique, detailed cross-sectional images of the arterial wall not previously obtainable *in vivo* by any other technique and is more sensitive than angiography in the detection of atherosclerosis. Intravascular ultrasound images of atherosclerotic wall abnormalities have the potential to greatly augment the understanding of the anatomy and pathophysiology of coronary disease.

For interventional applications, ultrasound analysis of lesion characteristics offers many potential advantages. Evaluation of the "normal" reference segment used for device sizing constitute an important emerging application for intravascular imaging. Post-procedure, intravascular ultrasound often yields smaller luminal size measurements than angiography and greater stenosis severity. These differences likely reflect augmentation of the "apparent" angiographic diameter by extra-luminal contrast within cracks, fissures or dissection planes. New ultrasound instruments under development combine an imaging transducer with an interventional device, permitting on-line guidance during the procedure. Although the clinical value of routine ultrasound imaging following mechanical revascularization has not been tested by randomized trials., it seems likely that this new imaging modality will provide valuable insights into diverse phenomena such as abrupt occlusion and restenosis. As a consequence of refinements in equipment and knowlege derived from clinical investigations, we anticipate a major role for intravascular ultrasound in the diagnosis and therapy of coronary disease well into the next century.

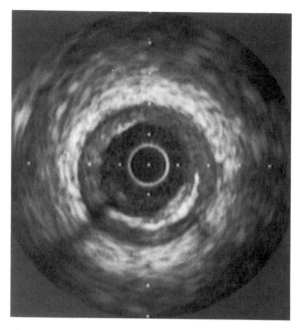

Figure 1 Intravascular ultrasound visualization of plaque morphology. The imaging catheter is seen as a dark circle in the center of the image surrounded by a white halo. The fine specular appearance in the lumen is produced by red blood cells in motion. The plaque within the vessel wall is variable and echogenicity, which is dependend upon lipid and fibrous tissue content.

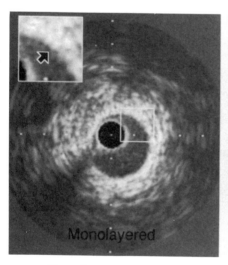
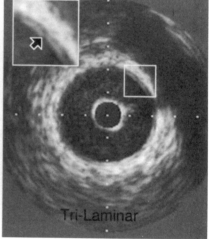

Figure 2 Normal wall morphology by intravascular ultrasound. In the left panel, a monolayered artery is visible without distinctive laminations. In the right hand frame a tri-laminar appearance is evident.

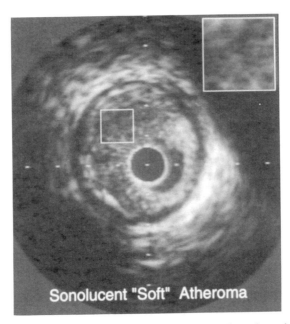

Figure 3 A sonolucent soft atheroma. In this case, the echogenicity of the plaque is less that that of the adventitia. This is characteristic of lipid-laden atheroma.

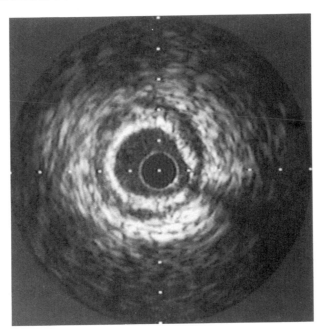

Figure 4 Fibrous plaque. In this example, the plaque is highly echogenic, but does not obscure (shadow) the underlying structure of the vessel wall. This is consistent with a fibrous plaque.

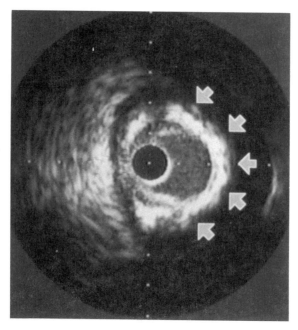

Figure 5 Calcified plaque. In this example, a highly echogenic plaque attenuates transmission of ultrasound energy resulting in a "shadowing" effect. (arrows). Tis is consistent with calcified plaque.

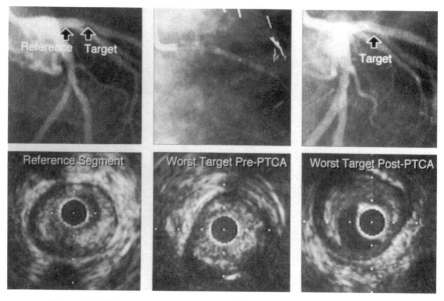

Figure 6 Diffuse coronary disease. In this example, both the "normal reference" segment and the target lesion contain extensive atherosclerosis. When a vessel is diffusely diseased, angiography tends to underestimate atherosclerosis severity.

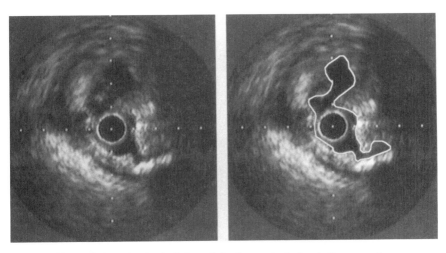

Figure 7 Complex luminal shape following angioplasty. In the example, a balloon has produced multiple fractures and tears in the plaque with an oddly shaped lumen. The right panel shows planimetry of the irregularly shaped lumen.

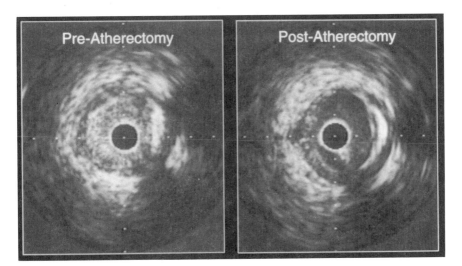

Figure 8 Intravascular ultrasound pre- and post-atherectomy. In this case, plaque removal is excellent.

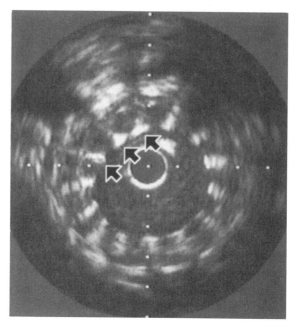

Figure 9 Underployed Palmaz Schatz Stent. In this example, three stent struts (arrows) are not fully expanded. Further balloon inflations at higher pressures resulted in complete stent apposition.

References

1. Topol EJ, Nissen SE. Our preoccupation with coronary luminology. the Dossociation between clinical and angiographic findings in ischemic heart disease. Circulation 92:2333-2342, 1995

2. Zir LM, Miller SW, Dinsmore RE, Gilber JP, Harthorne JW: Interobserver variability in coronary angiography. Circulation 53:627-632, 1976.

3. Vlodaver Z, Frech R, van Tassel RA, Edwards JE: Correlation of the antemortem coronary angiogram and the postmortem specimen. Circulation 47:162-168, 1973.

4. White CW, Wright CB, Doty DB, Hirtza LF, Eastham CL, Harrison DG, Marcus ML: Does visual interpretation of the coronary arteriogram predict the physiologic importance of a coronary stenosis? N Engl J Med 310:819-24,1984.

5. Waller BF: "Crackers, breakers, stretchers, drillers, scrapers, shavers, burners, welders, and melters": The future treatment of atherosclerotic coronary artery disease? A clinical-morphologic assessment . J Am Coll Cardiol 13:969-87, 1989.

6. Nissen SE, Grines CL, Gurley JC, Sublett K, Haynie D, Diaz C, Booth DC, DeMaria AN: Application of a new phased-array ultrasound imaging catheter in the assessment of vascular dimensions: In vivo comparison to cineangiography. Circulation 81(2): 660-666, 1990.

7. Nissen SE, Tuzcu EM, De Franco AC: Coronary Intravascular Ultrasound: Diagnostic and Interventional Applications. In: Topol EJ ed. Update to Textbook of Interventional Cardiology, W B Saunders, Philadelphia, PA, pages 207-222, 1994.

8. Nissen SE, Gurley JC, Grines CL, Booth DC, McClure R., Berk M, Fischer C, DeMaria AN: Intravascular ultrasound assessment of lumen size and wall morphology in normal subjects and coronary artery disease patients Circulation 84(3):1087-1099, 1991.

9. St. Goar FG, Pinto FJ, Alderman EL, Fitzgerald PJ, Stinson EB, Billingham ME, Popp RL. Detection of coronary atherosclerosis in young adult hearts using intravascular ultrasound, Circulation 86(3):756-763, 1992.

10. Fitzerald PJ, St. Goar FG, Connolly AJ, Pinto JF, Billingham ME, Popp RL, Yock PG: Intravascular ultrasound imaging of coronary arteries. Is three layers the norm? Circulation 86(1):154-158, 1992.

11. Tobis JM, Mallery J, Mahon D, Lehmann K, Zalesky P, Griffith J, Gessert J, Moriuchi M, McRae M, Dwyer ML, et al: Intravascular ultrasound imaging of human coronary arteries in vivo. Analysis of tissue characterizations with comparison to in vitro histological specimens. Circulation 83(3):913-926, 1991.

12. Nissen SE, De Franco AC, Raymond RE, Franco I, Eaton G, Tuzcu EM: Angiographically Urecognized Disease at "Normal" Reference Sites: A risk Factor for Sub-Optimal Results After Coronary Interventions. Circulation 88(4)I:412A, 1993.

13. Glagov S, Weisenberg E,Zarins CK et al: Compensatory Enlargement of Human Coronary Arteries. N Engl J of Med 316:1371-1375, 1987.

14. White CJ, Ramee SR, Collin TJ, Jain A, Mesa JE: Ambiguous coronary angiography: clinical utility of intravascular ultrasound. Cathet Cardiovasc Diagn 26(3):200-203, 1992.

15. Tuzcu EM, Hobbs H, Rincon G , Bott-Silverman C , De Franco AC, Robinson K, McCarthy P, Stewart R, Guyer S, Nissen SE: Occult and Frequent Transmission of Atherosclerosis Coronary Disease with Cardia Transplantation.. Circulation 1995; 91: 1706-1713

16. DeFranco AC, Tuzcu E, Abdelmeguid A, Lincoff AM, Brown D, Bernardi M, Ellis SG, Whitlow PL, Sutton JM, Casale PM, Raymond RE, Topol EJ, Nissen SE: Intravascular Ultrasound Assessment of PTCA Results: Insights into the Mechanisms of Balloon Angioplasty. J Am Coll Cardiol 1993, 21 (2):485A.

17. Popma JJ, Mintz GS et al Clinical and Angiographic outcome after Directional coronary Atherectomy. A qualitative and Quantitative Analysis Using Angiography and Intravascular Ultrasound. Am J Cardiol 72(13) 55E-64E

18. DeFranco AC, Tuzcu EM, Moliterno DJ, Raymond RE, Franco I, Guyer S, Ellis SG, Whitlow PL, Nissen SE: "Directional" Coronary Atherectomy Removes Atheroma More Effectively from Concentric than Eccentric Lesions: Intravascular Ultrasound Predictors of Lesional Success. Journal American College of Cardiology, Special Issue, February 1995;137A:730-3.

19. Tuzcu EM, Berkalp B, De Franco AC, Ellis SG, Whitlow PW, Franco I, Raymond RE, Nissen SE The Dilemma of Diagnosing Coronary Calcification: Angiography vs. Intravascular Ultrasound. J Am Coll Card, 1995, 27:832-838

20. Kovach JA, Mintz GS, Pichard AD, Kent KM, Popma JJ, Satler LF, Leon MB: Sequential intravascular ultrasound characterization of the mechanism of rotational atherectomy and adjunct balloon angioplasty. J Am Coll Cardiol 22:1024-1032, 1993.

21. Columbo A., Hall, P. et al Results of intravascular ultrasound guided coronary stenting without subsequent anticoagulation. J Am Coll Card: 335A:1994.

3.

QUANTITATIVE ANALYSIS OF LESION MORPHOLOGY BY COMPUTERIZED TECHNIQUES

G. B. John Mancini, M.D., F.R.C.P.(C), F.A.C.C.
Professor and Head of Internal Medicine
University of British Columbia and
Vancouver Hospital and Health Sciences Centre

Gilles Hudon, M.D., Head, Department of Radiology, Montreal Heart Institute, Associate Professor, Department of Radiology, University of Montreal

INTRODUCTION

The purpose of this chapter is to outline the development and application of a computerized method that provides quantitative indexes of lesion irregularity. The rationale for developing this methodology was based on a need to complement visual analysis methods and caliper based methods which are more commonly used to assess lesion complexity. The method allows one to assign continuous, numerical values to shape characteristics that define luminal roughness. This approach allows for more refined analysis and greater sensitivity in detecting subtle changes in lesion characteristics that cannot be quantitated adequately by categorical, visually-based methods.

BACKGROUND

Traditional methods of coronary artery disease description such as percent stenosis, number of diseased vessels, and lesion distribution have not been found to vary significantly between different ischemic cardiac syndromes and are only weak predictors of cardiac events (1-3). Coronary lesion morphology, however, varies between stable and unstable patients; complex lesions that have rough or irregular borders are found more often in clinically unstable situations (4-10). Increased roughness also predicts the development of myocardial infarction: a study by Ellis *et al* showed that irregular lesions were associated with a greater than fourfold increased risk for development of myocardial infarction for any degree of percent stenosis (11). The same study ranked lesion roughness as the most predictive feature for development of myocardial infarction, ahead of percent stenosis. Another study, by Freeman *et al*, found that complex coronary morphology, evidence of coronary thrombus, and the presence of multi-vessel disease were predictive of in-hospital cardiac events (12). Thus, lesion morphology may be the most important angiographically detectable feature of a coronary stenosis that is associated with clinical manifestations.

Complex lesions are usually defined qualitatively by irregular or hazy borders, outpouchings within a narrowed segment (presumed ulcerated plaque), intraluminal lucencies (indicating thrombus formation) and sharp leading or trailing edges associated with a lesion. Evidence that angiography can differentiate between complex and simple stenoses has been demonstrated with postmortem angiographic analysis (13). Most studies to date have used only qualitative assessments of morphology, which are subject to inter- and intraobserver variability inherent in visual inspection (14,15). Further, lack of standardization between laboratories, and the absence of a rigorous indexing system to grade lesions and detect subtle changes in response to therapy are also problematic. The most widely used qualitative classification system is that defined by Ambrose, which classifies lesions into 4 discrete morphology types (8). Previous attempts to quantitate lesion morphology have been hampered by cumbersome methodology and the inability to reliably detect all manifestations of a complex lesion (16).

METHOD

Angiograms are projected on a cine viewer(Vanguard Instruments, model XR-15, Melville, NY) optically coupled to a video camera. At 2.4:1 optical magnification, the video signal was digitized at 512 x 512 x 8 bit resolution onto a digital angiographic computer (ADAC Laboratories, model DPS-4100C, Milpitas, CA). Images are magnified twofold using bilinear interpolation. The operator determines the lesion of interest from preselected cine frames by placing a variable sized circle around the appropriate segment of the artery. Every effort is made to minimize the amount of normal artery included in the portion analyzed since inclusion of variable amounts of normal artery could bias results and increase variability.

The automatic edge detection portion of the program, previously described (17), was enhanced by the addition of a sequential edge linking technique which provides spatial sampling of sufficient density to characterize complex arterial borders (18). The sequential edge linking algorithm uses the known, undersampled edge points as a template to generate very detailed, contiguous pixel edges all along the magnified arterial border. These additional edge points are selected based on their expected pixel intensities and locations interpolated from the known edge points surrounding them. After detailed edge detection was completed, each border of a given lesion was analyzed individually using vector and fractal analysis techniques described below.

Curvature of a circle is defined as the inverse of the radius of that circle; as the radius decreases the curvature value increases. Any point along a continuous curve may be thought of as lying on the perimeter of a circle and its curvature may be calculated using vector analysis with standard Frenet-Serret formulas (19, 20). These formulas show that curvature is directly proportional to the rate of change of the tangent vector to the curve with respect to the arc length of the curve. Tight bends are associated with high curvature values and a straight line has a curvature value of 0. Arterial borders may be treated as continuous curves and their shape may be described by plotting the curvature valueat each point along the edge. This function is known as a "curvature signature". The angiographic catheter is assumed to have smooth, straight borders and therefore its edges should have curvature values of zero. Deviations from zero are assumed to reflect all factors contributing to image noise. Therefore, to account for image noise and difference in image quality, the curvature signature of the arterial edge was divided by the standard deviation of the curvature of the catheter edges to yield a normalized curvature signature. Curvature peaks of arterial edges were only considered significant when values were greater than 2 standard deviations of the catheter curvature values. Such peaks were felt to represent true irregularities of the arterial border.

Morphometric parameters (Figures 1 & 2)

Five morphometric parameters were calculated, 4 derived from the normalized curvature signature, and 1 based on the concept of fractal analysis (21). Parameters were determined individually for each border of an arterial lesion segment. The use of these parameters as shape descriptors was previously validated by substituting various mathematical functions for arterial borders (18):

1. *Peaks/cm:* defined as the number of curvature peaks outside ± 2 standard deviations, per centimeter of lesion length.
2. *Summed maximum error/cm:* the sum of the maximum normalized curvature value occurring at each significant peak, corrected for lesion length.
3. *Integrated error/cm:* the summation of areas under the curvature signature for each significant peak, corrected for lesion length.
4. *Number of major features/cm:* determined using pattern recognition when examining the curvature signature of a border. A "feature" was defined as a bulge or indentation along the edge of a lesion which

corresponds to groupings of three curvature peaks (a "triplet") of alternating sign along the curvature signature, *i.e.* frompositive to negative to positive, or from negative to positive to negative (Figure 1). The number of features is obtained by summing the number of triplets thus defined and correcting for lesion length.

5.   *Scaled edge length ratio:* (Figure 2) calculated using a simplification of fractal analysis. True fractal analysis uses multiple ruler sizes to measure the length of the same border and takes the slope of the line resulting from the plot of the logarithm of the measured length vs. the logarithm of the ruler length as a descriptor of border roughness (21) . The scaled edge length ratio parameter used in this study equals the ratio of 2 measured lengths of the same arterial border using different ruler sizes. The 2 lengths were chosen empirically for this study. The first length (L1) was measured using a ruler length of 2 pixels on the digitized angiogram. The second length (L2) was measured using a ruler length of 1/2 the maximum diameter of the normal arterial segment. For irregular borders, L1 is greater than L2 since a smaller ruler is able to measure more of the edge detail. The scaled edge length ratio equals L1 divided by L2. As lesion roughness increases, L1 increases out of proportion to L2 and, therefore, the scaled edge length ratio also increases.

An example of the finalized borders from the automatic edge detection program and curvature signature for the edges are shown in Figure 3. Note that one edge is relatively smooth but the other is quite complex with a number of significant curvature peaks.

58

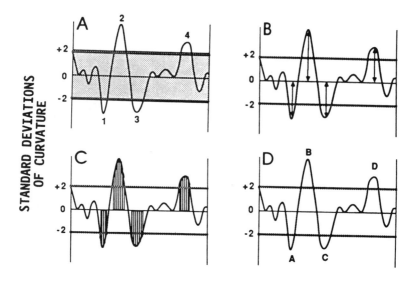

FIGURE 1.   PANEL A: Curvature signature of an arterial border
demonstrating *peaks per centimeter*.   Standard deviations of
curvature are plotted on the ordinate, with a cutoff of +2
standard deviations (shaded area).   Peaks in the curvature
signature beyond ± 2 SD "normal" range are considered
significant (labelled 1-4).   In all panels the x-axis
represents lesion length.   PANEL B: Analysis of curvature
signature showing *summed maximum error*.   Maximum values at
each curvature peak (*arrows*) are added together to obtain
this parameter.   PANEL C: *Integrated curvature error* is
calculated by finding all regions of the curvature signature
which extend beyond the +2SD lines, integrating under the
curve in these regions, and summing these values (*shaded
areas*).   PANEL D: The *number of major features* is extracted
from analysis of triplet patterns of significant positive-
negative-positive or negative-positive-negative curvature
peaks.   Two features are found in this curvature signature,
labelled *ABC* and *BCD*. (Reproduced with permission from
reference #22.)

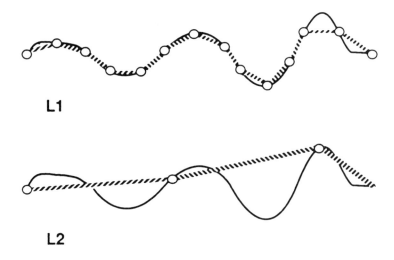

L1

L2

FIGURE 2: The *scaled edge length ratio* is the ratio of two measured lengths of the same arterial border (L1/L2) using different ruler sizes. L1 is determined using a ruler length of two pixels, L2 is calculated with a ruler length of one-half the arterial diameter of the normal segment. (Reproduced with permission from reference #22).

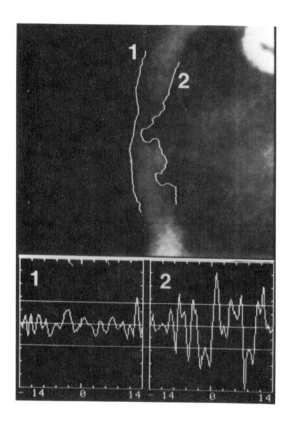

FIGURE 3: A digital image with automatically determined artery edges and corresponding curvature signatures for a complex coronary lesion in a patient with unstable angina. Edge 2 shows numerous complex features. (Reproduced with permission from reference #22).

Reproducibility

The quantitative analysis was found to be
highly reproducible for all of the parameters
(Table 1). The correlation coefficients for both
intra- and interobserver variability ranged
between 0.79 and 0.96 and none of the mean
differences were significantly different from 0.0
(all p values were >0.05).

TABLE 1:   Intra- and interobserver variability of
morphometric parameters:

PARAMETER	r value	mean difference
INTRAOBSERVER VARIABILITY		
PEAKS/CM	0.93	0.44 + 0.90
SUMMED MAXIMUM		
ERROR/CM	0.96	1.37 + 2.59
INTEGRATED ERROR/CM	0.98	-7.6 + 16.1
NUMBER OF FEATURES/CM	0.83	0.07 + 0.55
SCALED EDGE		
LENGTH RATIO	0.90	.002 + 0.014
INTEROBSERVER VARIABILITY		
PEAKS/CM	0.94	0.55 + 0.88
SUMMED MAXIMUM		
ERROR/CM	0.93	1.56 + 3.46
INTEGRATED ERROR/CM	0.94	10.4 + 25.6
NUMBER OF FEATURES/CM	0.79	0.0 + 0.71
SCALED EDGE		
LENGTH RATIO	0.86	.009 + 0.016

Mean difference is expressed as mean + standard deviation.
r value = correlation coefficient. All p values are >0.05
for mean difference vs. 0.0. (Reproduced with permission
from reference #22).

CLINICAL APPLICATIONS

Unstable Angina

Two groups of patients were analyzed, those
with chronic stable angina and those with
unstable angina.

Four of the 5 morphometric parameters were
found to be significantly different between the
unstable and stable angina patients (Table 2).
There were approximately one and one half the
number of significant peaks/cm between the

62

unstable and stable angina patients, 4.29±2.19
versus 2.69±2.36, p=0.0056. Roughly twice the
mean value for summed maximum error/cm was found
in the unstable cohort, 15.42±10.57 versus
8.43±8.91, p=0.0018, as was the case for
integrated error/cm 112.5±94.8 versus 51.7±61.9,
p=0.0008. Also significantly different were the
number of major features/cm (bulges and
indentations) detected, unstable angina 0.82±0.83
versus stable 0.37±0.62, p=0.0069. The scaled
edge length ratio was not different between the
2 groups, unstable angina 1.089±0.039 versus
stable angina 1.068±0.0021, p=0.0841.
Collectively, these data indicate quantifiably
greater lesion complexity in the unstable angina
population.

TABLE 2:   Morphometric differences between stable and
unstable angina.

	UNSTABLE ANGINA n=59	STABLE ANGINA n=20	p*
PEAKS/CM	4.29 ± 2.19	2.69 ± 2.36	0.0056
SUMMED MAXIMUM ERROR/CM	15.42 ± 10.57	8.43 ± 8.91	0.0018
INTEGRATED ERROR/CM	112.5 ± 94.8	51.7 ± 61.9	0.0008
NUMBER OF FEATURES/CM	0.82 ± 0.83	0.37 ± 0.62	0.007
SCALED EL RATIO	1.089 ± 0.039	1.068 ± 0.021	0.0841

Data are mean ± standard deviation. MAX = maximum. Each
lesion was evaluated by taking the average of the parameters
calculated from its 2 edges (*Mann - Whitney test).
(Reproduced with permission from reference #22).

    The stable and unstable angina groups were
also compared using traditional methods of
coronary artery disease description, including
lesion distribution, percent diameter stenosis,
minimum diameter and the qualitative morphology
classification scheme defined by Ambrose.
Unstable angina patients were found to have a
significantly greater percent diameter stenosis
(76.2 ± 13.7 vs 49.2 ± 21.4%, p < 0.0001) and
smaller minimum luminal diameter (0.74 ± 0.44 vs
1.79 ± 0.78 mm, p < 0.0001). When the groups

were compared using the Ambrose morphology classification scheme no statistically significant difference was found by Chi-Square analysis (P=0.7239) although the expected trend of more complex lesions in the unstable angina group was evident.

Each of the quantitative parameters was compared to both percent diameter stenosis and minimum diameter using linear regression analysis after combining the 2 cohorts (Table 3). No significant correlation was found between the morphometric parameters and these measures of luminal narrowing, showing the method's independence from traditional assessments of lesion severity.

Table 3: Correlations with traditional methods of coronary artery disease description.*

	r vs %sten	r vs min. diam
PEAKS/CM	.0703	-.0978
SUMMED MAX. ERROR/CM	.01524	-.0556
INTEGRATED ERROR/CM	.0453	-.0329
NUMBER OF FEATURES/CM	.0730	-.0373
SCALED EL RATIO	.0995	-.0946

n = 79 - the analysis was performed after combining the 2 populations. *all r values are associated with p values $\geq$ 0.39. (Reproduced with permission from reference #22.)

The two groups were compared graphically to determine the amount of overlap for each parameter between the stable and unstable angina patients (Figure 4). An analysis was performed to determine a cutoff value for differentiating stable from unstable lesions for each of the 4 parameters which were found to be significantly different between the two groups. The cutoff values were chosen to maximize the concordance while keeping the sensitivity and specificity within 10% of one another (Table 5). For these 4 parameters the cutoff values yielded sensitivities ranging from 71.2% to 79.7%, specificities from 65.0% to 70.0%, and concordance rates of 70.9% to 77.2%. The best results were obtained with the peaks/cm parameter (cutoff value of 2.7: sensitivity = 79.7%, specificity = 70.0% and concordance = 77.2%) for differentiating unstable from stable angina lesions.

Post-lysis Reocclusion

Early reocclusion after successful thrombolysis is an important limiting factor in the efficacy of this treatment for acute myocardial infarction. The ability to identify patients at increased risk for rethrombosis could concievably improve the stratification of patient management after thrombolysis. To date, no clinical or angiographic variable has been shown consistently to predict ischemic events after thrombolysis. Previous studies in patients treated with streptokinase reported that a residual high-grade stenosis could predict the occurrence of early ischemic events (23-26). However, Ellis et al. failed to show any significant difference in stenosis severity, evaluated through quantitative coronary angiography, between patients with and without recurrent ischemia in a large population of patients that had received human recombinant tissue-plasminogen activator (rt-PA) (27).

An example of the borders from the automatic edge detection program and curvature signature for the edges is shown in Figure 5. The five morphometric parameters described were calculated for each edge of each lesion for both reocclusion and no-reocclusion groups in two orthogonal views, when biplane analysis was feasible, or in only one view when single plane quantitative analysis was performed.

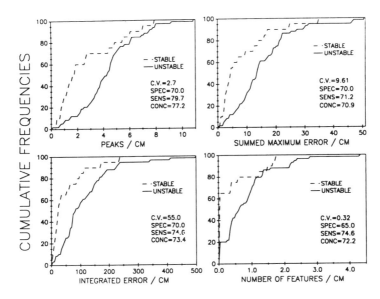

FIGURE 4: Plots of the cumulative frequencies at different values for the parameters to distinguish between the stable and unstable angina patients. The y axis gives the cummulative percentage of the lesions in each group associated with an index value ≤ to the value on the x axis. The cut-off or critical value (C.V.) is generally seen at the value on the x-axis where the two curves are most divergent. SPEC = specificity, SENS = sensitivity, CONC = concordance. See text for definition of these terms. (Reproduced with permission from reference #22).

TABLE 4: Cutoff values to differentiate stable from unstable angina lesions.

		Sensitivity	Specificity	Concordance
Peaks/cm	≥ 2.7	79.7%	70.0%	77.2%
Summed Max. Error/cm	≥ 9.61	71.2%	70.0%	70.9%
Integrated Error/cm	≥ 55	74.6%	70.0%	73.4%
Number of Features/cm	≥0.32	74.6%	65.0%	72.2%

See text for definition of terms. (Reproduced with permission from reference #22.)

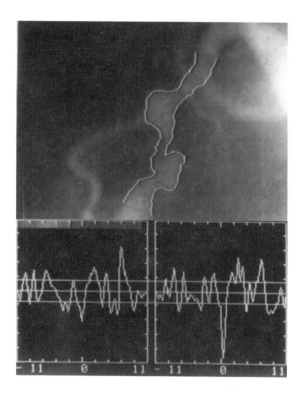

Figure 5: Proximal right coronary artery with a long and highly complex, post-lysis lesion that eventually reoccluded. The curvature plots are shown beneath the arterial image with its superimposed edges. The left plot corresponds to the left edge and the right plot corresponds to the right edge. The x-axis signifies length and the y axis signifies mormalized curvature values. The central, horizontal, straight line corresponds to a curvature value of zero (ie a segment that is perfectly smooth would have zero curvature). The horizontal bars on either side are $\pm$ 2 standard deviations for the curvature analysis of the catheter shaft (not shown), presumed to be straight and smooth. These bars represent the curvature value extremes that could be accounted for solely by image noise. The curvature signature peaks extending beyond these boundaries represent true morphological features of the arterial edges from which are based the mathematical roughness indexes. (Reproduced with permission from reference #28.)

No significant difference between the two groups was found with respect to the traditional quantitative parameters of stenosis severity either in single plane (minimum diameter, percent diameter stenosis) or in biplane analysis (minimal cross-sectional area, percent cross-sectional area stenosis). There was a trend suggesting that more severe lesions occurred in the reocclusion group (Table 5). In contrast, length was found to be significantly ($p<.05$) greater in the reocclusion group. Thrombus was visually recognized in 4 cases (16%) of reocclusion and in 14 (24%) cases of no-reocclusion group (difference not significant). When the groups were compared by the Ambrose morphology classification scheme, percentage of patients with reocclusion was significantly higher in patients with more complex lesions (Ambrose code I (smooth, concentric): 12.5%; IIa (smooth, ecentric): 19.1%; IIb (irregular edges, ecentric): 37.5%, III (serial lesions): 55.6%; $p<.05$).

Table 5: Quantitative angiographic parameters describing the 90 minute post-thrombolysis appearance of infarct-related lesions.

	REOCCLUSION	NO REOCCLUSION
Minimum diameter (mm)	0.82 + 0.35	0.87 + 0.89
% diameter stenosis	72 + 10	67 + 14
Minimal cross-sectional area (mm^2)	0.88 + 0.61	0.92 + 0.90
% cross-sectional area	88 + 7	85 + 11
Length (mm)	12.2 + 5.0	10.0 + 4.2*

p <.05, all data in tables presented as mean + S.D. (Reproduced with permission from reference #28.)

Four of the five quantitative morphometric parameters were found to be significantly higher in patients with reocclusion (Table 6). When normalized by the length, the differences in parameters of vector analysis between the two groups were no longer significant (Table 6).

68

Table 6: Quantitative roughness measurements describing the
90 minute post-thrombolysis appearance of infarct-related
lesions.

	REOCCLUSION	NO REOCCLUSION	P
Scaled EL ratio	1.15 + 0.10	1.09 + 0.08	.006
Peaks	98 + 40	80 + 41	.031
Summed maximum error	406 + 218	329 + 219	n.s.
Integrated error	334 + 186	257 + 196	.041
Features	37 + 27	23 + 17	.037
Peaks/centimeter	8.3 + 2.5	8.0 + 2.6	n.s.
Summed maximum error/centimeter	34.4 + 17.9	32.7 + 16.0	n.s.
Integrated error/centimeter	281 + 136	255 + 146	n.s.
Features per centimeter	3.2 + 2.1	2.4 + 1.7	n.s.

(Reproduced with permission from reference #28.)

By stepwise logistic regression analysis,
length (p < .03) and the number of features/cm (p
< .04) were independent predictors of
reocclusion. When stepwise regression analysis
was applied to the mean value of each parameter
from all edges, the scaled edge length ratio
parameter was the only independent predictor of
reocclusion (p < .03).

Data from the unstable angina study were
used to establish optimal cutoff or threshold
values that distinguished between patients with
stable and unstable angina. These cutoff values
were prospectively applied to the postthrombolytic lesions. Table 7 shows that with
respect to the peaks/cm, summed maximum error/cm,
the integrated error/cm, and the features/cm
indexes, a minority of the lesions in this study
had morphological features similar to patients
with chronic, stable angina (2.4 - 13.1%). When
these indexes were similar to those of lesions in
chronic, stable angina, reocclusion rarely
occurred. The rest of the lesions had indexes
indicating greater complexity. Of these,
approximately 30% reoccluded. With respect to
the scaled edge length ratio, however, 40% of
lesions had relatively normal values and the
majority of these (76%) did not reocclude. 40%
of lesions with high scaled edge length ratios
reoccluded (p<.03).

Table 7: Distribution of lesions with respect to critical threshold values* for each quantitative index.

	OCCLUSION	NO REOCCLUSION	Sen	Sp	PV
PEAKS/CM[a]					
< 2.7	0	2			
> 2.7	25	57	100%	3%	32%
SUMMED MAXIMUM ERROR/CM[a]					
< 9.61	0	4			
> 9.61	25	55	100%	7%	35%
INTEGRATED ERROR/CM[a]					
<55	0	4			
>55	25	55	100%	7%	35%
FEATURES PER CM[a]					
<0.32	2	9			
>0.32	23	50	92%	15%	38%
SCALED EL RATIO[b]					
<1.07	5	29			
>1.07	20	30	80%	49%	58%

* Critical threshold values were determined from reference #8 and are those values shown to best distinguish between lesions associated with stable and unstable angina. a = n.s., b = p < .03 (Fischer's Exact Test). Sn = sensitivity, Sp = specificity, PV = positive predictive value of a high roughness index. (Reproduced with permission from reference #28.)

The sensitivity, specificity and predictive values were also generated by using threshold or cutoff values generated solely from the data obtained from the post-lytic lesions investigated in this study. Table 8 shows the results using these criteria and demonstrates that featues/cm, scaled edge length ratio and length had statistically significant distributions with sensitivities ranging between 76-84%, specificities ranging between 47-54% and predictive values ranging between 57-62% for predicting reocclusion.

70

Table 8: Distribution of lesions with respect to critical threshold values* for each quantitative index.

	REOCCLUSION	NO REOCCLUSION	Sen	Sp	PV
PEAKS/CM[a]					
< 4.28	2	12			
≥ 4.28	23	47	92%	20%	42%
SUMMED MAXIMUM ERROR/CM[a]					
< 17.5	5	20			
≥ 17.5	20	39	80%	34%	35%
INTEGRATED ERROR/CM[a]					
<126	4	20			
≥126	21	39	84%	34%	35%
FEATURES PER CM[b]					
<0.83	6	29			
≥0.83	19	30	76%	49%	57%
SCALED EL RATIO[c]					
<1.066	4	28			
≥1.066	31	21	84%	47%	58%
LENGTH[d]					
<9.05	5	32			
≥9.05	20	27	80%	54%	62%

===
* In contrast to Table 8, the critical, threshold values in this table are derived solely from the post-lytic lesions analyzed in this study. a = n.s., b = p < .03, c = p < .006, d = p < .004 (Fischer's Exact Test). Sn = sensitivity, Sp = specificity, PV = positive predictive value of a high roughness index or length. (Reproduced with permission from reference #28.)

DISCUSSION

Problems are associated with qualitative assessment of morphology due to the subjective nature of the process. There is a lack of standardization in interpretation between different laboratories and no rigorous indexing system exists to grade lesions or detect subtle changes in response to therapy. Most previous studies using qualitative descriptions of morphology require that each lesion be assigned to a discrete morphology type (4-10). The method described above allows all parameters of a lesion to be derived in continuous scale fashion and therefore avoids the problem of assigning a lesion to a predetermined category. Use of this method would allow uniformity in clinical trials and provide a rigorous and perhaps more sensitive system for grading change in lesion morphology. Another major problem with subjective visual inspection of coronary lesions is the inherent potential for inter- and intraobserver variability (14,15). The program described showed excellent reproducibility as evidenced by low inter-and intraobserver variability for all of the parameters.

Previous quantitative assessments of lesion morphology have been few in number. Wilson *et al* used an "ulceration index" to describe lesion roughness (16). The method, however, is cumbersome, since it relies on hand tracing of arterial borders. In addition, the ulceration index was dependent upon measurement of 2 separate luminal diameters within a lesion, a problem which was avoided in the present study since each edge is initially examined separately for individual shape characteristics. All parameters are, therefore, independent of lesion stenosis. Probably the most important difficulty with the Wilson approach is that it detects only complex lesions with areas of plaque ulceration within a narrowed segment. The current methodology is applicable to all lesion morphologies and does not require specific characteristics for analysis.

The importance of complicated stenoses, those with plaque rupture, ulceration or hemorrhage in the pathogenesis of acute thrombosis and myocardial infarction is well known. Pooled data from 5 necropsy studies showed that 292 episodes of acute thrombosis were associated with 265 complicated stenoses, a prevalence of 91% (29-33). Postmortem angiography was found to have a sensitivity of 88% and specificity of 79% in defining complicated stenoses on the basis of an irregular border or intraluminal lucencies (13,34), suggesting that these lesions may be detected before the development of thrombosis and potentially modified to reduce the risk of future cardiac events. A recent study using qualitative morphology analysis to compare stable and unstable patients found that evidence of coronary thrombus had a sensitivity of only 42% and evidence of complex lesion morphology (defined as haziness, smudging or irregular lesion margins) had a sensitivity of only 44% in detecting lesions from unstable angina patients (35). In our study the quantitative parameters peaks/cm, summed maximum error/cm, integrated error/cm and number of features/cm gave sensitivities of 71.2% to 79.7%, while maintaining specificities of 65.0% to 70.0%. This compares favorably to the above mentioned study (35) in which the combination of 2 criteria (intracoronary thrombus and complex morphology) yielded a sensitivity of 70% and a specificity of 79%.

Although 4 of the 5 quantitative morphometric parameters tested were found to be significantly different between stable and unstable angina populations, no statistically significant difference was found between the unstable and stable angina patients when the qualitative classification scheme of Ambrose was used even though a trend toward greater lesion complexity was noted in the unstable group. This may have resulted from the relatively small sample size of the stable angina group, but serves to emphasize that this quantitative method appears to be more sensitive for detecting differences even between small groups of patients. The method is also better suited for detecting subtle changes that might be induced by therapy with thrombolytic, antiplatelet or lipid-lowering agents since the parameters are derived in a continuous, noncategorical fashion.

The one parameter which did not show a difference between the stable and unstable angina patient was the scaled edge length ratio. The calculation of this parameter was based on the concept of fractal analysis and was thus conceptionally different from the other 4 parameters which were calculated using curvature analysis. The failure of this parameter to differentiate between the 2 groups of patients may have been due to not choosing the optimal ruler lengths to maximize differences in border measurements or our inability to apply the more formal method of fractal analysis due to computer limitations. Hopefully future refinements of this concept will also prove useful in defining complex lesion morphology.

Rethrombosis after successfull thrombolysis occurs with all thrombolytic agents at a rate ranging between 2-46% (26,36,37). Reocclusion may cause recurrent ischemia or reinfarction, but it may also be silent. In a large population of patients, reocclusion was associated with worsened infarct zone regional wall motion even in patients with asymptomatic rethrombosis (38). This may be explained by experimental studies that showed an influence of maintained reperfusion in the infarct-related artery on the long-term healing of the myocardium after infarction (39,40). Thus, both symptomatic and asymptomatic reocclusion are linked to higher in-hospital and long-term complication rates. For this reason, in patients at high risk of reocclusion, more aggressive post-lytic monitoring and/or therapy may be necessary. Unfortunately, so far no clinical or angiographic parameter has been shown consistently to be predictive of reocclusion.

It has been noted that occlusive coronary thrombi are often associated with ulcerated or fissured atherosclerotic plaques (38,39,41). Moreover, Levine and Fallon found that these complicated lesions may be identified by angiography because of irregular borders, outpouchings with narrowed segments or intraluminal luciencies (40). Thus, complex morphology is now considered to be an important and perhaps the most important angiographic feature related to the prognostic significance of coronary lesions. However, qualitative assessment of complex lesions has proved to have a sensitivity of only 44% in predicting unstable coronary syndromes and/or infarction (42). Moreover, in different studies of the role played by lesion morphology in promoting unstable coronary syndromes, different qualitative criteria have been employed. The lack of a standard and precise indexing system to analyze lesion morphology motivated us to develop a quantitative, computerized analysis method for determining coronary lesion roughness.

Our data are concordant with very recent work showing that stenosis severity does not correlate with reocclusion (43,44). Although residual coronary stenoses were a little more severe in the reocclusion group, no statistical difference was demonstrated in this study. In contrast, we found that stenosis length was significantly greater in the reocclusion group.

Lange et al. reported that stenosis length was the most significant predictor of post-infarction angina (42). In contrast, Ellis et al. did not show any difference in length of residual coronary lesions between patients with and without reocclusion after thrombolysis (27). This was also true in a study performed in the Global Utilization of Streptokinase and t-PA for Occluded Coronary Arteries (GUSTO) Study (43). Despite these discrepancies, there are several reasons for considering lesion length as a plausible risk factor for reocclusion. In experimental studies, anterograde flow decreases for any given percent diameter stenosis as the stenosis length increases (45,46). Moreover, long stenoses represent larger atherosclerotic plaques with a potentially larger, fissured surface area. Both of these factors could easily promote platelet adhesion, thrombosis and either partial or total reocclusion. This possibility is supported by this study which shows that lesion length is the most important predictor of reocclusion. Although four of the five morphometric parameters were significantly higher compared with the no reocclusion group, no differences were seen between the two groups when these were normalized by lesion length, (Table 6). Perhaps even more important is to emphasize that the failure to identify length as a possible determinant of reocclusion in the GUSTO Study (43) may have been due to the method used to measure length. The lengths reported in that study were 16mm on average whereas the lengths reported in our study were in the 10 to 12mm range. It is likely, therefore, that the GUSTO analysis merely used the usual quantitative approach to measuring lesions which includes

variable and sometimes substantial reference
sement lengths that are smooth and featureless.
Our mehtodology specifically avoids inclusion of
the smooth, reference segment to avoid "dilution"
of the quantitative analysis, including length
measurement, of the roughened part of the lesion.

While perhaps not the primary factor, edge
roughness is still a contributing risk factor for
reocclusion. This is supported by our univariate
analysis showing that the scaled edge length
ratio (a parameter that is independent of length)
is greater in the reocclusion group. It is
further supported by the two multiple regression
analyses. The first, incorporating the roughness
indexes from each arterial edge as independent
observations, showed that both length and the
number of features (invaginations and
evaginations) per centimeter were independently
correlated with reocclusion. The second
regression analysis, utilizing an average of the
roughness indexes obtained from each arterial
edge, showed that the scaled edge length ratio
was a determinant of reocclusion.

In the previous study in which this
quantitative method was employed, cutoff values
for each of the parameters were defined for
differentiating stable and unstable lesions (22).
If we compare those values with the values of the
parameters found in the current study, very few
lesions can be considered "normal" (Table 7).
That is, infarct-related lesions early after
successful thrombolysis are a particular set of
complex lesions, whose morphology appears to be
quite different from that of "stable" lesions and
even more complex than lesions found in patients
with unstable angina. This is explained
reasonably by the fact that they all are plaques
with recent endothelial injury, plaque rupture or
ulceration (47-50). Table 8 also shows that low
roughness indexes were seldom associated with
reocclusion and that the scaled edge length ratio
was the best criterion in predicting reocclusion.
It had a sensitivity of 53% and a specificity of
76%.

It is worth noting that intracoronary
thrombus was angiographically identified in 16%

of patients with reocclusion and in 24% of patients without reocclusion (difference not significant). Recently, Reher et al. found intracoronary thrombus, defined as abrupt vessel cutoff with irregular margins or intraluminal filling defect in a patent vessel, to be present significantly more often (43%) in patients with prolonged rest angina without myocardial infarction than in patients with stable angina (14%) (29). In our study, patients with acute myocardial infarction and successful initial thrombolysis were studied, thereby constituting a distinctly different group of patients than the group studied by Reher et al. This may account for the low incidence of angiographically detected intracoronary thrombi. Thus, the mere presence of intracoronary thrombus in such patients is not a good predictor of recurrent occlusive thrombosis after thrombolysis. Our results are compatible with those of Ellis et al (27) as well as those of the GUSTO Study (43) and of the UNASEM Study (Unstable Angina Study Using Eminase, 44). But this should not be misinterpreted to mean that the majority of post-lysis lesions are free of clot. On the contrary, the marked irregularity of these lesions is likely to be a result of residual mural clot, as opposed to intraluminal clot. The angiographic appearance of the latter constituted the major requirement of our definition for the presence of clot. Mural clot does not yield a sufficiently characteristic angiographic appearance and may only be inferred to be present when irregular lumen boundaries in this type of patient cohort are detected. In general, however, irregular lumen borders are not necessarily caused solely by clot. Therefore, the mere presence of irregular luminal edges was not considered sufficient for designating the presence of clot.

The results of a recent study by Davies et al (49) demonstrated that high ulceration index (16) was associated with reocclusion after successful recanalization with streptokinase. The ulceration index showed a 58% sensitivity in prediction of reocclusion which is similiar to our 53% sensitivity when using the scaled edge length ratio applied prospectively (Table 7). However, we report higher sensitivities (between

76 and 84%) when criteria based only on post-lytic lesions are considered (Table 8). In contrast to our study, lesion length was not associated with reocclusion in the study of Davies et al. However, that study did not use automated edge detection methods to calculate length and the ulceration index reflects only relative lesion diameters within stenoses. The approcach used in our study is more general and can mathematically quantitate roughness of each arterial edge independently. That is, the values are not dependent on lesion diameters. Moreover, our analyses were based on films obtained 90 minutes, not 1 to 8 days, after thrombolysis.

In summary, this method provides an objective and quantitative description of morphology which differentiates stable from unstable angina patients as well as post-lysis lesions that remain patent or re-occlude. Major advantages include the ease and rapidity with which analysis may be performed, lack of reliance on expert users, excellent reproducibility, avoidance of subjective visual inspection, independence from traditional methods of coronary artery disease description such as percent stenosis or minimum diameter, and the ability to assess lesion morphology in a continuous scale fashion rather than assigning lesions to discrete categories. This type of analysis can give uniformity and power to trials studying the effects of interventions on coronary lesions in an attempt to alter patient prognosis. Given the potential importance of coronary morphology in predicting the clinical behavior of a lesion even in settings other than unstable angina or post-lysis reocclusion (52-54), a more rigorous and quantitative approach will probably be mandated in future clinical trials studying this aspect of coronary disease.

REFERENCES

1.   Friesinger GC, Page II, Ross RS: Prognostic significance of coronary arteriography. Trans Assoc Am Physicians 1970;83:78-92.
2.   Cass Principle Investigators and their Associates: Myocardial infarction and mortality in the coronary

artery surgery study randomized trial. New Engl J Med 1984;310:750-8.

3.   Alison HW, Russel RO, Mantel JA, Kouchoukos NT, Moraski RE, Rackley CE: Coronary anatomy and arteriography in patients with unstable angina pectoris. Am J Cardiol 1978;41:204-9.

4.   Sanasa M, Cernigliaro C, Bolognese L, Bongo SA, Rossi L, Rossi P: Angiographic morphology and response to therapy in unstable angina. Clin Cardiol, 1988;11;121-6.

5.   Lo YS, Cutler JE, Blake K, Wright AM, Kron J, and Swerdlow CD: Angiographic coronary morphology in survivors of cardiac arrest. Am Heart J 1988;115;781-5.

6.   Ambrose JA, Winters SL, Arora RR, Haft JI, Goldstein J, Rentrop KP, Gorlin R, Fuster V: Coronary angiographic morphology in myocardial infarction: a link between the pathogenesis of unstable angina and myocardial infarction. J Am Coll Cardiol 1985;6;1233-8.

7.   Ambrose JA, Craig E, Mosen H, Borrico S, Gorlin R, and Fuster V: Angiographic demonstration of a common link between unstable angina and non-Q wave acute myocardial infarction. Am J Cardiol 1988;61:244-7.

8.   Ambrose JA, Winters SL, Stern A, Eng A, Teichholz LE, Gorlin R, and Fuster V: Angiographic morphology and the pathogenesis of unstable angina pectoris. J Am Coll Cardiol 1985;5:609-16.

9.   Taus RH, Levin DC Boxt LM, Meyerowicz MF, Harrington DP: Angiographic stenosis morphology: a new way to interpret arteriograms. Radiology 1985;157:67 (abstr).

10. Lekakis J, Pistevos A, Rokas S, Moulopoulos S: Coronary morphology in unstable angina: study in one vessel disease. Circulation 1986;74:II-480.

11. Ellis S, Alderman EL, Cain K, Wright A, Bourassa M, Fisher L, and the Participants of the Coronary Artery Surgery Study. Morphology of left anterior descending coronary territory lesions as a predictor of anterior myocardial infarction: a CASS registry study. J Am Coll Cardiol 1989; 13: 1481-1491.

12. Freeman MR, Williams AE, Chisholm RS, Armstrong PW: Intracoronary thrombus and complex morphology in unstable angina: relation to timing of angiography and in-hospital cardiac events. Circulation 1989;80:17-23.

13. Levin DC, Fallon JT: Significance of the angiographic morphology of local-ized stenoses: histopathologic correlations. Circulation 1982;66:316-20.

14. Zir LM, Miller SW, Dinsmore RE, Zilbert JP, Harthorne JW: Interobserver variability in coronary angiography. Circulation 1976; 53:627-32.

15. DeRown TA, Murray JA, Owen W: Variability in the analysis of coronary angiograms. Circulation 1977;55:324-8.

16. Wilson RF, Myrl HD, White CW: Quantitative angiographic morphology and coronary stenoses leading to myocardial infarction or unstable angina. Circulation 1986;73:286-93.

17. Mancini GBJ, Simon SB, McGillem MJ, LeFree MT, Friedman HZ and Vogel RA: Automated quantitative coronary

arteriography: Morphologic and physiologic validation *in vivo* of a rapid digital angiographic method. Circulation 1987;75:452-60.

18. Simon SB, LeFree MT, McGillem MJ, Kalbfleisch SJ, Anselmo EG, Sitomer J, DeBoe SF, Ellis S, Mancini GBJ: Automated morphometric analysis of coronary artery lesions: an extension of quantitative coronary arteriography. Computers in Cardiology 1988; 347-50.

19. Speigel MR: Vector Analysis. New York: Schawm Publishing Co., 35-8, 1959.

20. Mancini GBJ, DeBoe SF, Anselmo E, Simon SB, LeFree MT, and Vogel RA: Quantitative regional curvature analysis: an application of shape determination for assessment of segmental left ventricular function in man. Am Heart J 1987;113:326-34.

21. Mandelbrot BB: Fractals: Form, Chance and Dimension. Freeman, 33, 1977.

22. Kalbfleisch SJ, McGillem MJ, Simon SB, DeBoe SF, Pinto IMF, Mancini GBJ. Automated quantitation of indexes of coronary lesion complexity. Comparison between patients with stable and unstable angina. Circulation 1990; 82: 439-447.

23. Serruys PW, Wijns WW, Van Den Brand M, Ribeiro V, Fioretti P, Simmons ML, Kooijman CJ, Rieber JHC, Hugenholtz PG. Is transluminal coronary angioplasty mandatory after successful thrombolysis? Quantitative coronary angiographic study. Br Heart J 1983; 59: 257-65.

24. Harrison DG, Ferguson DW, Collins SM, Skorton DJ, Ericksen EE, Kioschos JM, Marcus ML, White CW. Rethrombosis after reperfusion with streptokinase: importance of geometry of residual stenosis. Circulation 1984; 69: 991-999.

25. Gash AK, Spann JF, Sherry S, Delber AD, Carabello BA, McDonough MT, Mann RH, McCann WD, Gault GH, Gentzler RD, Kent RL. Factors influencing reocclusion after coronary thrombolysis for acute myocardial infarction. Am J Cardiol 1986; 57: 1754-177.

26. Badger RS, Brown BG, Kennedy JW, Mathey D, Gallery CA, Bolson EL, Dodge HT. Usefulness of recanalization to luminal diameter of 0.6 millimeter or more with intracoronary streptokinase during acute myocardial infarction in predicting "normal" perfusion status, continued arterial patency and survival at one year. Am J Cardiol 1987; 59: 519-522.

27. Ellis SG, Topol EJ, George BS, Kereiakes DJ, Debowey D, Sigmon KN, Pickel A, Lee KL, Califf RM. Recurrent ischemia without warning. Analysis of risk factors for in-hospital ischemic events following successful thrombolysis with intravenous tissue plasminogen activator. Circulation 1989; 80: 1159-1165.

28. de Cesare NB, Ellis SG, Williamson PR, Deboe SF, Pitt B, Mancini GBJ: Early reocclusion after successful thrombolysis is related to lesion length and roughness. Cor Art Dis 1993;4:159-166.

29. Chapman T: Morphogenesis of occluding coronary artery thrombosis. Arch Pathol 1965;80:256-61.

30. Friedman M, Van den Bovenkamp GJ: Pathogenesis of

coronary thrombus. Am J Pathol 1965;48:19-44.

31. Ridolfi RL, Hutchins GM: Relationships between coronary artery lesions and myocardial infarcts: ulceration of atherosclerotic plaques precipitating coronary artery thrombosis. Am Heart J 1977;93:468-86.

32. Falk E: Plaque rupture with severe preexisting stenosis precipitating coronary thrombosis: characteristics of coronary atherosclerotic plaques underlaying fatal occlusive thrombi. Br Heart J 1983;50:127-34.

33. Davies MJ, Thomas A: Thrombosis and acute coronary lesions in sudden cardiac ischemic death. N Engl J Med 1984;310:1137-40.

34. Levin DC, Gardiner GA: Complex and simple coronary artery stenoses: a new way to interpret coronary angiograms based on morphologic features of lesions. Radiology 164;675-80, 1987.

35. Reher R, Disciascio G, Vetrovec G, Cowley M: Angiographic morphology of coronary artery stenoses in prolonged rest angina: Evidence of Intracoronary Thrombosis. J Am Coll Cardiol 1989;14:1429-39.

36. Califf RM, Topol EJ, Stack RS et al: Evaluation of combination thrombolytic therapy and timing of cardiac catheterization in acute myocardial infarction: Results of thrombolysis and angioplasty inmyocardial infarction - Phase 5 randomized trial. Circulation 1991;83:1543-56.

37. Verstraete M, Arnold A, Brower RW, Collen D, de Bono DP, De Zwaan C, Erbel R, Hillis WS, Lennane RJ, Lubsen J, Mathey D, Reid DS, Rutsch W, Scartel M, Schofer J, Serruys PW, Simoons ML, Uebis R, Vahanian A, Verheugt FWA, von Essen R. Acute coronary thrombolysis with recombinant human tissue-type plasminogen activator: initial patency and influence of maintened infusion on reocclusion rates. Am J Cardiol 1987; 60: 231-237.

38. Ohman EM, Califf RM, Topol EJ, Candela R, Abbottsmith C, Ellis S, Sigmon KN, Kereiakes D, George B, Stack R, and the TAMI Study Group. Consequences of reocclusion after successful reperfusion therapy in acute myocardial infarction. Circulation 1990; 82: 781-791.

39. Myers DW, Nohara R, Abendschein DR, Saffitz JE, Sobel BE, Bergmann SR. Compromise of beneficial effects of reperfusion of myocardium supplied by vessels with critical residual stenosis. J Am Coll Cardiol 1988; 11: 1078-1086.

40. Wilson JL, Ramanathan KB, Ingram LA, Miruis DM. Effects of residual stenosis on infarct size and regional transmural myocardial flow after reperfusion. Am Heart J 1988; 116: 1523-1529.

41. Gold HK, Leinbach RC, Garabedian HD, Yasuda T, Johns JA, Grossbard EB, Palacios I, Collen D. Acute coronary reocclusion after thrombolysis with recombinant human tissue-type plasminogen activator: prevention by a maintenance infusion. Circulation 1986; 73: 347-352.

42. Lange RA, Cigarroa RG, Hillis LD. Angiographic characteristics of the infarct-related coronary artery in patients with angina pectoris after myocardial infarction. Am J Cardiol 1989; 64: 257-260.

43. Reiner JS, Lundergan CF, van den Brand M, Boland J,

thompson MA, Machecourt J, Py A, Pilcher GS, Fink CA, Burton JR, Simoons ML, Calif RM, Topol EJ, Ross AM: Early angiography cannot predict postthrombolytic coronary reocclusion: Observations from the GUSTO angiographic study. J Am Coll Cardiol 1994;24:1439-44.

44. Bar FW, Raynaud P, Renkin JP, Vermeer F, de Zwaan C, Wellens HJJ: Coronary angiographic findings do not predict clinical outcome in patients with unstable angina. J Am Coll Cardiol 1994;24:1453-9.

45. Feldman RL, Nichols WW, Pepine CJ, Conti CR. Hemodynamic significance of the length of a coronary arterial narrowing. Am J Cardiol 1978; 41: 865-871.

46. Feldman RL, Nichols WW, Pepine CJ, Conti CR. Hemodynamic effects of long and multiple coronary arterial narrowings. Chest 1978; 74: 280-285

47. Horie T, Sekiguchi M, Hirosawa K. Coronary thrombosis in the pathogenesis of acute myocardial infarction: Histopatological study of coronary arteries in 108 necropsied cases using serial section. Br Heart J 1978; 40: 153-161.

48. Ridolfi R, Hutchins G. The relationship between coronary artery lesions and myocardial infarcts: Ulceration of atherosclerotic plaques precipitating coronary thrombosis. Am Heart J 1977; 93: 468-486.

49. Falk E. Plaque rupture with severe pre-existing stenosis precipitating coronary thrombosis: Characteristics of coronary atherosclerotic plaques underlying fatal occlusive thrombi. Br Heart J 1983; 50: 127-134.

50. Levin D, Fallon J. Significance of the angiographic morphology of localized coronary stenoses: Histopathologic correlations. Circulation 1982; 66: 316-320.

51. Davies SM, Marchant B, Lyons JP, Timmis AD, Rothman MT, Layton CA, Bascon R: Irregular coronary lesion morphology after thrombolysis predicts early clinical instability. J Am Coll Cardiol 1991;18:669-74.

52. Nagatomo Y, Nakagawa S, Koiwaya Y, Tanaka K: Coronary angiographic ruptured atheromatous plaque as a predictor of future progression of stenosis. Am Heart j 1990;119:1244-53.

53. Alderman EL, Corley SC, Fisher LD, Chaitman BR, Faxon DP, Foster ED, Killip T, Sosa JA, Bourassa MG: Five-year angiographic follow-up of factors associated with progression of coronary artery disease in the coronary artery surgery study (CASS). J Am Coll Cardiol 1993;22:1141-54.

54. Lesperance J, Theroux, Hudon G, Waters D: A new look at coronary angiograms: Plaque morphology as a help to diagnosis and to evaluate outcome. Int J Card Imag 1994;10:75-94.

4.

INTRAVASCULAR ANGIOSCOPY IN THE ANALYSIS OF STENOSIS MORPHOLOGY AND COMPOSITION: THERAPEUTIC IMPLICATIONS

by

Steven Feld, MD
From the Shaare Zedek Hospital, Jerusalem, Israel

and

Richard W. Smalling, MD, PhD
The University of Texas Health Science Center, Houston, Texas

I. INTRODUCTION

Progress in percutaneous coronary intervention since successful balloon angioplasty was first introduced in 1977 by Andreas Grüntzig [1] has enabled interventional cardiologists to treat patients at increased risk for complication with a high degree of success [2,3]. Newer device technology often aided by intravascular imaging has become increasingly employed in transcatheter interventions involving complex lesion morphology. The precise role of the newer diagnostic and therapeutic interventional devices currently employed for coronary stenoses remains to be defined [4]. Intravascular angioscopy can provide high-quality, three-dimensional, color imaging of endovascular surface morphology contributing to our understanding of the pathophysiology of coronary artery disease. The clinical utility of angioscopy for the individual patient will depend, however, on the ability to identify pathologic findings that impact on interventional strategy and result in an improvement in procedural and long-term outcome. A logical extension of the current angioscopic systems would be their incorporation into a therapeutic device permitting lesion-specific therapy to be delivered under direct visualization.

Historical Development

Cardiovascular angioscopy began in 1913 with unpublished experimental work by Lawrence Rhea and I. C. Walker who attempted to visualize the interior of the canine heart by means of a rigid 'cardioscope' inserted via thoracotomy (Fig. 1) . Their efforts met with limited success due to their inability to obtain a blood-free field of view [5]. Improved visualization during intraoperative cardioscopy was accomplished by placing the lens in

84

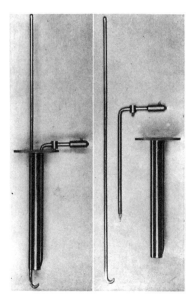

Figure 1: The first cardioscope used by Rhea and Walker in 1913 contained an electric light and knife designed for the treatment of mitral stenosis. A reset lens provided inadequate visualization of the cardiac structures. Reproduced with permission [5].

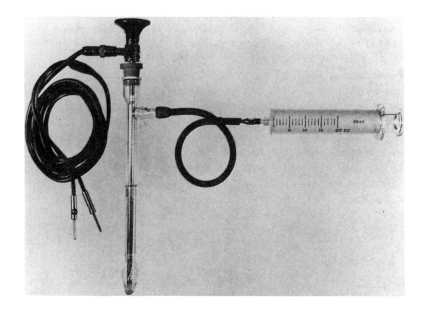

Figure 2: This early cardioscope had a transparent inflatable balloon at the distal end of a glass carrier which was apposed to the object of interest. Improved visualization permitted live photographs and sketches of intracardiac structures. Reproduced with permission [7].

direct contact with intracardiac structures [6] or by means of saline filled transparent balloons attached to the end of the early instruments which displaced blood from the field of view (Fig. 2) [7,8]. Advancements in fiberoptic technology leading to the development of miniaturized, flexible optical fibers with superior imaging capability heralded the onset of modern angioscopy. Prototypic fiberoptic angioscopes were successfully used during surgery to examine peripheral and coronary vessels [9-11]. In 1983, Spears et al. [9] were the first to report detailed coronary anatomy obtained from a flexible angioscope (prototype Olympus ultrathin 1.8 mm fiberscope) inserted intraoperatively through side branches of vein grafts and advanced across the distal anastomoses into the native coronary arteries. Shortly thereafter, they performed angioscopy during cardiac catheterization from the brachial artery with successful visualization of atheromatous plaque in patients with proximal occlusion of the right coronary artery [12]. The angioscope was successfully advanced to the tip of the guiding catheter in 3 of 5 patients and imaging facilitated by hand injection of saline through the guiding catheter. Refinements in technology led to the development of smaller, more flexible angioscopes with improved resolution and the capability of maintaining coaxial alignment during navigation of tortuous coronary segments. Direct visualization of complex coronary stenoses has contributed significantly to our understanding of unstable coronary syndromes by identifying histopathologic features not seen on angiography [13-15]. The significant disruptive effects of coronary angioplasty on surface morphology were also readily apparent to the chagrin of many interventionalists. Angioscopy has proven valuable in discerning the etiology of abrupt closure [16,17] and in predicting outcome following intervention [18-20].

II. DESCRIPTION OF ANGIOSCOPIC EQUIPMENT

Two percutaneous coronary angioscopic systems with high resolution imaging were intensively investigated in the U.S. The Microvision® system (Advanced Cardiovascular Systems) introduced in 1987 consisted of a triple lumen catheter with conventional over-the-wire coronary balloon design that could accommodate a 0.014" angioplasty wire. The third lumen contained an illumination bundle and 2000 imaging fibers. Tip deflection after rotation or withdrawal of a specially designed guidewire with curved tip facilitated circumferential imaging of the coronary lumen. This angioscope was capable of imaging distal coronary lesions with a fair degree of success, however a number of drawbacks in product design became apparent. First, the balloon was non-compliant requiring precise sizing of the vessel. A larger arterial diameter or changes in arterial lumen following intervention could lead to inadequate vessel occlusion that would impair visualization. Moreover, advancement of the angioscope for imaging multiple sites within the same vessel required deflation and re-inflation of the balloon with the potential for vascular injury due to the relatively high inflation pressure (3 atm) required. Over-the-wire exchanges for diagnostic imaging were cumbersome and resolution with 2000 imaging fibers was suboptimal.

The ImageCath® (Baxter Healthcare) became available in 1991 and is the only coronary angioscope currently marketed in the U.S. Advantages of this system are its monorail design which is considerably more 'user-friendly' for imaging before and after intervention and the superior imaging capability that was achieved by incorporating 3000 miniaturized individual optical fibers into an imaging bundle that measures 0.6 mm in diameter. The 4.5F (1.5 mm) flexible coronary ImageCath® angioscope (Fig. 3) consists of an outer polyethylene delivery catheter 125 cm in length with a compliant balloon at its distal end and an inner catheter containing the imaging bundle and illumination fibers. The optical bundle tracks over a 0.014" angioplasty wire in a monorail fashion and can be advanced independently up to 5 cm from the tip of the delivery catheter (Fig 4). The outer delivery catheter is also guided in a monorail fashion by the same angioplasty wire. Both the outer catheter shaft and the distal tip containing the optical bundle measure 1.5 mm allowing for delivery with an 8F conventional coronary

86

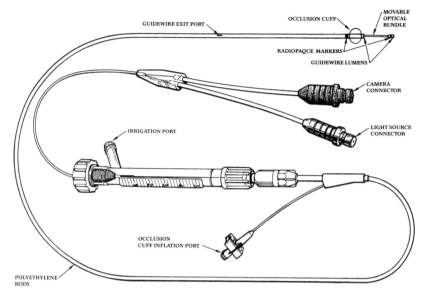

Figure 3: Schematic drawing of the Baxter ImageCath® Coronary Angioscope.
Courtesy Baxter Healthcare Corp.

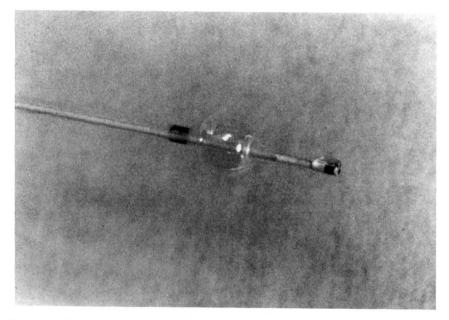

Figure 4: Distal end of the ImageCath® Coronary Angioscope's delivery catheter and
movable optical bundle. Courtesy Baxter Healthcare Corp.

guiding catheter. Cuff occlusion is accomplished with very low pressure inflation (<1 atm) due to the soft, extremely distensible synthetic latex (Kraton) balloon material. During imaging following balloon occlusion, a continuous infusion of flush solution exits the distal lumen of the outer catheter to provide a clear, blood-free field of view. A 300 Watt Xenon adjustable light source delivers high-intensity atraumatic illumination. Light travels to the tip of the ImageCath angioscope by illumination fibers which form a concentric ring around the imaging bundle to provide uniform lighting. Images are focused on the optical bundle by means of a gradient index (GRIN) lens that provides a 55° field of view and a greater than 0.5 mm depth of field. Individual imaging fibers are internally reflective and transmit one picture element (pixel) in a coherent fiberoptic bundle. The more imaging fibers present in the optical bundle, the sharper the resolution, but the larger and less flexible the device. While device size may not be an important consideration for examination of larger peripheral arteries, the competing interests of resolution and device flexibility are of paramount concern for inspection of the coronary anatomy. The angioscope is considerably stiffer than a balloon dilatation catheter. The independently mobile imaging bundle of the ImageCath measures only 0.6 mm in diameter with a bend radius of 5 mm providing greater flexibility for navigation of tortuous coronary segments. Other desirable features for increasing the likelihood of successful circumferential imaging of the vessel wall, such as torque transmission and tip deflection, are not present. The images transmitted by the optical fibers are too small for the naked eye to appreciate and are magnified by a high-resolution, miniaturized, charge couple device video camera for immediate display on a color television monitor. We prefer to record angioscopic images on broadcast-quality 3/4" videotape for later review, although the camera output may also be recorded onto a Super-VHS cassette. We strongly advocate simultaneous recording of angioscopic and fluoroscopic images by means of a video mixer resulting in a composite "picture-in-picture" image (Fig 5E). This permits angiographic localization of the optical bundle within the coronary vessel during subsequent review of the angioscopic images.

III. TECHNIQUE OF CORONARY ANGIOSCOPY

The technique of coronary angioscopy will be described in detail for the Baxter ImageCath®, which is the only angioscopic catheter available in the US. Experienced interventional cardiologists will find the procedure simple and straight-forward and can expect to encounter few complications [20-22].

Safety

The risks associated with angioscopy include those common to other percutaneous techniques involving instrumentation of the coronary arteries, such as groin complications, endothelial denudation, coronary spasm or dissection, myocardial infarction and arrhythmias. Only a single death has been attributed to coronary angioscopy, although ventricular fibrillation occurs in approximately 2% of patients [22]. One of forty consecutive patients in our series who underwent angioscopy for unstable coronary syndromes developed ventricular fibrillation during imaging of a proximal right coronary artery (RCA) stenosis. [18]. The patient was resuscitated and the interventional procedure completed successfully. It is likely that angioscopy results in more profound myocardial ischemia than balloon angioplasty. During angioscopy, balloon occlusion occurs proximal to the lesion being imaged. More importantly, coronary occlusion is coupled with vigorous flushing that removes oxygen-containing blood from the field of view and impairs collateral filling of the myocardium rendered ischemic. Den Heijer and coworkers [21] have documented that the onset of angina following balloon inflation occurs significantly sooner with angioscopy than with angioplasty. In their consecutive series of 100 patients who underwent angioscopy, two patients developed ventricular fibrillation during excessively prolonged imaging of their RCA stenoses [21]. We now limit the duration of ischemia to no more than 30-40 seconds per pass depending on the location of the lesion and the extent of coronary disease in the non-imaged coronary vessels. Intimal damage is probably a common occurrence aggravated by repetitive passes of the angioscope within the coronary lumen [23]. Angiographic deterioration of successfully dilated coronary stenoses following angioscopy [24] and angioscopic evidence of progressive coronary dissection within the first hour following PTCA [25] have been reported. The temporal sequence of events suggests that in these patients the deleterious changes observed at the site of angioplasty may have been aggravated by the angioscopic procedure itself, rather than representing purely evolutionary changes that follow balloon-mediated vascular injury. However, angiographically apparent coronary dissection occurred in less than 3% of 1746 angioscopic procedures performed at 27 European centers and rarely led to myocardial infarction or emergency CABG [22]. In a recent multicenter study, no complications were reported in 122 successful angioscopic procedures [20]. Stenosis at the site of angioscopic balloon inflation has not been observed on quantitative coronary angiography performed 6 months after angioscopy in 33 patients [26].

Choice of Vessel

Choosing an appropriate target lesion for angioscopic investigation should be planned ahead of time as part of the overall strategy for coronary intervention. Since balloon inflation proximal to the optical bundle is required to provide a blood-free field of view, ostial or very proximal lesions cannot be imaged effectively. The flexible angioscope is stiffer than a balloon dilatation catheter and extremely tortuous vessels or those with an acute bend should also be avoided. Appropriate target vessels for angioscopy include relatively straight or moderately tortuous segments that are at least 2.5 mm in diameter.

Preparation

Following inspection of the equipment, aspiration of air from the angioscopic balloon and lumen using a 20 cc syringe containing diluted contrast is performed in a similar manner to the negative preparation applied to standard PTCA balloons. The enclosed 1 cc syringe is attached to the balloon gate valve after being filled with 0.5 - 0.8 cc of diluted contrast depending on vessel size. The optical bundle is then connected to the video camera and light cable surrounded by a transparent sterile sleeve. The optical bundle is held close to a white sterile gauze and white balancing and focusing of the camera is performed. The irrigation port for the outer delivery catheter is connected to a power injector containing warmed saline or lactated Ringer's solution. The catheter is flushed at a rate of 20-40 ml/min while the hemostatic valve of the Y-connector is adjusted to permit free movement of the optical bundle without entry of air bubbles or leak of flush solution.

Procedure

Following engagement of the coronary ostium with a standard 8F guiding catheter and navigation of a 0.014" angioplasty guidewire as distally as possible to provide added support, the imaging bundle and outer delivery catheter are advanced over the guidewire in a monorail fashion under fluoroscopic guidance to a position just proximal to the coronary stenosis. Warmed saline is then infused at 20-40 ml/min via the power injector and gradual hand inflation of the balloon proceeds until a blood-free field of view is obtained. The fiberoptic bundle is advanced slowly under fluoroscopy while angioscopic images are observed on the television monitor and recorded on videotape. We often attempt to cross the stenosis, except in the presence of a large, protruding thrombus or in the event that resistance is felt by the operator and the image indicates that the optical bundle is advancing against tissue. Images are also recorded during careful withdrawal of the optical bundle. If resistance is encountered during withdrawal, it is imperative that the operator not attempt a forceful pullback of the imaging bundle. This may result in the formation of a wire loop between the optical bundle and the delivery catheter causing entrapment. Instead the imaging bundle should be advanced, the balloon deflated, and the delivery catheter withdrawn. Imaging should last no longer than 30-40 seconds, but may be repeated if adequate circumferential visualization of the lesion is not accomplished on first pass.

IV. ANGIOSCOPIC FINDINGS

Clinical Presentation

Acute coronary syndromes result from thrombus formation, platelet aggregation, and dynamic vasoconstriction at the site of plaque rupture leading to a cyclic alteration of the coronary flow pattern often heralding temporary or permanent coronary occlusion [27]. Local and systemic factors at the time of plaque rupture influence the stability of the growing thrombus producing a clinical spectrum of unstable coronary syndromes [28,29]. Patients with acute myocardial infarction are significantly more likely to have evidence of plaque rupture and thrombus formation on pathological examination than patients with either unstable angina or sudden cardiac death. A non-occlusive platelet-rich thrombus was found in 29% of patients with unstable angina, whereas an occlusive thrombus containing fibrin was present in 69% of patients with fatal acute myocardial infarction on autopsy [30]. Sherman et al. [13] performed angioscopy during coronary bypass surgery in 20 patients with stable and unstable angina. None of the ten patients with stable angina had complex plaque or thrombus present, whereas all three patients with accelerated angina had ulcerated plaques, but not thrombus, and all seven patients with rest angina had thrombus present on angioscopy. Mizuno et al. [14] performed percutaneous angioscopy in 31 patients with acute coronary syndromes and noted thrombus present in all but two patients. Patients with unstable angina were frequently observed to have grayish-white (platelet-rich) non-occlusive thrombi. By contrast, all patients with acute myocardial infarction had red thrombi which were frequently occlusive and likely contained fibrin mixed with erythrocytes and platelets. In a multicenter study of 120 patients undergoing coronary angioplasty, White et al. [20] reported that 74% of patients with unstable angina and 15% of patients with stable angina (p <0.001) had thrombus present on angioscopy. In our angioscopic series of 40 high-risk patients with unstable coronary syndromes and complex lesion morphology on angiography who underwent percutaneous intervention, we observed that patients with rest angina or recent myocardial infarction had thrombus present on angioscopy significantly more frequently than patients with crescendo angina (55% vs 13%, p <0.05) [18]. In a recent study, thrombus was universally present in patients with postinfarction angina, but uncommonly found in patients who were symptom-free after recent infarction [31]. Moreover, angiography has consistently underestimated the presence of intracoronary thrombus identified on angioscopy [13-15,18-21,31-36]. Thrombi may appear as red, white, or mixed red-white masses protruding into or occluding the vascular lumen or as textured red patches adherent to the underlying vessel surface that cannot be dislodged by flush solution (mural thrombi). Representative angioscopic findings in our series of unstable patients are shown in figure 5. Angiographic evidence of preexisting intracoronary thrombus has consistently been shown to be among the strongest predictors of unsuccessful angioplasty and abrupt closure [2,37]. White et al. [20] reported that angioscopic thrombus was strongly associated with in-hospital PTCA complications, even though most thrombi were not detected on angiography. Long term outcome may also be adversely affected by the presence of thrombus. Thrombus formation is the initial response to vascular injury which promotes cellular recruitment and extracellular matrix deposition leading to restenosis [38,39]. We found that thrombus present on angioscopy before or after coronary intervention was significantly associated with adverse outcome during six-month clinical follow-up [18].

Complex, ruptured or ulcerated plaques are frequently observed in patients with unstable coronary syndromes [40]. These are often yellow in appearance with red or brown staining from intramural hemorrhage or associated mural thrombus [13,18,33,40,41]. By contrast, patients with stable angina usually have yellow-white atheroma with a smooth luminal surface whose appearance is similar to that of the non-stenotic arterial segments [13,19,33]. In one study, the frequency of yellow plaque was similar in post-infarct patients and those with stable or unstable angina, but patients with ruptured yellow plaque had a greater thrombus burden [40]. In patients with chronic ischemic heart disease, Mizuno and co-workers reported that patients with yellow plaque were more likely to experience an acute coronary event during one year of follow-up than patients with white lesions on angioscopy [41]. Experimentally, plaques containing abundant soft, extracellular lipid deposits and a thin fibrous cap are prone to rupture and more thrombogenic than hard fibrous plaques [42]. Yellow plaque is the underlying substrate in acute myocardial infarction and recent coronary occlusion [43,44]. Itoh et al. [19] observed that patients with stable angina and solely white plaque were more prone to restenosis following PTCA than patients with yellow plaque. In one patient with angioscopic white plaque who underwent simultaneous intravascular ultrasound, an echogenic lesion was noted leading the authors to speculate that white plaque may be composed of hard, fibrous tissue. Restenotic lesions, whose histology is characterized by a neointimal fibroproliferative response to vascular injury, also have a white, smooth appearance on angioscopy [45].

Coronary Intervention

We performed intravascular imaging in sixty consecutive high-risk patients with unstable coronary syndromes and complex lesion morphology on angiography who underwent interventional therapy [18]. Forty patients had angioscopy, 46 patients had intravascular ultrasound and 26 patients had both procedures performed. All patients had off-line biplane QCA of the target lesion both pre- and post-intervention and were followed clinically for 1 year. The major findings of this study were that unstable clinical presentation (rest angina, myocardial infarction, or the recent use of thrombolytic therapy) or angioscopic correlates of plaque instability (ruptured plaque or thrombus) were significantly associated with recurrent ischemia during follow-up. The only multivariate predictors of adverse outcome were angioscopic findings of plaque rupture with obvious disruption of surface morphology before intervention or the presence of thrombus. Intramural hemorrhage, intimal flaps, tissue remnants, and minor dissection are frequently observed on angioscopy after balloon or laser angioplasty and rotational or directional atherectomy [18,21,32, 34,46-50]. These common angioscopic findings are not readily apparent on angiography, but do not appear to be associated with adverse clinical outcome [18]. Although angioscopy is more sensitive than angiography at detecting dissection, angiographically apparent dissection may be missed on angioscopy when significant post-procedural luminal surface disruption is present [32]. Nonetheless, angioscopy can accurately distinguish dissection from thrombus formation as the cause of procedural abrupt vessel occlusion leading to specific therapy [16-17]. In our series, 51% of patients with post-procedural angioscopy required a subsequent coronary intervention before completion of the procedure. This included repeat or adjunctive angioplasty, larger device size or new device, or the use of intracoronary thrombolytic therapy [18]. Although other researchers have also found angioscopy to be useful in guiding therapy during coronary intervention [51], the impact of angioscopy on improving outcome would depend on results from a controlled trial.

In our experience, the majority of patients with rest angina or acute or recent MI had thrombus visible in the index lesion by angioscopy. Interestingly, use of IC urokinase did not seem to make any difference in acute or long term outcome (see Table 2). Given the encouraging results of the EPIC trial [52], especially in patients with acute ischemic symptoms, it is likely that vigorous antiplatelet interventions such as the 7E-3 antiplatelet antibody will be more helpful than thrombolytics in this patient subset.

92

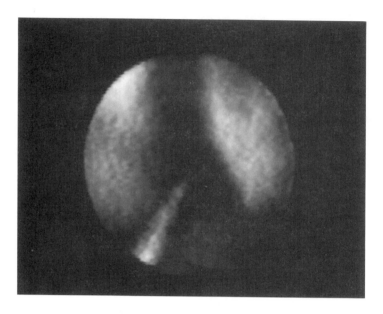

Figure 5A: Protruding thrombus

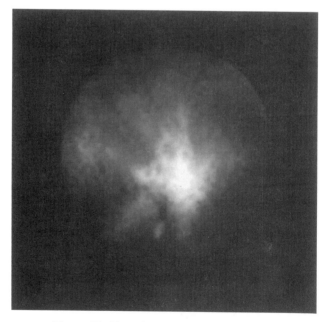

Figure 5B: Thrombus overlying a ruptured plaque

93

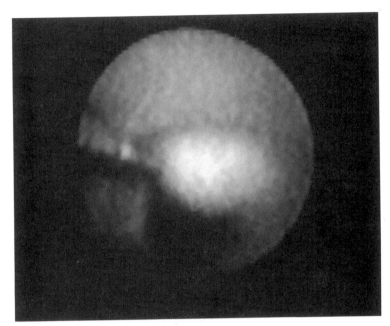

Figure 5C: Yellow atheroma

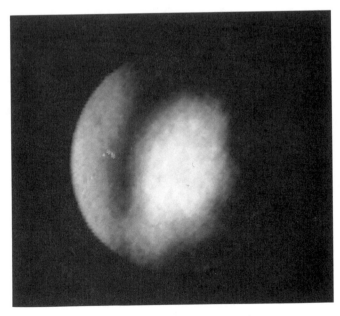

Figure 5D: Flap following directional atherectomy

94

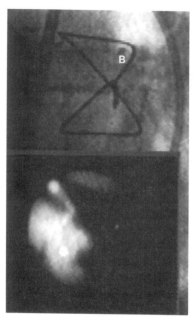

Figure 5E: Simultaneous "picture-in-picture" recording of a tissue remnant protruding through a stent articulation site (below) and the location of the angioscope during imaging (above). "B" indicates the position of the inflated angioscope balloon.

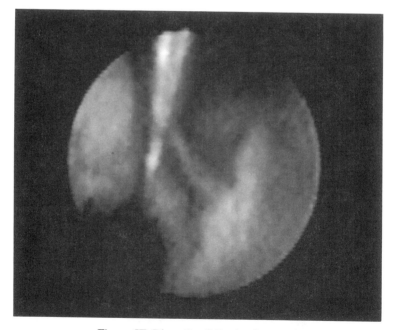

Figure 5F: Dissection following laser ablation

Comparative Findings During Intravascular Imaging

Angioscopy is more sensitive than angiography in detecting pathological features such as plaque rupture, intimal flaps, and thrombus present on the luminal surface, but insensitive in the assessment of deep dissection of the arterial wall. Intramural pathology is best identified with intravascular ultrasound, which is superior to angiography in determining the presence and extent of vessel calcification and dissection. In some studies involving small numbers of patients, the presence of major dissection on IVUS following angioplasty was associated with restenosis [53,54]. In larger studies including recent prospective trials, lesion morphology identified on IVUS following angioplasty or other percutaneous interventions was not predictive of restenosis or clinical events [55-57]. In our series that included 46 patients with post-procedural IVUS, none of the qualitative or quantitative parameters investigated were associated with recurrent ischemia [18]. Intravascular ultrasound assessment of residual plaque burden after angioplasty or other transcatheter interventions has been associated with restenosis in some larger studies [53,55,], but not others [54,56]. The precise relationship between angioscopic plaque color and composition is not known. On histological examination of atherosclerotic lesions, there is considerable variability in plaque composition among different lesions or within the same lesion. Most plaques contain both hard collagenous and soft atheromatous components, with the former predominating. In unstable coronary syndromes, a significant atheromatous component is usually present [42]. On angioscopy, some observers have reported that yellow plaque is more common in unstable coronary syndromes, whereas white plaque predominates in stable angina and in restenotic lesions [13,33,41,45]. The frequency of yellow plaque was not associated with clinical presentation in our patients [18], nor in a large series of patients with stable and unstable coronary syndromes reported by Baptista et al. [40] from the Thoraxcenter. In a single patient evaluated by angioscopy and IVUS, white plaque appeared echogenic leading Itoh et al. [19] to speculate that white plaque contains hard, fibrous tissue, whereas yellow plaque is composed of soft, atheromatous material. In our series, 26 patients underwent both angioscopy and IVUS imaging (Table 1). We found that of the 20 patients with yellow plaque on preprocedural angioscopy, 11 (55%) were soft (echolucent). Of the 6 patients with white plaque, 5 (83%) were hard (echogenic) and all were event-free on follow-up [18]. Although fibrocalcific lesions are more likely to be present when white plaque is observed during angioscopy, a yellow plaque color does not appear to indicate plaque composition.

V. CONCLUSION

Coronary arteriography remains the gold standard for the diagnosis of coronary artery disease and for evaluation of interventional therapy. Intravascular imaging can accurately identify intraluminal and intramural histopathologic features not routinely visualized on angiography improving our ability to diagnosis and treat cardiovascular disease. Angioscopy is a safe procedure easily performed by an interventional cardiologist that provides excellent visualization of the arterial surface. Angioscopic findings during coronary intervention may provide prognostic information and influence therapeutic strategy.

TABLE 1

Stenosis Characteristics Associated with Acute or Chronic Adverse Outcomes

    Thrombus detected by angioscopy

    Plaque rupture detected by angioscopy

Stenosis Characteristics not Associated with Acute or Chronic Adverse Outcomes

    Severity of calcification by IVUS

    Minimal lumen diameter aby QCA or IVUS

    Presence of intraluminal flaps by angioscopy

    Lesion eccentricity by IVUS

    Presence of dissection by IVUS or angioscopy

TABLE 2:   **ANGIOSCOPY AND OUTCOME**
                       FOLLOWING INTERVENTION

	NO. OF PATIENTS	EVENT FREE	ADVERSE OUTCOME	P VALUE
PRE-PROCEDURE (N=33)				
Plaque Rupture	10	3 (30%)	7 (70%)	<0.005
Thrombus	13	5 (38%)	8 (62%)	<0.01
(+) Urokinase	7	3 (43%)	4 (57%)	NS
(-) Urokinase	6	2 (33%)	4 (67%)	NS

TABLE 3. SIGNIFICANCE OF PLAQUE COLOR OBSERVED ON ANGIOSCOPY BEFORE CORONARY INTERVENTION

	NO. OF PATIENTS	YELLOW PLAQUE	WHITE PLAQUE	P VALUE
CLINICAL PRESENTATION				NS
Crescendo Angina	13	9 (69%)	4 (31%)	
Rest Angina	7	6 (86%)	1 (14%)	
Acute MI	13	12 (92%)	1 (8%)	
COMPOSITION ON IVUS				NS
Soft Plaque	12	11 (92%)	1 (8%)	
Hard Plaque	14	9 (64%)	5 (36%)	
CLINICAL OUTCOME				<0.07
Event Free	22	16 (73%)	6 (27%)	
Adverse	11	11 (100%)	0 (0%)	

VI. REFERENCES

1. Grüntzig AR, Senning A, Siegenthaler WE. Nonoperative dilatation of coronary-artery stenosis. Percutaneous transluminal coronary angioplasty. N Engl J Med 1979;301:61-8.
2. Ryan TJ, Bauman WB, Kennedy JW, et al. Guidelines for percutaneous transluminal coronary angioplasty. J Am Coll Cardiol 1993;22:2033-54.
3. Detre K, Holubkov R, Kelsey S, et al. One-year follow-up of the 1985-1986 National Heart, Lung, and Blood Institute's Percutaneous Transluminal Coronary Angioplasty Registry. Circulation 1989;80:421-8.
4. Holmes D Jr, Myler R, Kent K, et al. National Heart, Lung, and Blood Institute Percutaneous Transluminal Coronary Angioplasty Registry as a standard for comparison of new devices: when should we use it, and what should we compare? Circulation 1991;84:1828-30.
5. Cutler EC, Levine SA, Beck CS. The surgical treatment of mitral stenosis: experimental and clinical studies. Arch Surg 1924;9:689-821.
6. Allen DS, Graham EA. Intracardiac surgery - a new method. JAMA 1922;79:1028-30.
7. Harken DE, Glidden EM. Experiments in intracardiac surgery. II. Intracardiac visualization. J Thorac Surg 1943;12:566-72.
8. Bolton HE, Bailey CP, Costas-Durieux J, Gemeinhardt W. Cardioscopy - simple and practical. J Thorac Surg 1954;27:323-9.
9. Spears JR, Marais HJ, Serur JR, et al. In vivo coronary angioscopy. J Am Coll Cardiol 1983;1:1311-4.
10. Grundfest WS, Litvack F, Sherman T, et al. Delineation of peripheral and coronary detail by intraoperative angioscopy. Ann Surg 1985;202:394-400.
11. Chaux A, Lee ME, Blanche C, et al. Intraoperative coronary angioscopy. J Thorac Cardiovasc Surg 1986;92:972-6.
12. Spears JR, Spokojny AM, Marais HJ. Coronary angioscopy during cardiac catheterization. J Am Coll Cardiol 1985;6:93-7.
13. Sherman CT, Litvack F, Grundfest W, et al. Coronary angioscopy in patients with unstable angina pectoris. N Engl J Med 1986;315:913-9.
14. Mizuno K, Satomura K, Miyamoto A, et al. Angioscopic evaluation of coronary-artery thrombi in acute coronary syndromes. N Engl J Med 1992;326:287-91.
15. Siegel RJ, Ariani M, Fishbein MC, et al. Histopathologic validation of angioscopy and intravascular ultrasound. Circulation 1991;84:109-117.
16. Sassower MA, Abela GS, Koch JM, et al. Angioscopic evaluation of periprocedural and postprocedural abrupt closure after percutaneous coronary angioplasty. Am Heart J 1993;126:444-50.
17. White CJ, Ramee SR, Collins TJ, Jain SP, Escobar A. Coronary angioscopy of abrupt occlusion after angioplasty. J Am Coll Cardiol 1995;25:1681-4.
18. Feld S, Ganim M, Vaughn WK, et al. Utility of angioscopy and intravascular ultrasound in predicting outcome following coronary intervention. (abstr) Circulation 1995 (In press).
19. Itoh A, Miyazaki S, Nonogi H, Daikoku S, Haze K. Angioscopic prediction of successful dilatation and of restenosis in percutaneous transluminal coronary angioplasty. Significance of yellow plaque. Circulation 1995;91:1389-96.
20. White CJ, Ramee SR, Collins TJ, Escobar AE, Karsan A, Shaw D, Jain SP, Bass TA, Heuser RR, Teirstein PS, Bonan R, Walter PD, Smalling RW. Coronary Thrombi Increase PTCA Risk:Aangioscopy as a ClinicalTool. Circulation (In press).
21. Den Heijer P. Coronary angioscopy. The Hague, The Netherlands:Drukkerij Opmeer; 1994:9-142.
22. Lablanche JM, Geschwind H, Cribier A, et al. Coronary angioscopy safety survey: European multicenter experience. (abstr) J Am Coll Cardiol 1995:154A.
23. Lee G, Beerline D, Lee MH, et al. Hazards of angioscopic examination: documentation of damage to the arterial intima. Am Heart J 1988;116:1530-6.
24. Alfonso F, Hernandez R, Goicolea J, et al. Angiographic deterioration of the previously dilated coronary segment induced by angioscopic examination. Am J Cardiol 1994;74:604-6.
25. Den Heijer P, Van Dijk RB, Hillege HL, Pentinga ML, Serruys PW, Lie KI. Serial angioscopic and angiographic observations during the first hour after successful coronary angioplasty: a preamble to a multicenter trial addressing angioscopic markers for restenosis. Am Heart J 1994;128:656-63.
26. Hamon M, Lablanche J-M, Bauters C, McFadden EP, Quandalle P, Bertrand ME. Effect of balloon inflation in angiographically normal coronary segments during coronary angioscopy: a quantitative angiographic study. Cathet Cardiovasc Diagn 1994;31:116-21.

100

27. Willerson JT, Golino P, Eidt J, Campbell WB, Buja LM. Specific platelet mediators and unstable coronary artery lesions. Experimental evidence and potential clinical implications. Circulation 1989;80:198-205.
28. Badimon L, Chesebro JH, Badimon JJ Thrombus formation on ruptured atherosclerotic plaques and rethrombosis on evolving thrombi. Circulation 1992;86[suppl III]:III-74-III-85.
29. Willerson JT, Campbell WB, Winniford MD, et al. Conversion from chronic to acute coronary artery disease: speculation regarding mechanisms. Am J Cardiol 1984;54:1349-54.
30. Kragel AH, Gertz SD, Roberts WC. Morphologic comparison of frequency and types of acute lesions in the major epicardial coronary arteries in unstable angina pectoris, sudden coronary death and acute myocardial infarction. J Am Coll Cardiol 1991;18:801-8.
31. Tabata H, Mizuno K, Arakawa K, et al. Angioscopic identification of coronary thrombus in patients with postinfarction angina. J Am Coll Cardiol 1995;25:1282-5.
32. Den Heijer P, Foley DP, Escaned J, et al. Angioscopic versus angiographic detection of intimal dissection and intracoronary thrombus. J Am Coll Cardiol 1994;24:649-654.
33. Mizuno K, Miyamoto A, Satomura K, et al. Angioscopic coronary macromorphology in patients with acute coronary disorders. Lancet 1991;337:809-12.
34. Ramee SR, White CJ, Collins TJ, Mesa JE, Murgo JP. Percutaneous angioscopy during coronary angioplasty using a steerable microangioscope. J Am Coll Cardiol 1991;17:100-5.
35. McFadden E, Bauters C, Hamon M, et al. Sensitivity and specificity of angiographic markers for thrombus: a prospective comparison with angioscopy. (abstr) J Am Coll Cardiol 1995:154A.
36. Teirstein PS, Schatz RA, DeNardo SJ, Jensen EE, Johnson AD. Angioscopic versus angiographic detection of thrombus during coronary interventional procedures. Am J Cardiol 1995;75:1083-7.
37. Detre KM, Holmes DR, Holubkov R, et al. Incidence and consequences of periprocedural occlusion. The 1985-1986 National Heart, Lung, and Blood Institute percutaneous transluminal coronary angioplasty registry. Circulation 1990;82:739-50.
38. Fuster V, Badimon L, Badimon JJ, Chesebro JH. The pathogenesis of coronary artery disease and the acute coronary syndromes. N Engl J Med 1992;326:242-50.
39. Schwartz RS, Holmes DR Jr, Topol EJ. The restenosis paradigm revisited: an alternative proposal for cellular mechanisms. J Am Coll Cardiol 1992;20:1284-93.
40. Baptista J, de Feyter P, di Mario C, Roelandt JRTC, Serruys PW. Yellow plaques and vessel morphology prior to coronary intervention. A study using intracoronary angioscopy. (abstr) J Am Coll Cardiol 1995:280A.
41. MiatkeT, Arakawa K, Satomura K, et al. Efficacy of angioscopic findings for prediction of cardiac events in patients with chronic ischemic heart disease. (abstr) J Am Coll Cardiol 1995:428A-9A.
42. Falk E. Why do plaques rupture? Circulation 1992;86[suppl III]:III-30-III-42.
43. Hosokawa H, Suzuki T. Coronary angioscopy in patients with acute myocardial infarction undergoing direct balloon angioplasty. (abstr) J Am Coll Cardiol 1994:364A.
44. Alfonso F, Goicolea J, Hernandez R, et al. Angioscopic findings during coronary angioplasty of coronary occlusions. J Am Coll Cardiol 1995;26:135-41.
45. White CJ, Ramee SR, Mesa JE, Collins TJ. Percutaneous coronary angioscopy in patients with restenosis after coronary angioplasty. J Am Coll Cardiol 1991;17:46B-9B.
46. Uchida Y, Hasegawa K, Kawamura K, Shibuya I. Angioscopic observation of the coronary luminal changes induced by percutaneous transluminal coronary angioplasty. Am Heart J 1989;117:769-76.
47. Siegel RJ, Chae J-S, Forrester JS, Ruiz CE. Angiography, angioscopy, and ultrasound imaging before and after percutaneous balloon angioplasty. Am Heart J 1990;120:1086-90.
48. Nakamura F, Kvasnicka J, Uchida Y, Geschwind HJ. Percutaneous angioscopic evaluation of luminal changes induced by excimer laser angioplasty. Am Heart J 1992;124:1467-72.
49. Larrazet FS, Dupouy PJ, Rande J-LD, Hirosaka A, Kvasnicka J, Geschwind HJ. Angioscopy after laser and balloon coronary angioplasty. J Am Coll Cardiol 1994;23:1321-6.
50. Eltchaninoff H, Cribier A, Koning R, et al. Comparative angioscopic findings after rotational atherectomy and balloon angioplasty. (abstr) J Am Coll Cardiol 1995:95A.
51. Mirecki FJ, Sharaf BL, Williams DO. Intracoronary angioscopy impacts clinical decision making in patients with acute coronary syndromes. (abstr) J Am Coll Cardiol 1994:170A.
52. The EPIC Investigators. Use of a Monoclonal Antibody Directed Against the Platelet Glycoprotein IIb/IIIa Receptor in High-Risk Coronary Angioplasty. N Engl J Med 1994;330:956-61

53. Jain SP, Jain A, Collins TJ, Ramee SR, White CJ. Predictors of restenosis: a morphometric and quantitative evaluation by intravascular ultrasound. Am Heart J 1994;128:664-73.
54. Tenaglia AN, Buller CE, Kisslo KB, Phillips HR, Stack RS, Davidson CJ. Intracoronary ultrasound predictors of adverse outcomes after coronary artery interventions. J Am Coll Cardiol 1992;20:1385-1390.
55. Mintz GS, Chuang YC, Popma JJ, et al. The final % cross-sectional narrowing (residual plaque burden) is the strongest intravascular ultrasound predictor of angiographic restenosis. (abstr) J Am Coll Cardiol 1995:35A.
56. Peters RJG, PICTURE Study group (Post Intra Coronary Treatment Ultrasound Result Evaluation). Prediction of the risk of angiographic restenosis by intracoronary ultrasound imaging after coronary balloon angioplasty. (abstr) J Am Coll Cardiol 1995:35A-6A.
57. Ferguson JJ. Meeting highlights. Circulation 1995;91:2111-2.

5.

COMPUTERIZED THREE-DIMENSIONAL INTRAVASCULAR RECONSTRUCTION

RR Heuser, MD, T Laas, B Prebil, DB Reid, MD

The development of digital image processing for intravascular ultrasound (IVUS) has advanced significantly over the last five years. Various computerized imaging techniques described in the literature have brought a new and unique method for visualizing two-dimensional IVUS of coronary arteries and other vascular structures to the cardiac catheterization suite.[1–11] Early development focused on computerized cross-sectional viewing of two-dimensional IVUS images, whereas three-dimensional modeling was based on software algorithms developed for multiplanar and three-dimensional modeling of images provided by computerized tomography (CT) and magnetic resonance imaging (MRI). This early work allowed researchers to present heuristic three-dimensional modeling while newer algorithms were in development for IVUS.

The first, near-real-time IVUS post-scan image processor was developed utilizing the Intel i860 microprocessor chip as the host central processing unit (CPU) with 32 megabytes of random access memory (RAM). A commercial digital frame grabber and medium-sized mass storage drive were added to provide storage for several hundred two-dimensional digital images that were acquired in sequential order during manual or motorized pullback on the IVUS catheter. Early efforts to develop the technique for three-dimensional modeling were limited to short-segment acquisition, usually 128 frames of image data that measured 256 x 256 square. Cross-sectional viewing was limited to a fixed axis of rotation for longitudinal views, and three-dimensional surface modeling was based solely on algorithms developed for CT and MRI modeling techniques.[12]

The development of application-specific ultrasound processing software (ASUP) was announced after multiple research sites presented positive results for post-scan processing of two-dimensional IVUS images. New two- and three-dimensional algorithms were developed for cost-effective, off-the-shelf microprocessors and peripheral devices. Development of each new algorithm was instrumental in advancing the awareness two-dimensional IVUS systems and the application of post-scan two- and three-dimensional processing.[13] Current workstations provide for interactive three-dimensional heuristic modeling, real-time multiplanar reprocessing of cross-sectional views, and on-line assessment of various therapeutic techniques.

The Concept Of Digital Imaging Processing With IVUS Hardware Requirements

Current minimum requirements include a 100-MHz Intel Pentium microprocessor or equivalent CPU, 64 megabytes of RAM, high-resolution 30-frame-per-second image frame grabber, a 2-gigabyte SCSI hard drive, and a 1-gigabyte optical disk drive for archival storage.

Image acquisition is accomplished by direct video interface with the IVUS system or SVHS tape unit for postprocedure analysis. A constant and smooth pullback of the IVUS catheter is required to obtain uniform data for post-scan processing. Several manual and motorized pullback techniques have appeared in the literature since 1991. It was determined that a motorized system is necessary for precise measurements, while analysis of manual pullbacks was deemed adequate for routine two-dimensional IVUS review and three-dimensional modeling.

Image Processing Algorithm Requirements

As advancements were made in the development of application-specific software algorithms for IVUS image processing and viewing, each provided a unique array of two- and three-dimensional image analysis not available on standard IVUS systems. By acquiring IVUS images during the pullback of the imaging catheter, multiple two-dimensional cross-sectional images could be stacked in a format similar to CT and MRI image sets. Post-scan computer-based viewing could include basis frame-by-frame two-dimensional review or real-time 30-frame-per-second cine review. Cross-sectional sagittal views could be created to provide infinite angular cross slicing of two-dimensional image data. Three-dimensional modeled images could be created by an efficient edge-tracking algorithm that provides for image pixel segmentation, interpolation between image frames, and image frame stacking for real-time 360-degree viewing over the entire length of the pullback. These unique image processing algorithms allowed the system operator to perform real-time multiplanar reformatting with unlimited viewing angles of two-dimensional image data, a feature not available on the standard IVUS system.

Modern developments in the IVUS three-dimensional algorithm have provided for surface volume rendering that includes soft tissue gray-scale display and a combination of volume and gray-scale display during heuristic viewing. Current graphic display technology has aided the development of display features that permit interactive three-dimensional modeling from arbitrary angles. The processing speed of the Intel 100-MHz Pentium has improved the rendering time from earlier workstation models by a factor of five, while reducing the cost of previous systems by a factor of two.

On-Line And Long-Term Archival Storage

Early models of three-dimensional workstations provided for the acquisition and storage of approximately 128 frames of two-dimensional IVUS data. By adjusting the acquisition frame rate of the image frame grabber, the system could acquire and store an image set from a 10- to 15-mm segment of vessel. Current systems provide acquisition and storage for approximately 2,048 two-dimensional frames with variable frame acquisition rates. Today, a motorized pullback of 1 mm/s with an acquisition rate of 30/fps can store a 68-mm-long segment and provide for real-time, interactive display of the acquired data set.

As a result of the increased size of digital data files, larger, faster hard disk drives are now required to optimize storage and fast image set loading for review and post-scan processing. A similar requirement exists for long-term archive storage. High-capacity, high-speed SCSI hard drives for on-line digital image storage are now augmented with read, write, erasable SCSI optical disk drives for cost-effective image file management and long-term archival storage. As the speed of CPU processors increases, the need for additional RAM and larger disk drives will continue to grow.

The Utility of Three-Dimensional Heuristic Modeling of Coronary Vessels

As the application of two-dimensional IVUS imaging advanced from research tool to clinical modality, interventionists unfamiliar with two-dimensional IVUS experienced difficulties reconstructing the overall view of the coronary segment in question during clinical review. Many expressed the need for a fast, near-real-time reviewing system capable of two-dimensional image playback and cross-sectional remodeling. Further review led system developers to model three-dimensional data sets in a heuristic fashion to aid physicians unfamiliar with two-dimensional IVUS cross-sectional viewing. Early developers defined a need for real-time, high-resolution interactive display of two-dimensional IVUS in coronary arteries and suggested that three-dimensional heuristic modeling would aid ongoing development efforts in directional atherectomy, PTCA, and stent deployment.

Figure 1 provides a typical illustration of successful stent deployment as disclosed by three dimensional IVUS. The patient, a 66-year-old female, suffered an acute lateral wall myocardial infarction 6 months before presentation and underwent emergent angioplasty of the circumflex and left main junction and placement of a Gianturco-Roubin Flex-Stent® (Cook Inc., Bloomington, IN, USA). Restenosis of the stent necessitated deployment of a 3.0 Palmaz-Schatz stent (Johnson & Johnson Interventional Systems Co., Warren, NJ) inside the Gianturco-Roubin device. IVUS images of final stent positioning were obtained using a 2.9F ultrasound device, which demonstrated an excellent outcome.

108

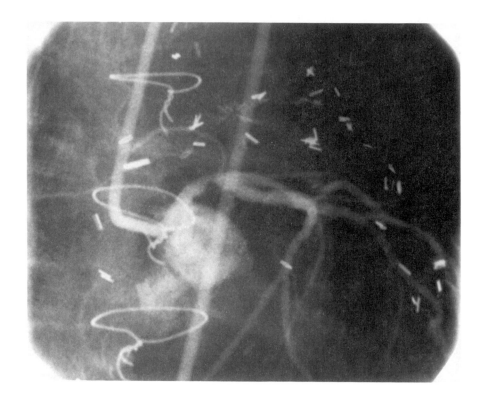

Figure 1. (a) Angiographic image of left main stenosis.

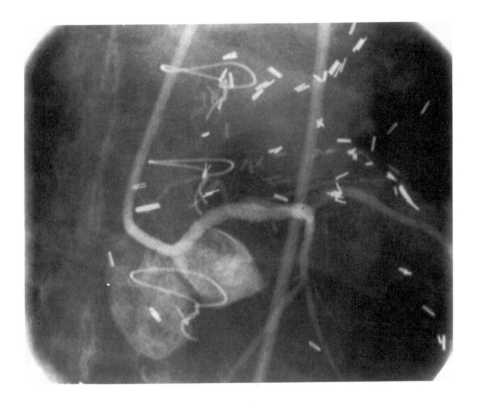

Figure 1. (b) Angiographic image of left main stenosis following Palmaz-Schatz stent placement.

110

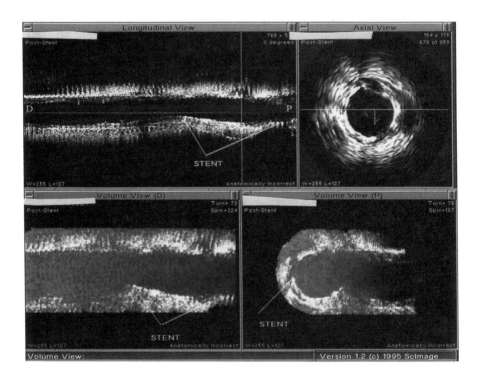

Figure 1. (c) IVUS images showing final stent placement. Axial and volume views indicate good stent/wall apposition. Although longitudinal view demonstrates tapering of the distal portion of the stent, it is the same diameter as the distal vessel.

Figure 2 outlines a series of images illustrating inadequate stent expansion with poor stent/wall apposition. Such views enable the clinician to redilate the stent until proper deployment is achieved.

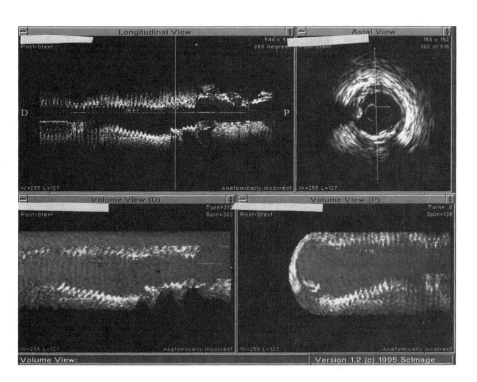

Figure 2. Longitudinal, axial, and volume views of poor stent/wall apposition in proximal ostial left anterior descending artery.

Current and Future Clinical Applications

To date, the majority of interventional cardiologists rely on angiography for road mapping and dynamic image assessment during diagnostic and therapeutic procedures. However, angiography has been shown to underestimate the degree of residual stenosis following atherectomy and stent deployment. IVUS has proved an excellent complement to angiography by verifying cross-sectional lumen dimension, tortuosity or narrowing of access vessels, aneurysms, and residual stenosis following atherectomy and PTCA.[14,15] It has aided the assessment of intimal flaps and dissections. Figure 3 comprises a series of IVUS images from a 64-year-old male patient presenting with intermittent claudication of the left thigh and buttock. Angiography demonstrated an ulcerative atheromatous plaque with a dissection just proximal to the iliac bifurcation. Three-dimensional IVUS confirmed the diagnosis and a Palmaz 204 stent was deployed. Postdeployment IVUS images of the stented artery indicated exclusion of the ulcer and dissection. Figure 4 highlights the ability of three-dimensional IVUS to evaluate aneurysm for endoluminal grafting.

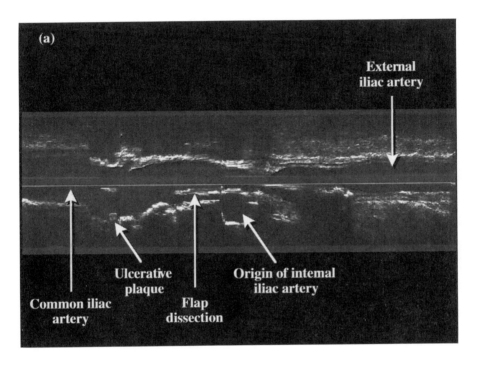

Figure 3. (a) Prestent longitudinal scan indicating flap dissection just proximal to the iliac bifurcation.

114

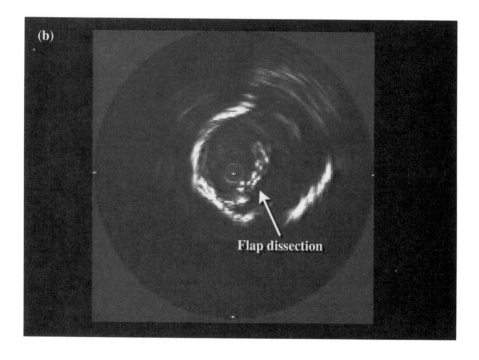

Figure 3. (b) Axial image presenting another view of dissection.

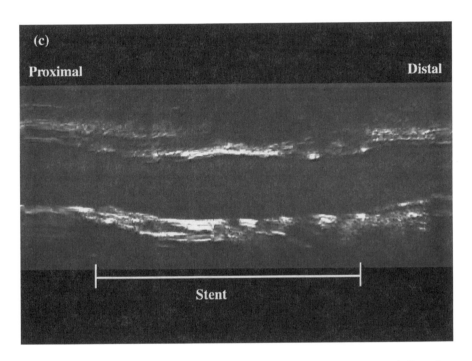

Figure 3. (c) Poststent longitudinal cross section demonstrating resolution of dissection.

116

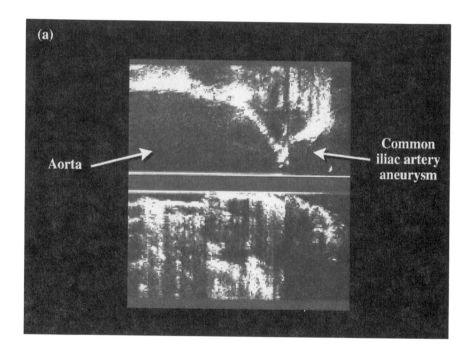

Figure 4. (a) A longitudinal view of an abdominal aortic aneurysm with waisting at the common iliac artery origin.

117

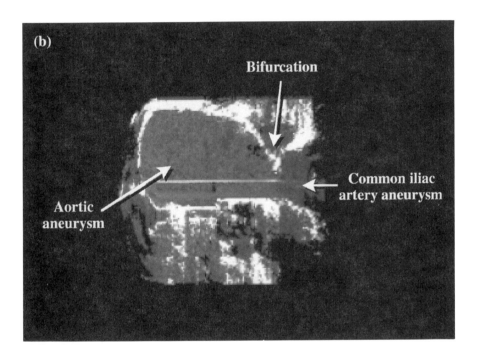

Figure 4. (b) Volume view.

More recent developments have provided for real-time IVUS imaging during stent placement and deployment. This technique places the IVUS imaging wire within the lumen of the deployment catheter, enabling the clinician to accurately guide the placement and expansion of the stent via two-dimensional IVUS. More advanced computerized image processing permits real-time image processing that displays an interactive view of the full-length of the balloon and stent during deployment.

The use of on-line computerized image processing with IVUS for the placement of endoluminal grafts (ELG) is in the investigative stage at several facilities throughout the world. IVUS provides a very accurate cross-sectional view of the ELG for localization and deployment of the device.[19]

Although the cost of IVUS systems and catheters continues to hamper widespread use in clinical cardiology, the flexibility of this modality and the ability to adapt it to various therapeutic devices suggests that future applications for IVUS are growing.

References

1   Wickline SA, Sobel BE. Ultrasonic tissue characterization: prospects for clinical cardiology. J Am Coll Cardiol 1989;14:1709–1711.

2.   Yock PG, Linker DT. Intravascular ultrasound. Looking below the surface of vascular disease. Circulation 1990;81:1715–1718.

3.   Tobis JM, Mahon D, Moriuchi M, et al. Intravascular ultrasonic imaging. Texas Heart Inst J 1990;17:181–189.

4.   Potkin BN, Bartorelli AL, Gessert JM, et al. Coronary artery imaging with intravascular high-frequency ultrasound. Circulation 1990;81:1575–1585.

5.   Nishimura RA, Edwards WD, Warnes CA, et al. Intravascular ultrasound imaging: in vitro validation and pathologic correlation. J Am Coll Cardiol 1990;16:145–154.

6.   Nissen SE, Grines CL, Gurley JC, et al. Application of a new phased-array ultrasound imaging catheter in the assessment of vascular dimensions. In vivo comparison to cineangiography. Circulation 1990;81:660–666.

7.   Tabbara M, White R, Cavaye D, Kopchok G. In vivo human comparison of intravascular ultrasonography and angiography. J Vasc Surg 1991;14:496–504.

8.   Tobis JM, Mallery J, Mahon D. Intravascular ultrasound imaging of human coronary arteries in vivo. Analysis of tissue characterizations with comparison to in vitro histological specimens. Circulation 1991;83:913–926.

9.   St. Goar FG, Pinto FJ, Alderman EL, et al. Intravascular ultrasound imaging of angiographically normal coronary arteries: an in vivo comparison with quantitative angiography. J Am Coll Cardiol 1991;18:952–958.

10.   Keren G, Pichard AD, Kent KM, et al. Failure or success of complex catheter-based interventional p[procedures assessed by intravascular ultrasound. Am Heart J 1992;123:200–208.

11.   Hodgson JMB, Reddy KG, Suneja R, et al. Intracoronary ultrasound imaging: Correlation of plaque morphology with angiography, clinical syndrome and procedural results in patients undergoing coronary angioplasty. J Am Coll Cardiol 1993;21:35–44.

12.   Rosenfield K, Kaufman J, Pieczek A, et al. Real-time three dimensional reconstruction of intravascular ultrasound images. Am J Cardiol 1992;70:412–415.

13.   Raya SP, Udupa JK, Barrett WA. A PC-based three-dimensional imaging system: algorithms, software, and hardware considerations. Computerized Med Imaging Graphics 1990;14:353–370.

14.   Lee D-Y, Eigler N, Luo H, et al. Effect of intracoronary ultrasound imaging on clinical decision making. Am Heart J 1995;129:1084–1093.

15.   Mudra H, Klauss V, Blasini R, et al. Ultrasound guidance of Palmaz-Schatz intracoronary stenting with a combined intravascular ultrasound balloon catheter. Circulation 1994;90:1252–1261.

16.   Mintz GS, Pichard AD, Kovach JA, et al. Impact of preintervention intravascular ultrasound imaging on transcatheter treatment strategies in coronary artery disease. Am J Cardiol 1994;73:423–430.

17.   Tobias JM, Mahon DJ, Goldberg SL, et al. Lessons from intravascular ultrasonography: observations during interventional angioplasty procedures. J Clin Ultrasound 1993;21:589–607.

18.   Laskey WK, Brady ST, Kussmaul WG, et al. Am Heart J 1993;125:1576–1583.

19.   Heuser RR, Reynolds GT, Papazoglou C, Diethrich EB. Endoluminal grafting for percutaneous aneurysm exclusion in an aortocoronary saphenous vein graft: the first clinical experience. J Endovasc Surg 1995;2:81–88.

6.

CORONARY STENOSIS MORPHOLOGY: IMPORTANCE OF LESION LENGTH, STENOSIS ECCENTRICITY, SEVERITY AND CORONARY BLOOD FLOW IN CLINICAL DECISION MAKING

Morton J. Kern, M.D.; Thomas J. Donohue, M.D.; Richard G. Bach, M.D.

Department of Internal Medicine, Division of Cardiology, J.G. Mudd Cardiac Catheterization Laboratory, St. Louis University Health Sciences Center, 3635 Vista Avenue at Grand, St. Louis, Missouri

Introduction

The morphology of a stenosis has a profound impact on the physiologic significance of the lesion. Blood flow through a coronary narrowing is affected by several factors, some of which were described over a century ago by Poiseuille [1]. These factors include vessel size, lesion length, area of stenosis, and inlet and exit angle. Stenosis morphology may also be altered in a dynamic manner under conditions of vasodilator or vasoconstrictor stimuli. Serial stenoses of a fixed morphology also produce disturbance of blood flow to a greater degree than a more severe single stenosis. In this section, stenosis morphology and its impact on coronary blood flow will be addressed. Because of the limitations of angiography, the measurable aspects of stenosis morphology in patients are restricted to relative area reduction, length, eccentricity, and an estimate of thrombotic involvement. Studies of coronary blood flow during interventions in patients analyzed in relation to stenosis morphology have been facilitated by Doppler angioplasty guidewire measurements.

Physiologic significance of stenosis morphology

Assessment of stenosis severity using pressure-flow characteristics: The study of coronary blood flow in assessing functional severity of a stenosis raises basic conceptual questions on how the severity of a coronary stenosis should be defined. In geometric terms, the relative percent diameter or area stenosis is related to the relative hemodynamic variables of the pressure gradient-flow (velocity) relationship. However, the absolute stenosis dimensions and the relation of pressure gradient-volumetric flow may be a more accurate gauge of stenosis severity. In most experimental studies, volumetric flow measured by Doppler probes is assumed equivalent to velocity flow if the vessel cross-sectional area is constant. Gould and Kelley [2] found that, across the average range of stenoses from 45-78% diameter narrowing (mean 68%) with concomitant reductions in stenosis cross-sectional area of 78-95% (mean 91%), an asymmetric coronary stenosis produced by an external constrictor in a canine model yielded changes in coronary blood flow ranging from 45-90ml/min. Under basal conditions, coronary flow velocity at rest was 19 ± 6 cm/sec and coronary volume flow was 25 ± 7ml/min. During maximal vasodilatation, although the stenosis eccentricity changed in comparison to the rest arteriograms, the mean cross-sectional area remained constant at 0.40 ± 0.61mm². The stenosis severity could be described by two curvilinear relationships: pressure-velocity and pressure-volume flow (Figure 1).

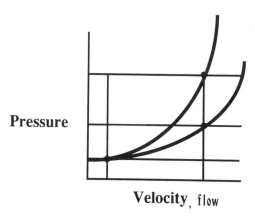

Pressure

Velocity, flow

Figure 1: Pressure-flow velocity relations of two coronary stenoses of similar angiographic severity but different resistance to blood flow. Both lesions have the same resting flow velocity and pressure. At high flow, the lesion characterized by the top curve has twice the pressure gradient as the lesion in the bottom curve. Which change will be associated with ischemia? (Reproduced with permission from reference #37.)

An early transient and very small decrease in cross-sectional area had no hemodynamic consequences. Under these experimental conditions, there was a significant change in the size of the normal vessel on either side of the stenosis with a stable divergence angle at the distal end of the stenosis. During vasodilatation, the cross-sectional area of the proximal arterial segment increased from 4.98 to 5.87mm² and distal vessel cross-sectional area increased from 4.44 to 4.97mm² (with standard deviations of approximately 1mm²). These changes in cross-sectional area of the normal vessel resulted in an increase in the relative percent diameter stenosis from 68 to 71% and percent area stenosis from $91 \pm 0.4\%$ to $92 \pm 0.3\%$ ($p < 0.001$)

associated with a 22% increase in the coefficient of pressure loss. As coronary flow increased, the pressure gradient also increased along the family of quadratic relationships as shown on Figure 1.

The pressure-flow curve increases during hyperemic coronary blood flow for two reasons: 1) increasing the separation coefficient (i.e., more energy [pressure] loss due to friction) at high blood flow, and 2) increasing the relative severity of percent stenosis. In the experimental animal [3], during maximal coronary blood flow (occurring approximately 10 seconds after intracoronary papaverine), a significant but very small reduction in minimal stenosis area from 0.39 to 0.36mm² associated with the dilatation of normal segments, produced an even greater relative percent diameter stenosis.

Coronary flow reserve: influence of distal bed vasodilation to flow across stenoses: Coronary flow reserve is the ability to augment flow over baseline values in response to a hyperemic stimulus and should be incorporated into any assessment of lesion morphology (Figures 2A,2B).

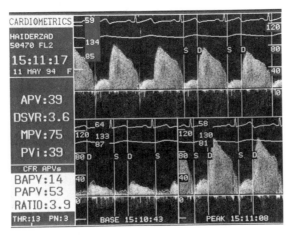

Figure 2A: Spectral coronary flow velocity signals used in the calculation of coronary vasodilatory reserve. The display screen is split into top and bottom which is then subdivided into left and right panels. (TOP SECTION) Continuous phasic flow velocity during hyperemia. The velocity scale is 0-120cm/sec. Electrocardiogram and arterial pressure are the top two tracings. S and D indicate systolic and diastolic periods. The heart rate and systolic and diastolic pressures are shown as the numbers in the gray box at the upper left corner of the flow panel. (BOTTOM left and right panels) Coronary flow velocity at baseline and at peak hyperemia are shown in the lower panel of the split screen. The same velocity scale is used in the upper panel. APV=average peak velocity; DSVR=diastolic/systolic velocity ratio; MPV=maximal peak velocity; PVi=peak velocity integral. Coronary vasodilatory reserve is calculated from basal average peak velocity (BAPV) of 14cm/sec and peak average peak velocity (PAPV) of 53cm/sec to produce a coronary vasodilatory reserve ratio of 3.9 (shown in the lower far left light gray panel).

124

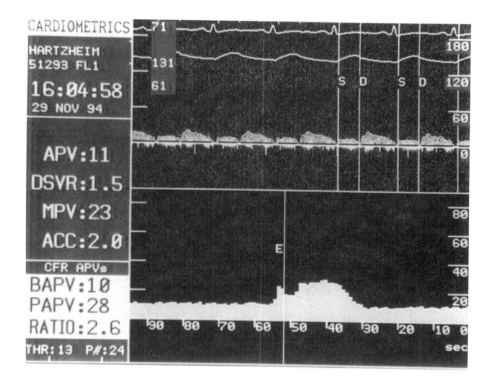

Figure 2B: Coronary flow velocity and reserve is also displayed as a continuous trend plot of average peak velocity (lower panel of split screen). The trend plot scale of average peak velocity is from 0-80cm/sec. The time axis is over 90 seconds. The vertical line marked E is the event marker for injection of intracoronary adenosine. Coronary hyperemia with intracoronary adenosine lasts approximately 30 seconds and rapidly returns to baseline values after injection. The coronary reserve in this individual was lower at 2.6 ratio (abbreviations as in Figure 1A).

Clinically significant stenoses, traditionally defined by diameter stenosis > 60%, impair coronary hyperemia and coronary flow reserve (Figure 3).

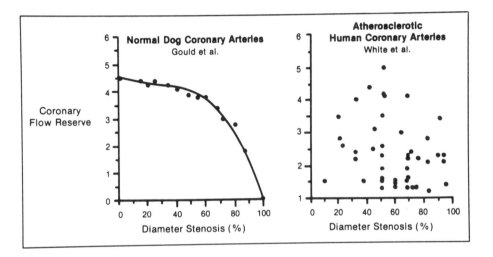

Figure 3: (LEFT PANEL) Effect of progressive constriction on hyperemic flow in the left circumflex artery to intracoronary injection of Hypaque in a single dog. Percent constriction by diameter is shown on the horizontal axis. Flow after Hypaque injection, expressed as the ratio of hyperemia to baseline flow values (coronary flow reserve), is shown on the vertical axis. (Reproduced with permission from Gould KL, Lipscomb K, Hamilton GW. Physiologic basis for assessing critical coronary stenosis: instantaneous flow response and regional distribution during coronary hyperemia as measures of coronary flow reserve. Am J Cardiol 1974;33:87-94.) (RIGHT PANEL) Relation between the measured percentage of vessel-diameter stenosis for the most severe lesion assessed from the coronary angiogram and the coronary flow reserve obtained from Doppler catheter velocity recordings at the time of open heart surgery. (Reproduced with permission from reference #29.)

The compensatory changes which occur in distal coronary vascular beds during progressive coronary narrowing must be considered when assessing coronary blood flow across a stenosis. Gould et al [4] studied the pressure-flow relationships in 157 different stenoses in 9 open chest dogs measuring coronary flow, aortic pressure, and post-stenotic distal coronary pressure during progressive coronary vasoconstriction or narrowing. Hyperemia was produced using intracoronary radiographic contrast media. This landmark study showed that the pressure-flow relationships and hydraulic resistance of stenoses do not become abnormal and do not alter resting flow nor elicit compensatory changes for coronary narrowings of ≤60% diameter of the vessel. In this model, compensatory vasodilatation of the distal coronary vascular bed is able to maintain near normal resting flow for intermediate lesions between 60 and 85% diameter stenosis. In general, post-stenotic vasodilatory failure occurs for lesions >85% diameter. Ischemia, however, may occur with less severe degrees of stenosis since coronary vasodilatory reserve exists in a continuum across the myocardium [4].

Although theoretically compelling, the concept of impaired coronary flow reserve has not been clinically employed in the assessment of stenoses in patients with coronary artery disease until recently. Earlier studies used large 3F Doppler catheters obtaining data only proximal to a stenosis. Normal hyperemic flow could occur in a vessel with a severe stenosis due to pre-stenotic side branch dilation. Post-stenotic coronary flow reserve differs from proximal coronary flow reserve as measured with angioplasty Doppler guidewires [5-7]. Coronary flow reserve is also impaired under conditions in which microcirculatory compromise may exist. Coronary flow reserve has been reported to be abnormal in patients with left ventricular hypertrophy due to hypertension, aortic stenosis, or hypertrophic cardiomyopathy. In addition, coronary flow reserve is compromised in patients with syndrome X, diabetes mellitus, or other small vessel disease entities. Coronary flow reserve in regions of myocardial infarction is likewise compromised due to the scar tissue and impaired vascular bed. In addition, the percent diameter stenosis by angiography in patients does not reproduce the precise area reductions of experimental models and, in part, this explains the poor correlation between lesion and severity coronary flow reserve except in the extreme cases (Figure 3).

Coronary blood flow: volumetric vs velocity data: Assessing stenosis significance may differ when gauging blood flow changes by flow velocity as compared to volume flow. Because of increases in the normal arterial segment diameter in experimental studies, the relative increase in flow velocity was less than the relative increase in <u>volumetric</u> flow. The differences between volumetric and velocity flow during vasodilatation are approximately 30% with maximal volumetric flow relatively greater than velocity occurring at the peak hyperemic phase. The duration of hyperemic flow is also correspondingly shorter when velocity is used as a measure of flow changes because, although flow velocity rapidly returns to baseline values, volumetric flow remains somewhat elevated with a larger arterial diameter than the control value.

When comparing data expressing lesion severity, the pressure gradient-velocity relation may indicate a marked worsening of stenoses while the pressure gradient-volume flow relation indicates only a mild exacerbation of the same stenosis after coronary vasodilatation [1]. The approach to accurate stenosis characterization depends on the understanding of hemodynamic severity and the acceptance of concepts related to either velocity or volumetric flow.

Stenosis severity: pressure-velocity (P-V) or pressure-volume (P-Q) flow relationship: For any given stenosis, the pressure-velocity relationship has a steeper curvilinear relationship than pressure-volume flow (Figure 4).

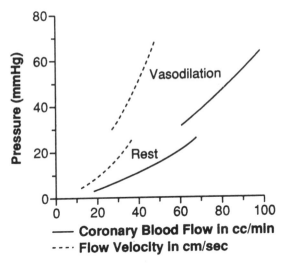

Figure 4: Relation of stenosis pressure gradient to coronary volume flow and to flow velocity. Both volumetric flow and velocity flow (solid and dashed lines) demonstrate steeper slopes after vasodilation. The gradient-velocity relation shows a much more prominent increase in slope, illustrating that it is more sensitive to more severe relative percent stenosis caused by vasodilation on either side of the stenotic segment. (Modified from reference #2.)

This effect occurs in the experimental models because the vessel dimensions on either side of a stenotic segment vasodilate. The relative percent stenosis thus increases with velocity flow failing to increase proportionally with volumetric flow due to the increase in cross-sectional area of the normal adjacent segment [8,9]. The relative percent stenosis traditionally used in clinically assessment of stenosis severity is the dominant geometric influence of the pressure-velocity relationship. A worsening of relative percent stenosis is associated with a worsening hemodynamic definition (steeper slope) when examining the pressure-velocity relationship. The pressure-velocity relationship appears most appropriate to compare stenosis severity in different sized vessels, normally carrying different volumetric flows such as great vessels versus smaller coronary arteries (Figure 5A).

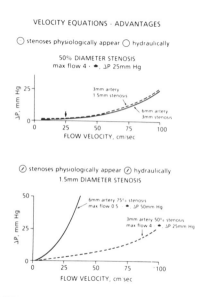

Figure 5A: (UPPER PANEL) Relation of pressure gradient (ΔP) and arterial flow velocity in the normal unstenosed part of the artery for physiologically equal stenoses (50% diameter) in a small artery with a diameter of 3mm (dashed line) and in a large artery with a diameter of 6mm (solid line). The arrow indicates the normal value for coronary flow velocity at rest (25cm/sec). (LOWER PANEL) Similar relation for physiologically unequal stenoses of 1.5mm absolute diameter in the small (dashed line) and the large (solid line) artery. (Reproduced with permission from reference #9.)

Estimates of relative percent stenosis and the pressure-velocity analysis are useful for comparing the consequences of stenosis in different sized arteries in broad categorical terms. Two stenoses of equal percent diameter narrowing in different sized arteries will show the same pressure gradient and flow reserve regardless of the magnitude of normal vessel cross-sectional area (Figure 5B).

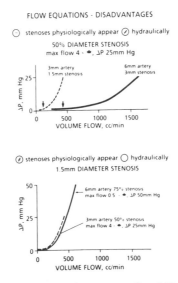

Figure 5B: (UPPER PANEL) Relation of pressure gradient (▲P) and arterial volume flow for physiologically equal stenoses in a small (dashed line) and a large (solid line) artery. The arrows represent normal volume flow at rest in each of these two arteries, corresponding to a flow velocity at rest of 25cm/sec. (LOWER PANEL) Similar relation for physiologically unequal stenoses of 1.5mm absolute diameter in the small (dashed line) and large (solid line) artery. (Reproduced with permission from reference #9.)

In contrast to the pressure-velocity relationship, the pressure-volume flow relationship has a less steep slope for a similar stenosis. The pressure-flow volume relation for a given stenosis at rest changes only slightly during hyperemia due to vasodilatation of the pre- and post-stenotic normal vessel segment. Thus, in the pressure-volume flow analysis, a slight worsening of percent stenosis due to altered geometry at high flows causes <20% increase in the pressure gradient over the predicted gradient (from fluid dynamic equations) in the absence of epicardial vasodilatation. The dominant geometric influence on the pressure-volume flow relation is the absolute stenosis dimension, not the relative percent narrowing.

There is no requirement for normalization of absolute cross-sectional area of the stenosis to the normal reference area. Since small arteries transport lower volumes for any given pressure, the pressure-volume flow (P-Q) relation will appear steeper and hence worse for smaller vessels when compared to a larger vessel with the same percent diameter stenosis having the same physiologic consequences on distal blood flow. The P-Q relation is inappropriate for comparing severity of stenoses in different size arteries. Therefore, stenosis severity defined by a P-Q relation which causes organ dysfunction in a small experimental animal cannot be extrapolated to a corresponding larger artery in a patient. For example, a stenosis diameter of 2mm in a coronary artery which is normally 3mm in diameter is not physiologically severe, but a 2mm stenosis diameter in a 15mm diameter artery is a physiologically severe stenosis [1,8]. The P-Q relation is useful for comparing physiologic affects of an intervention on volumetric blood flow or comparing the geometric severity of a stenosis before and after an intervention in the same vessel.

Comparing coronary blood flow after changing stenosis morphology: Volumetric flow measurements may be useful when comparing geometric severity of stenoses before interventions, such as the response to administration of nitroglycerin in the same stenosis in the same artery after an intervention. However, when assessing pre- and post-interventional responses, coronary volume flow and pressure in the distal bed may improve or deteriorate as a result of the intervention. The volume flow that normally passes through the artery is an unknown factor prior to the intervention. To address the effects of a stenosis on volume flow requires reference to the volume flow and pressure gradient relation. To substitute flow velocity for volume flow, the vessel cross-sectional area at the site of Doppler velocity measurements is used to estimate volume flow. Proper application of the pressure-flow velocity relationships examining changes after stenosis intervention should provide an accurate assessment of the physiologic impact of the intervention.

For the physiologic assessment of stenosis severity, two standard assumptions are made [9]:

1)   Pressure and flow should be measured with systems providing satisfactory phasic information in which diastolic gradient and flow can be acquired. Quantitative angiography has limitations for precisely assessing translesional flow and pressure.

2)   When comparing a stenosis to itself before and after an intervention, the flow volume-pressure gradient relationship appears to be useful since velocity may be influenced by vessel diameter. If vessel diameter is incorporated into the assessment, then the pressure-velocity relationship can be used.

Variable lesion geometry in experimental studies: Coronary blood flow in the setting of variable stenosis geometry during coronary vasodilatation in awake dogs has been examined in the classic work by Gould and Kelley [2]. Quantitative coronary arteriography of 51 coronary stenoses in chronically instrumented intact animal models was used to define geometric changes in the stenosis after coronary vasodilators. The results of the experiments indicated that the increased hemodynamic severity (i.e., post-stenotic pressure and flow loss) of coronary stenoses at high coronary blood flows can be entirely and quantitatively explained by vasodilatation of the artery on either side of a fixed stenosis with slightly worsened percent diameter narrowing and modestly greater pressure loss disturbing coronary flow. Of importance, significant passive stenosis narrowing did not occur and the exit geometry of the stenosis did not change after coronary vasodilators. Changes in coronary flow velocity were 30-40% less than changes in volume flow, thereby producing a significant error regarding relative flow reserve unless changes in arterial diameter were also determined [1].

Four mechanisms have been postulated to account for fixed coronary stenosis changing during vasodilatory states within the coronary circulation. These 4 mechanisms include:

a.   Vasodilatation of the normal coronary segment adjacent to the stenotic region

b.   Further stenotic narrowing due to decreased intraluminal distending pressure after vasodilators as proposed by Santamore et al [8], Walinsky et al [10], Swartz et al [11], and Logan [12].

c.   Arterial smooth muscle vasodilatation of the stenotic segment in response to large vessel vasodilators by Brown et al [13] and Doerner et al [14].

d.   Turbulence induced by lesion conformation changes in the stenotic segment resulting in potential energy losses manifested as decrease in pressure reducing coronary blood flow without changing stenosis geometry [15].

e.   Coronary stenosis narrowing during exercise or vasoactive conditions may also contribute to ischemia [15A].

Critically severe stenoses have been reported to be associated with a decrease in coronary blood flow in the presence of distal dilatation attributed to fall in flow with passive collapse of the stenotic segment [8,11] (Figure 6).

132

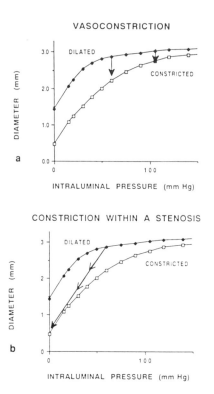

Figure 6: (a) The two lines show the effects of vasoconstriction at two levels of intraluminal pressure. Lowering the intraluminal pressure results in a greater decrease in vessel dimensions with vasoconstriction. (b) In a stenotic artery, the initial intraluminal pressure is decreased by the effects of the atherosclerotic plaque. This initial decrease in intraluminal pressure makes constriction more effective. More importantly, localized vasoconstriction decreased the intraluminal pressure. As the vessel constricts, the pressure decrease leads to further vessel shortening. Thus, the constriction is along a decreasing pressure line. The combination of an initial decrease in intraluminal pressure plus the pressure decreases as the vessel constricts causes exaggerated constriction within the stenosis. (Reproduced with permission from Santamore WP, Corin WJ. New concepts regarding constriction within a stenosis: influence of intraluminal pressure changes. Trends Cardiovasc Med 1992;2:189-196.)

Passive collapse has been questioned as a primary force since passive narrowing increases the stenosis severity leading to a further fall in intraluminal pressure, thus promoting further passive collapse until complete cessation of flow, a finding not present in the majority of animal and human studies. The stenosis geometry and its consequences on flow are intimately linked.

Controversy exists regarding the degree to which altered coronary blood flow to vasodilators may be the result of changing configuration of the stenosis due to elastic components. Santamore et al [8] examined pressure-flow relationships in an open chest anesthetized animal model with coronary stenosis in response to intracoronary isoproterenol, nitroglycerin, methoxamine, and vasopressin. Isoproterenol and nitroglycerin increased flow and decreased coronary resistance. Methoxamine and vasopressin decreased coronary flow and increased coronary resistance. These findings occurred in the absence of a significant stenosis. After partial coronary constriction, isoproterenol decreased coronary pressure, produced a 23% decrease in coronary resistance, and a 22% decrease in flow associated with an increase in stenotic resistance. Nitroglycerin decreased coronary pressure, but increased distal coronary resistance 29% with only a 1% increase in flow associated with a 38% increase in stenotic resistance. Passive changes in the stenotic area caused by coronary pressure changes were postulated as a mechanism for the alterations of stenotic resistance. In an in vitro carotid preparation similar findings were observed. A change in stenotic resistance was associated with radiographic analysis in an experimental carotid artery preparation which demonstrated that the pressure dependency of stenotic resistance is an additional factor that should be considered in patients being treated with coronary artery disease. Dynamic coronary stenoses as postulated by Gould et al [9] and Santamore et al [8] indicated that small changes in the diameter of the stenosis would have a large impact on the hemodynamic significance.

Length and diameter of stenosis and flow: The length of a stenosis, its absolute diameter, and size of normal arterial lumen influence, to variable and inter-related degrees, the hemodynamic severity of a stenosis [9,16, 17]. Lipscomb and Hooten [18] indicate that the 3 most important determinates of the pressure gradient in descending order are:

a.   The diameter of the stenosis
b.   Flow rate
c.   Absolute length of stenosis

The principal determinant of the arterial pressure-flow relation is thus the relative diameter reduction of the normal vessel caused by the stenosis. As noted earlier, stenoses of an unequal absolute diameter that produce identical percent reduction of luminal diameter have identical gradient-flow velocity, but not volumetric flow, relationships [9]. Stenoses of equal absolute diameters that cause different percent reduction in vessel diameter yield very different pressure-flow relationships.

134

The technique of inducing experimental coronary stenosis will also determine the physiologic response. A 50% stenosis of 5mm (external constrictor) or more in length, reduced peak reactive hyperemia between 30 and 50% [17]. In contrast, a 7mm long fixed rigid stenosis implanted as in the model of Gewirtz et al did not reduce maximal hyperemia [19]. The clinical significance of a 50% stenosis thus may rest on the pressure-flow relationship generated by that lesion. Brown et al [20] found that in 50 individual stenoses with intermediately severe stenoses (30-70%), 27/50 lesions failed to exhibit a statistically significant change in stenosis flow resistance in response to nitroglycerin-induced hyperemia. Many coronary stenoses of mild to moderate severity may be rigid in configuration. The pressure-flow relations under conditions of coronary vasodilatation thus may differ for fixed versus dynamic components of the stenosis.

The study of Sabbah et al [21] demonstrated that length of a stenotic segment had little effect on the magnitude of reduction of coronary blood flow. Similar work by others demonstrated that doubling the length of a carotid stenosis in dogs caused a minor reduction in carotid blood flow and that increasing the length of a stenotic segment from 1-3mm produced no significant hemodynamic affect. Feldman et al [16,22], examining stenoses of 40-60% diameter in coronary arteries of dogs, demonstrated the length of the stenotic segment had a marked affect on coronary blood flow (Figure 7).

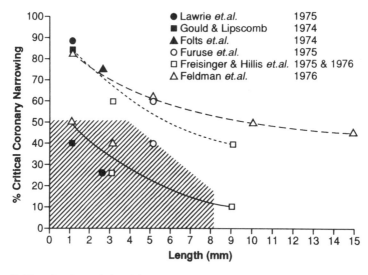

Figure 7: The role of stenosis length in the determination of critical coronary narrowing. Data at rest and during reactive hyperemia from several investigators are shown (horizontal axis). The reduction in diameter significantly altering flow is shown on the vertical axis. (Modified from reference #16.)

The length of a stenosis also impacts on the pressure gradient. For every diameter stenosis, a longer stenosis length has a steeper pressure gradient-flow relationship. The differences induced by stenosis length are minimal in the most severe and least severe cases (Figure 8).

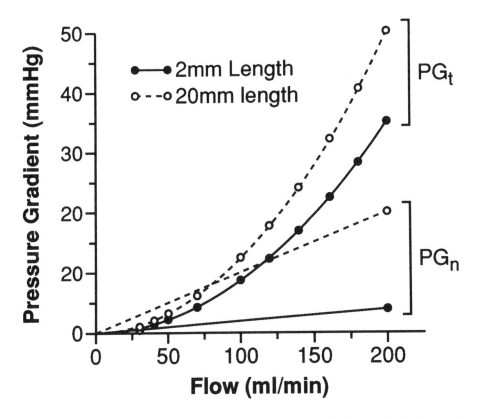

Figure 8: Relation of pressure gradient to flow plotted separately for the turbulent (PG_t) and nonturbulent (PG_N) components of the pressure gradient in stenoses 2 and 20mm long. The diameter of the stenoses is 1.3mm. Because the diameter affects PG_t and PG_N equally, the relation of PG_t to PG_N at each rate of flow is the same for stenoses of all diameter. (Reproduced with permission from reference #18.)

These findings should be considered when assessing coronary blood flow across stenoses in patients with diffuse disease or serially diseased segments.

Inlet geometry and shear stress: The entrance and exit angle to stenoses also contribute to turbulent flow and increasing post-stenotic pressure loss. Entrance angles of 90° produce little affect on 5mm stenoses in varying lengths of external constrictors placed on arteries [23]. Flow patterns through stenoses depend on the relative turbulence created by the configuration of the stenosis. Stenosis turbulence is translated to a Reynold's number as the product of velocity, diameter, blood density, and the inverse of blood viscosity. Reynold's numbers of < 2,000 are generally associated with minimal turbulence. Higher Reynold's numbers occur with greater degrees of stenoses exit angles, thus turbulence is directly related to stenosis morphology. The length of a stenosis has a greater affect on the non-turbulent than on the turbulent component of the pressure gradient. Because the non-turbulent component of flow is relatively more significant at low flow rates, a change in the length of stenosis will have a greater affect at low rather than high rates of coronary blood flow.

The stenosis inlet geometry alters shear rates of coronary blood flow. Abnormal shear rates of blood flow have been implicated in activation of atherosclerotic plaques and thrombosis leading to unstable angina or myocardial infarction. To assess stenosis inlet geometry on shear rates in regions proximal to the stenosis, Denardo et al [23] studied velocity profiles in asymmetric stenoses in canine aortas. Intermediate stenoses of 40 and 75% were tested, altering the inlet angulation from 45 to 90°. The investigators found that increasing the severity of stenosis and angulation resulted in a decrease in shear rate at the endothelial surface and significant increase in the maximal shear rate within the vessel lumen from 189 to 295 units in the region immediately upstream to the stenosis. These effects were less pronounced for lower Reynold's numbers. The authors concluded that stenosis inlet geometry had a significant impact on the flow conditions in the proximal region of the stenosis in relation to the Reynold's number which is directly related to coronary blood flow rate and has clinical importance for relating stenosis morphology to subsequent risk of vessel thrombosis.

Taeymans et al [24] found that coronary stenoses with average inlet angle > 25° and cross-sectional area > 75% reduction were at highest risk for thrombotic occlusion within 3 months after examination. An increased severity of inlet geometry caused development of low shear rates and blood flow separation at the endothelial surface in the region immediately proximal to the stenosis which established the milieu for thrombi generation at this location.

Influence of single and serial intermediately severe lesions: The extent to which normal coronary physiology is disturbed by a proximal coronary artery stenoses in the intermediate range remains controversial. Early canine experiments indicate that mild stenoses produced by externally applied coronary constrictor minimally reduced coronary reserve [19]. The impact of a 50% diameter coronary artery stenosis on regional myocardial blood flow and transmural distribution of blood flow was examined by Gewirtz et al [19] in 16 closed chest conscious pigs with an implanted 50% rigid coronary stenosis. Transmural endocardial and epicardial blood flow values did not differ significantly between the groups with 50% stenosis and the control group without stenosis. Basal endocardial to epicardial flow ratios were also similar. Maximal hyperemic transmural and endocardial and epicardial flow ratios increased to similar degrees. It is interesting to note that the 50% stenosis pressure gradient increased from 4 to 8, 11, and 21mmHg during infusions of 100, 200, and 400μg/min of intracoronary adenosine, corresponding to increases of regional coronary flow (ml/min/g) of 2.4, 3.7, and 5.1ml/min/g myocardial blood flow, respectively. Although these experiments may not be directly extrapolated to patient studies, these data demonstrated that in contrast to 50% stenoses formed with external coronary constrictors, fixed 50% stenoses within coronary vessels did not appear to reduce maximal myocardial hyperemic flow reserve.

The hemodynamics of multiple versus single intermediate stenoses in an experimental animal model have been studied [21]. An in vitro pulse duplicating system consisting of an acrylic mold of the aortic root of a calf with a coronary artery with serial 50% stenoses was constructed. Aortic, left ventricular, and post-stenotic pressures were measured in the test section with catheter-tipped micromanometers. Coronary flow was measured with a cannulating electromagnetic flow transducer. Sequential studies performed with one 2mm long arterial stenosis of 50%, two stenotic segments, and 3 stenotic segments were examined. A second series of experiments using 4mm long 50% stenoses and 6mm long 50% diameter stenoses were also performed at constant heart rate, stroke volume, and aortic pressure. The single 2mm 50% stenosis reduced coronary blood flow 6%. Three such stenoses in series reduced coronary blood flow 19%. These findings contrasted to a single 6mm long 50% stenosis which caused an 8% reduction of coronary flow. In a maximally dilated coronary bed, a greater reduction in coronary flow would occur in the presence of multiple short stenoses than in the presence of a single stenosis of equivalent length and diameter [25-27]. This phenomenon is postulated to be related to summation of turbulence and viscous friction forces above that occurring with a single severe lesion.

Clinical applications of coronary blood flow to assessment of lesion significance

Prediction of lesion physiology from arteriography: Quantitative angiography has been used for determining pressure-flow characteristics across coronary stenoses [3] applying classic fluid dynamic equations to tapering stenosis in vasoactive flexible coronary arteries in vivo [25-27].

138

Although quantitative coronary angiography is widely available, angiographically-derived parameters of translesional physiology have not been compared with those directly measured in the same patients having coronary artery disease. Tron et al [28] compared quantitative coronary angiographic prediction of translesional pressure and flow with directly measured pressure and flow responses. Quantitative coronary angiography, as determined by the DCI-ACA program (Philips, Shelton, CT), was compared to translesional pressure gradient data and pressure and flow velocity data obtained with a 2.7F fluid-filled tracking catheter and a 0.018" Doppler-tipped angioplasty guidewire (FloWire™, Cardiometrics, Inc., Mountain View, CA). Simultaneous measurements were obtained in 28 arteries from 25 patients. Mean diameter stenosis was $51\pm2.3\%$ (range 29-73%). No patient had left ventricular hypertrophy or valvular heart disease. There were 14 left anterior descending, 8 circumflex, and 6 right coronary artery stenoses studied. Stenotic flow reserve determined from the quantitative coronary angiography program, baseline and maximal gradients from the angiogram were determined and compared with coronary flow reserve, basal and maximal hyperemic gradients from direct measurements after production of coronary hyperemia with 12-18μg of intracoronary adenosine. Quantitative coronary angiographic-derived pressure gradients did not correlate with measured baseline or maximal hyperemic gradients ($r=0.1$; $p=0.13$) (Figure 9A).

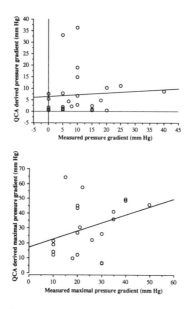

Figure 9A: Individual data for comparisons between quantitative coronary angiography (QCA)-derived and directly measured pressure gradients (top panel, $r^2=0.005$, $p=0.73$) and between QCA-derived and directly measured maximal pressure gradients (bottom panel, $r^2=0.1$, $p=0.13$). (Reproduced with permission from reference #28.)

No correlation was found between quantitative coronary angiographic predicted stenotic flow reserve and coronary flow reserve measured distal to the stenosis (r=0.02; p=0.46). Stenotic flow reserve and measured pressure gradient were not significantly correlated (Figure 9B).

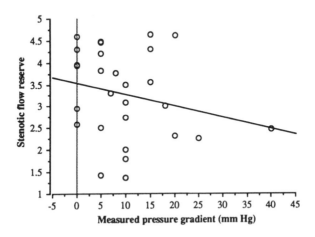

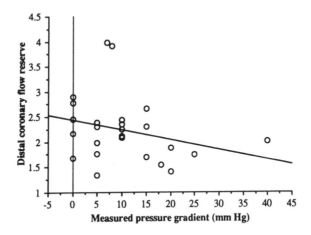

Figure 9B: Individual data for comparisons between measured pressure gradient and stenotic flow reserve (top panel, r²=0.1, p=0.23) and measured distal coronary flow reserve (bottom panel, r²=0.1, p=0.16). (Reproduced with permission from reference #28.)

The weak correlations between quantitative coronary angiography-derived and directly measured translesional physiology is likely due to several factors. Variations in 3-dimensional and intraluminal geometry are not appreciated by the angiographic technique. Flow velocity measurements were assumed at constant values and vasotonic activity and distal bed microvascular impairment was not included in the calculations. These results indicated that due to inherent limitations of angiography and theoretical assumptions of the physiologic state, quantitative coronary angiographic-derived parameters of translesional physiology particularly relevant for the assessment of lesions of intermediate severity do not correlate with directly measured translesional pressure and flow. Given these limitations, caution should be applied in extending the angiographic data to clinical decision making based on physiologically-derived parameters. Quantitative coronary angiographic-derived physiology may benefit from further refinement by input functions of physiologic variables.

The visual interpretation of coronary arteriograms is a poor predictor of physiologic lesion significance. Using intracoronary Doppler catheter measurements of coronary flow velocity reserve in the operating room, White et al [29] assessed the correlation between coronary hyperemia (using transient coronary artery occlusion) in 44 patients with stenoses ranging from 10-90% severity (Figure 3).

Based on coronary flow reserve (normal ≥ 3.5), underestimation of lesion severity occurred in 90% of vessels with >60% stenosis diameter by arteriography. Both under- and over-estimation of lesions with <60% stenosis were common. These results, combined with the high intraobserver and interobserver variability of standard angiographic lesion assessment [30], indicate that the physiologic affects of the most common coronary obstructions cannot be determined accurately by angiography.

Coronary blood flow velocity has not been routinely used in the assessment of coronary stenoses on a clinical basis for several reasons. Earlier 3F catheter size and proximal location of velocity measurements severely hampered the application of the technique and interpretation of coronary flow reserve. Only the more recent development of Doppler angioplasty guidewires has allowed measurement of flow velocity in the post-stenotic bed.

Post-stenotic coronary flow velocity reserve, quantitative coronary angiography, and myocardial perfusion imaging: Clinical decisions for coronary interventions are often based on the results of out-of-laboratory physiologic testing such as thallium perfusion myocardial imaging. Because the physiologic assessment of angiographically intermediate stenoses remains problematic, functional measurements of post-stenotic intracoronary flow velocity reserve may have utility in clinical decision making. However, a correlation between post-stenotic coronary flow reserve and hyperemic myocardial perfusion scintigraphic imaging was not previously identified. To correlate myocardial perfusion imaging with post-stenotic coronary flow reserve in patients with angiographically intermediate coronary stenosis, Miller et al [31] studied 33 patients. The angiographic percent diameter stenosis by quantitative coronary angiography was $56 \pm 14\%$ (range 20-84% diameter stenosis). Proximal and post-stenotic Doppler flow velocities were obtained at rest and during maximal hyperemia with intracoronary adenosine as previously reported [32]. Intravenous pharmacologic stress imaging was performed with adenosine in 20 patients and dipyridamole in 13 patients with technetium-99m sestamibi tomographic perfusion imaging within one week of coronary flow velocity studies. A Kappa statistic measuring the strength of correlation among the velocity imaging and quantitative coronary angiographic variables was computed. Quantitative coronary angiography stenosis severity and post-stenotic coronary flow velocity reserve of <2.0 were correlated in 20/27 patients (74%, Kappa=0.48). Perfusion imaging abnormalities and stenosis quantitative coronary angiographic severity were correlated in 28/33 patients (Kappa=0.63). Sestamibi imaging results agreed with basal transstenotic velocity ratios of <1.7 in 48% of patients (Kappa=0.17). The strongest correlation was noted between hyperemic post-stenotic flow velocity reserve and sestamibi perfusion imaging in 24/27 patients (89%, Kappa=0.78). All patients with abnormal distal hyperemic flow velocity values had corresponding reversible myocardial perfusion tomographic imaging defects. The high correlation between two different physiologic techniques to assess myocardial perfusion in the post-stenotic region suggests that clinical decisions can be made in the laboratory in a similar fashion to out-of-laboratory testing. The physiologic assessment of coronary stenoses, especially in lesions of angiographically intermediate severity, may be improved by the use of post-stenotic flow velocity measurements when perfusion imaging has not or cannot be performed.

A similar correspondence between post-stenotic coronary flow reserve and myocardial perfusion imaging has been described by Joye et al [32] who compared single photon emission computed tomographic thallium imaging to coronary flow reserve in 30 patients with intermediate coronary stenoses. The post-stenotic flow reserve and SPECT thallium studies were compared with blinded interpretations of the results. Coronary flow reserve of <2.0 was determined to be abnormal. The sensitivity, specificity and overall predictive accuracy of Doppler-derived coronary flow reserve with stress SPECT thallium-201 results were 94, 95, and 94%, respectively. The investigators indicated that selected patients with intermediate coronary stenoses can be assessed accurately by determination of post-stenotic flow reserve as a surrogate for SPECT thallium imaging, an especially important consideration for lesions of intermediate severity prior to coronary intervention.

To improve on coronary flow reserve, the slope of instantaneous hyperemic diastolic coronary flow velocity-pressure relationship has been proposed as a better index for the assessment of physiologic significance of coronary stenoses in humans (Figure 10).

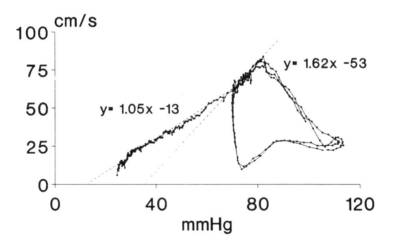

Figure 10: Flow velocity/pressure loops during maximal hyperemia. During mid-late diastole, a linear relation is observed, with an extrapolated zero-flow pressure of 37mmHg. However, during a long diastolic pause (cardiac arrest induced by the intracoronary injection of 3mg of adenosine), the pressure/flow velocity/pressure relation deviates considerably from the extrapolated curve. (Reproduced with permission from Serruys PW, Di Mario C, Meneveau N, de Jaegere P, Strikwerda S, de Feyter PJ, Emanuelsson H. Intracoronary pressure and flow velocity with sensor-tip guide wires: a new methodologic approach to assessment of coronary hemodynamics before and after coronary interventions. Am J Cardiol 1993;71: 41D-53D.)

Di Mario et al [33] examined the sensitivity and specificity of the simultaneous relationship between diastolic coronary flow velocity and aortic pressure during maximal hyperemia and coronary flow velocity reserve for detecting flow-limiting coronary stenoses. The instantaneous coronary flow velocity (using a Doppler guidewire) measured during maximal hyperemia induced with intracoronary papaverine was plotted against aortic pressure over the hyperemic period in 79 patients. The intraobserver variability was $0.4 \pm 11\%$. The instantaneous hyperemic diastolic velocity pressure relationship was significantly lower in arteries with $>30\%$ diameter stenosis than in normal or near normal vessels (0.7 ± 0.48 vs 1.73 ± 0.8cm/ sec/mmHg) ($p < 0.01$). In the stenosis group, both the instantaneous hyperemic pressure velocity and coronary flow reserve were significantly correlated. The investigators concluded that although the instantaneous pressure velocity relationship can distinguish arteries with and without coronary stenoses, the precision of the measurement requires refinement before clinical application. Coronary flow reserve had similar sensitivity and specificity in distinguishing normal and stenotic vessels and demonstrated similar correlations with minimal luminal cross-sectional area.

Translesional flow velocity for lesion assessment: Proximal flow through branching coronary vessels may be directed by stenosis resistance to pre-stenotic branch vessels of lower resistance (Figure 11).

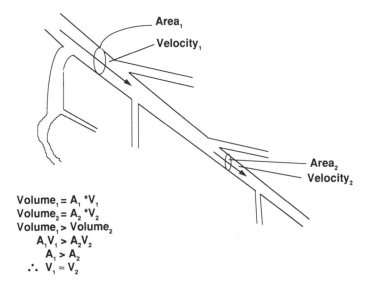

Figure 11A: Volumetric flow is equal to [mean velocity * cross-sectional vessel area] at any point in the artery. Since the arteries are branched systems, flow volume is reduced as it is distributed by branches. The cross-sectional area is likewise reduced over the course of the vessel, resulting in proximal to distal velocity ratios approaching 1. (Reproduced with permission from reference #36.)

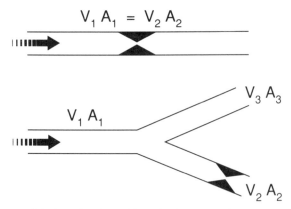

Figure 11B: Diagram of single (top) and branching tube (bottom) models. In the single tube, the continuity equation can be applied for proximal and distal flow. However, a resistance in the branching tube produces the diversion of flow to alter proximal and distal lesional flow values proportionally. (Reproduced with permission from reference #36.)

Under these conditions, proximal flow velocity may be greater than distal or post-stenotic flow. To assess the difference in proximal and post-stenotic flow velocity, Donohue et al [7] demonstrated that the proximal to distal flow velocity ratio (P/D) was related to translesional pressure gradients > 30mmHg in patients with coronary stenoses and side branch systems. Hemodynamically significant stenoses, independent of angiographic morphology, reduced post-stenotic flow relative to proximal flow velocity. P/D ratios > 1.7 were associated with translesional pressure gradients > 30mmHg in $> 90\%$ of left anterior descending coronary arteries (Figure 12).

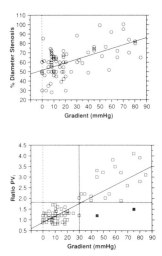

Figure 12: (TOP) Correlation between angiography (percent diameter stenosis) and translesional pressure gradients (mmHg). (BOTTOM) Correlation between the ratio of proximal to distal total velocity integral (ratio PV_i) and translesional pressure gradients (mmHg). The two solid squares represent the proximal right coronary artery stenoses occurring before any branch points. (Reproduced with permission from reference #7.)

In right coronary arteries, the proximal to distal flow velocity relationship was less significant due to the lack of side branches.

Post-stenotic flow velocity: The flow velocity findings distal to severe coronary stenoses demonstrate several common findings: 1) decrease in mean velocity (usually <20cm/sec) [for lesions with translesional gradients >30mmHg, a mean proximal:distal flow velocity ratio >1.7]; 2) an impaired phasic pattern of coronary flow; and 3) impaired distal coronary hyperemia (<2.0 x basal values). Figure 13 illustrates flow velocity before and after coronary angioplasty in a patient with multiple intermediate stenoses.

T.H. 43 yr old Male - 1 week post anterior MI LAD

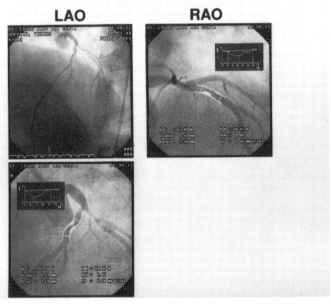

Figure 13A: Frames from a coronary cineangiogram in the left anterior oblique projection (LAO) and right anterior oblique projection (RAO) of the left anterior descending artery demonstrating a 60% diameter narrowing of the proximal segment by QCA in the "worse" projection.

146

T.H. 43 yr old Male - 1 week post anterior MI
RCA

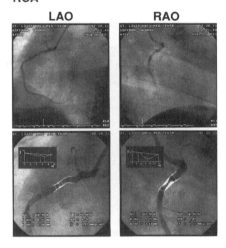

Figure 13B: Angiogram frames of the right coronary artery demonstrating the eccentric proximal lesion in the right anterior oblique (RAO) projection. Quantitative angiography in this projection revealed a percent diameter narrowing of 63%. The eccentric nature of the plaque was apparent from the left anterior oblique (LAO) view.

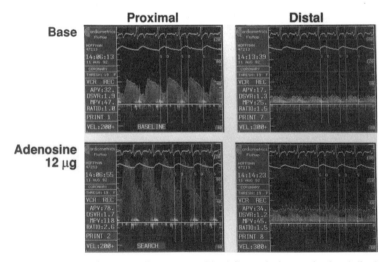

Figure 13C: Left anterior descending coronary blood flow velocity proximal and distal to the stenosis at baseline and during maximal hyperemia with 12mcg of intracoronary adenosine (flow velocity scale = 0-200cm/sec). The ratio of proximal to distal flow velocity is 1.9 prior to angioplasty. Distal hyperemia was impaired with a flow reserve ratio of approximately 1.42.

147

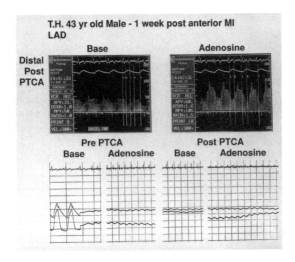

Figure 13D: Corresponding translesional gradient before and after angioplasty at baseline and during maximal hyperemia. (Bottom) Hemodynamic tracings show electrocardiogram, aortic pressure and distal coronary pressure (from the top of panel down, 0-200mmHg scale). Resting gradient is 40mmHg which widens to approximately 50mmHg at maximal hyperemia. Following angioplasty, baseline gradient is 8mmHg which widens to approximately 20mmHg during maximal hyperemia. The distal flow velocity spectral tracings are shown on the lower 2 panels which indicate an increase of the distal velocity equivalent to proximal velocity with restoration of the phasic flow signal and hyperemia of 2.1 times basal flow velocity in association with the reduction in the translesional gradient.

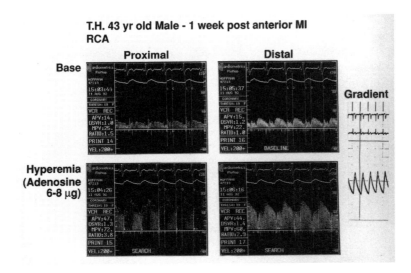

Figure 13E: Flow velocity data for the right coronary artery, proximal and distal to the eccentric stenosis. Proximal to distal flow velocity ratio was 0.9. Distal hyperemia was 2.9 x baseline flow. There was no translesional gradient at rest or during hyperemia in this artery. Angioplasty was not performed. (Reproduced wtih permission from reference #41.)

Normally, the diastolic component of flow velocity is nearly two times the systolic component with a normal diastolic to systolic velocity ratio (DSVR) of >1.8 for the left coronary artery. For severe lesions, a DSVR <1.4 is common. Maximal coronary hyperemia in normal patients and experimental animal models may be 3-5 x basal levels. In our and other laboratories, lower values (>2.5) have commonly been observed in patients with chest pain and angiographically normal arteries when measured using the Doppler guidewire. In recently (<1 year) transplanted hearts with angiographic normal arteries which are past the initial healing phase, coronary vasodilatory reserve ratios are usually >3.0. For severe coronary lesions, proximally measured flow velocity can detect nearly normal degrees of hyperemia due to augmentation of branch vessel flow, whereas flow velocity distal to severe stenoses is universally impaired. Impaired distal hyperemic flow velocity (<2.0) is reliably or highly correlated with abnormal scintigraphic perfusion imaging.

Blood flow in the branched artery system: The continuity equation of flow conservation states that in a continuous single tube, the volume of flow must be equal at any point along the tube [37,38]. Volume flow is equal to velocity of flow x cross sectional area (see Figure 11A).

However, in a branched tube, reduced distal flow compared to proximal flow occurs when flow is diverted away from the branch with a high resistance (due to a stenosis) to branches with lower resistances. The proximal/distal ratio will not apply in conduit arteries without branches or non-branching saphenous vein grafts where the continuity equation remains valid stating equality of volumetric flow (not flow velocity) at any point along the circuit (see Figure 11B) must occur.

In situations where arteries are single tube conduits without branches, such as proximal right coronary arteries or bypass grafts, the proximal and distal blood flow velocity will be affected equally and the transstenotic velocity ratio is not useful for predicting stenosis severity. In branching normal coronary vessels, proximal and distal velocity remains similar with a ratio of nearly 1. This relationship is postulated to occur since the flow volume and cross-sectional area of the epicardial conduits are both diminishing toward the distal myocardial regions. Thus, flow velocity remains relatively constant.

Characteristic blood flow in coronary arteries depends on the vessel measured, the function of the distal myocardial perfusion bed (infarction or ischemia), and factors related to microcirculatory impairment (left ventricular hypertrophy, diabetes, or hypertension). The use of coronary blood flow velocity in assessing the significance of lesion morphology has been limited. The ability to characterize flow modulation related to the contribution of stenosis morphology is limited by angiography.

Assessment of blood flow for interventional procedures: Morphologic considerations:

Coronary artery dissections: Significant coronary dissection is frequently encountered in the post-angioplasty angiogram. The effect of dissection on coronary blood flow is highly variable. A large flap producing a luminal lucency either parallel to or crossing (spiral) through the angioplasty site is generally considered an unsatisfactory result with a propensity to an abrupt serious ischemic event. Less severe grades of dissection are often considered satisfactory by qualitative angiographic assessment, but little objective quantification of the physiologic impact of a coronary dissection is available.

In patients undergoing coronary angioplasty, coronary dissections produce alterations of the flow velocity patterns which are readily identified, suggesting significantly impaired coronary lumina and flow. Such dissections can be stabilized by stenting, so recognition of flow limitation has substantial impact on management. After restoration of the angiographic appearance by stent placement, normalization of the distal flow velocity pattern is usually achieved. Recognition of abnormal distal coronary flow may assist in decision making for similar interventional procedures.

Assessment of serial lesions in a left anterior descending artery: A 57 year old man with insulin-dependent diabetes mellitus, hypertension and renal insufficiency developed unstable angina prior to planned renal transplantation [40]. Coronary arteriography demonstrated multiple severe left anterior descending coronary artery narrowings (Figure 14A, top panel). The left circumflex and right coronary arteries had mild, non-critical (<50%) diameter narrowings. Coronary angioplasty was performed with a 0.018" Doppler flowire and a 2.5mm angioplasty balloon. Sequential balloon inflations were performed for lesions A, B and C

150

(Figure 14A, top panel). Coronary flow velocity (Figure 14A, bottom left), obtained proximal to the left anterior descending lesion A was normal in phasic pattern (diastolic/systolic velocity ratio, DSVR = 1.9) and mean velocity (38cm/second). Coronary flow velocity beyond the lesion C was reduced to 18cm/second (mean velocity) with an abnormal DSVR of 1.2 (Figure 14A, bottom right).

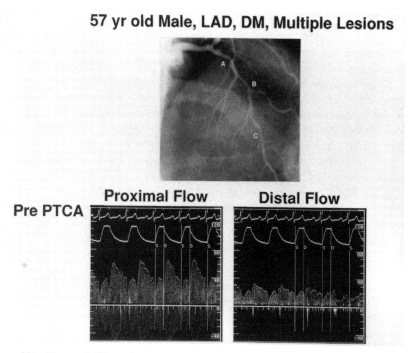

Figure 14A: (Top panel) Cineangiogram and coronary flow velocity proximal to lesion A (bottom left) and distally beyond lesion C (bottom right) before (pre-) angioplasty. Arrow shows location of distal flow measurements. Proximal flow velocity has normal phasic diastolic/systolic velocity ratio (DSVR, 1.9) and mean velocity (38cm/second). Distal flow velocity is abnormal with DSVR of 1.2 and mean velocity of 18cm/second. Velocity scale is 0-200cm/second. Electrocardiogram and arterial pressure are displayed at top of flow scale. Vertical lines mark systolic (S) and diastolic (D) flow periods. (Modified with permission from reference #39.)

The proximal-to-distal flow velocity ratio of 2.1 suggested a trans-arterial pressure gradient > 30mmHg. After the first series of balloon inflations for the 3 lesions, 2 areas of coronary dissection could be seen at locations B and C (Figure 14B, top panel left side, labelled D). The angiographic flow appeared adequate without ischemic electrocardiogram abnormalities or symptoms. However, distal coronary flow velocity had a new and abnormal systolic predominant flow pattern (DSVR 0.6) with an unchanged mean flow velocity (22cm/second) (Figure 14B, bottom left). Prolonged (5 minute) balloon inflations were then performed with mild angiographic improvement (Figure 14B, top middle panel) and only minimally improved distal flow velocity. The distal mean flow velocity was 16cm/second with a DSVR of 1.1 (Figure 14B, bottom middle panel). Because of the extensive dissection with impaired coronary flow velocity, 2 serial 2.5 x 20mm stents (Cook, Inc.) were inserted into locations B and C. Angiographic results were improved with residual evidence of dissection at lesion B (Figure 14B, top right). Distal flow velocity normalized with a mean velocity of 39cm/second and DSVR of 2.3 (Figure 14B, bottom right). With restoration of normal distal flow, further dilations and stent placements were deemed unnecessary.

57 yr old Male, LAD, DM, Multiple Lesions

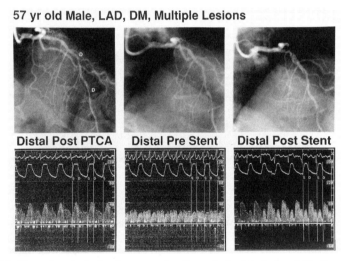

Figure 14B: Cineangiograms (top) and corresponding flow velocity data (bottom left) after coronary angioplasty (PTCA), before stent placement at dissected (D) regions (bottom middle) and after two serial stent implantations (bottom right). Distal flow velocity after serial balloon inflations showed abnormal systolic predominant flow pattern (DSVR 0.6, bottom left). Prolonged balloon dilations improved the DSVR, but did not normalize phasic flow (bottom middle). After stent placement, distal flow velocity is normal in both phasic pattern (DSVR 2.2) and is equivalent to proximal pre-procedural values (40cm/sec, bottom right). (Velocity scale is 0-200cm/second for pre-stent angioplasty panels and 0-300cm/second for post-stent velocity scale.) (Modified with permission from reference #39.)

These cases demonstrate that abnormal phasic patterns of coronary flow beyond significant lesions can be restored with angioplasty and then may revert to an abnormal pattern when flow-limiting dissections compromise the lumina. Based on angiography alone, a decision against a stent in the first case may have been made based on the LAO angiogram and low translesional gradient. Flow monitoring demonstrated abnormal flow in the absence of clinical or new angiographic findings. Similarly, the serial dissections were associated with marginal but acceptable angiographic results which could have been managed with observation and prolonged heparin therapy. The abnormal flow pattern was further physiologic evidence of limited flow which was normalized after serial stent placement.

Eccentric lesions: Eccentric stenoses present a dilemma for the clinician. These lesions are difficult to interpret angiographically due to limitations in obtaining viewing angles which delineate stenosis severity in orthogonal projections. Patients considered candidates for intervention will benefit by having objective translesional flow and pressure measurements before making a decision to proceed.

A 43 year old man had an acute anterior myocardial infarction with mild chest discomfort on hospital day 3 [41]. Coronary angiography demonstrated a 60% diameter narrowing in the proximal left anterior descending coronary artery and an eccentric 63% diameter narrowing of the proximal right coronary artery (Figures 13A,13B).

Intervention was deferred and a thallium-201 exercise test was performed on day 7 following infarction which revealed a small anterior and inferior apical reversible defect. Angioplasty was anticipated after translesional flow velocity assessment of both stenoses.

After administration of 10,000 units of IV heparin, flow velocity was measured with the 0.018" flowire (Cardiometrics, Inc., Mountain View, CA) and a translesional pressure gradient was measured with a 2.7 French tracking catheter (Target Therapeutics) as previously described [32,37].

Left anterior descending coronary lesion assessment: Flow velocity distal to the left anterior descending coronary stenosis was impaired with a proximal/distal mean flow ratio > 1.7 (average peak velocity proximal 32cm/sec, distal 17cm/sec, ratio 32/17 = 1.9). In addition, the phasic pattern of flow velocity was abnormal with diastolic/systolic velocity ratio of 1.3 (normal left coronary diastolic/systolic velocity ratio > 1.5) [7]. Distal hyperemia was also impaired [distal flow (hyperemic/basal) reserve = 1.42]. A 40mmHg gradient was obtained (with the tracker catheter) which increased to 48mmHg during maximal hyperemia (Figure 13C) (Table I).

Table I. Hemodynamic and Flow Velocity Data

	Base				Hyperemia				
	DSVR	MV	DV$_i$	Gradient	DSVR	MV	DV$_i$	Gradient	CVR
LAD: Pre-PTCA									
Proximal	1.9	32	25.1	-	1.7	78	54.1	-	2.21
Distal	1.3	17	14.0	40	1.2	31	20.3	48	1.42
P/D ratio	-	1.9	-	-	-	2.5	-	-	-
LAD: Post-PTCA									
Distal	1.5	33	25.0	8	1.6	60	49.0	20	1.96
P/D ratio	-	0.9	-	-	-	-	-	-	
RCA									
Proximal	1.1	14	9.1	-	1.3	47	30.5	-	3.35
Distal	1.2	15	10.6	0	1.4	44	30.8	5	2.90
P/D ratio	-	0.9	-	-	-	1.1	-	-	-

CVR=coronary vasodilatory reserve (hyperemic/basal DV); DSVR=diastolic/systolic velocity ratio; DV$_i$=diastolic flow velocity integral; MV=mean velocity (cm/sec); P/D=proximal to distal flow ratio. Gradients in mmHg. (Reproduced with permission from reference #41.)

Because of the significantly abnormal translesional flow dynamics, coronary angioplasty was successfully performed which reduced the stenosis to <30% diameter narrowing with restoration of normal distal phasic flow velocity patterns (diastolic/systolic ratio=1.6) and improvement of basal flow (mean velocity=33cm/ second) and distal hyperemia (distal flow reserve=1.96). The final gradient was 8mmHg at rest which increased to 20mmHg during maximal hyperemia (Figure 13D).

Right coronary lesion assessment: Proximal flow velocity was normal at baseline and after 8μg of intracoronary adenosine demonstrated a normal hyperemic response (Figure 13E).

The diastolic/systolic velocity ratio was within normal limits for the right coronary artery. Data were obtained before the origin of the posterior descending branch artery. Distal flow velocity was maintained (proximal/distal ratio=0.9) with the same phasic flow pattern. Distal coronary vasodilatory reserve was normal (hyperemia/basal mean velocity, 44/15=2.9). The translesional pressure gradient was zero. Angioplasty was not performed on this artery. The patient did well and was discharged home two days later on a routine post-myocardial infarction and angioplasty medical regimen.

Summary: Coronary blood flow is significantly affected by stenosis morphology. Although experimental studies emphasize the complexity of stenosis geometry to alterations of coronary blood flow, only limited morphologic characteristics of stenoses in patients can be defined by angiography. The precision of angiography for physiologic lesion assessment can be improved by measurement of translesional flow in the catheterization laboratory.

Using translesional flow velocity as a marker of physiologic significance, an objective determination of the need for intervention, especially important for a-ngiographically intermediate lesions, can be obtained. Given the frequently employed current strategy of non-invasive testing for functional assessment of coronary stenoses, patients with clinical syndromes suggesting need for coronary intervention may be spared unnecessary procedures by having lesions assessed with direct intracoronary flow dynamic measurements.

ACKNOWLEDGEMENT

The author wishes to thank Donna Sander for manuscript preparation.

156

REFERENCES

1. Poiseuille JLM. Recherches sur les causes du movement du sang dans les veins. J Physiol Pathol 1830;10:277; reproduced in Best CH (ed): The Physiologic Basis of Medical Practice, ed 8. New York, Williams & Williams Co, 1966, p 654.

2. Gould KL, Kelley KO. Physiological significance of coronary flow velocity and changing stenosis geometry during coronary vasodilation in awake dogs. Circ Res 1982;50:695-704.

3. Gould KL, Kelley KO, Bolson EL. Experiemental validation of quantitative coronary arteriography for determining pressure-flow characteristics of coronary stenosis. Circulation 1982;66:930-937.

4. Gould KL, Lipscomb K, Calvert C. Compensatory changes of the distal coronary vascular bed during progressive coronary constriction. Circulation 1975;51:1085-1094.

5. Segal J, Kern MJ, Scott NA, King SB III, Doucette JW, Heuser RR, Ofili E, Siegel R. Alterations of phasic coronary artery flow velocity in humans during percutaneous coronary angioplasty. J Am Coll Cardiol 1992;20:276-286.

6. Ofili EO, Kern MJ, Labovitz AJ, St. Vrain JA, Segal J, Aguirre F, Castello R. Analysis of coronary blood flow velocity dynamics in angiographically normal and stenosed arteries before and after endolumen enlargement by angioplasty. J Am Coll Cardiol 1993;21:308-316.

7. Donohue TJ, Kern MJ, Aguirre FV, Bach RG, Wolford T, Bell CA, Segal J. Assessing the hemodynamic significance of coronary artery stenoses: analysis of translesional pressure-flow velocity relations in patients. J Am Coll Cardiol 1993;22:449-458.

8. Santamore WP, Walinsky P. Altered coronary flow responses to vasoactive drugs in the presence of coronary arterial stenosis in the dog. Am J Cardiol 1980;45:276-285.

9. Gould KL. Dynamic coronary stenosis (special commentary). Am J Cardiol 1980;45: 286-292.

10. Walinsky P, Santamore WP, Wiener L, Brest AN. Dynamic changes in the hemodynamic severity of coronary artery stenosis in a canine model. Cardiovasc Res 1979;13:113-118.

11. Swartz JS, Caryle PF, Cohn JN. Effect of dilation of the distal coronary bed on flow and resistance in severely stenotic coronary arteries in the dog. 1979;42:219-224.

12. Logan SE. On the fluid mechanics of human coronary artery stenosis. IEEE Trans Biomed Eng 1975;22:327-334.

13.   Brown GB, Bolson E, Frimer M, Dodge HT. Angiographic distinction between variant angina and non-vasospastic chest pain (abstr). Circulation 1978;57,58(Suppl II):II-122.

14.   Doerner TC, Brown GB, Bolson E, Frimer M, Dodge HT. Vasodilatory effects of nitroglycerin and nitroprusside in coronary arteries - a comparative analysis (abstr). Am J Cardiol 1979;43:416.

15.   Berguer R, Hwang NHC. Critical arterial stenosis: a theoretical and experimental solution. Ann Surg 1974;180:39-50.

15A.   Klein LW, Segal BL, Helfant RH. Dynamic coronary stenosis behavior in classic angina pectoris: active process or passive response? J Am Coll Cardiol 1987;10:311-313.

16.   Feldman RL, Nichols WW, Pepine CJ, Conti CR. Hemodynamic significance of the length of a coronary arterial narrowing. Am J Cardiol 1978;41:865-871.

17.   Feldman RL, Nichols WW, Pepine CJ, Conetta DA, Conti CR. The coronary hemodynamics of left main and branch coronary stenosis: The effects of reduction in stenosis diameter, stenosis length and number of stenoses. J Thorac Cardiovasc Surg 1979;77:377-388.

18.   Lipscomb K, Hooten S. Effect of stenotic dimensions and blood flow on the hemodynamic significance of model coronary arterial stenoses. Am J Cardiol 1978;42:781-792.

19.   Gewirtz H, Williams DO, Most AS. Quantitative assessment of the effects of a fixed 50% coronary artery stenosis on regional myocardial flow reserve and transmural distribution of blood flow. J Am Coll Cardiol 1983;1:1273-1280.

20.   Brown BG, Josephson MA, Petersen RB, et al. Intravenous dipyridamole combined with isometric handgrip for near maximal acute increase in coronary flow in patients with coronary artery disease. Am J Cardiol 1981;48:1077-1085.

21.   Sabbah HN, Stein PD. Hemodynamics of multiple versus single 50 percent coronary arterial stenoses. Am J Cardiol 1982;50:276-280.

22.   Feldman RL, Nichols WW, Pepine CJ, Conti CR. Hemodynamic significance of the length of a coronary arterial narrowing. Am J Cardiol 1978;41:865-871.

23.   Denardo SJ, Yamada EG, Hargrave VK, Yock PG. Effect of stenosis inlet geometry on shear rates of blood flow in the upstream region. Am Heart J 1993;125:350-356.

24.   Taeymans Y, Theroux P, Lesperance J, Waters D. Quantitative angiographic morphology of the coronary artery lesions at risk of thrombotic occlusion. Circulation 1992;85:78-85.

25.   Logan SE. On the fluid mechanics of human coronary artery stenosis. IEEE Trans Biomed Eng 1975;22:327-334.

26. Vonruden WJ, Blaisdell FW, Hall AD, Thomas AN. Multiple arterial stenoses: effects on blood flow. Arch Surg 1964;89:307-315.

27. Sun Y, Most AS, Ohley W, Gewirtz H. Estimation of instantaneous blood flow through a rigid, coronary artery stenosis in anaesthetised domestic swine. Cardiovas Res 1983;17:499-504.

28. Tron C, Kern MJ, Donohue TJ, Bach RG, Aguirre FV, Caracciolo EA, Moore JA. Comparison of quantitative angiographically-derived and measured translesion pressure and flow velocity in patients with coronary artery disease. Am J Cardiol 1995;75:111-117.

29. White CW, Wright CB, Doty DB, Hiratza LF, Eatham CL, Harrison DG, Marcus ML. Does visual interpretation of the coronary arteriogram predict the physiologic importance of a coronary stenosis? N Engl J Med 1984;310:819-824.

30. Zir LM, Miller SW, Dinsmore RE, Gilbert JP, Harthorne JW. Interobserver variability in coronary angiography. Circulation 1976;53:627-632.

31. Miller DD, Donohue TJ, Younis LT, Bach RG, Aguirre FV, Wittry MD, Goodgold HM, Chaitman BR, Kern MJ. Correlation of pharmacologic ^{99m}Tc-sestamibi myocardial perfusion imaging with poststenotic coronary flow reserve in patients with angiographically intermediate coronary artery stenoses. Circulation 1994;89:2150-2160.

32. Joye JD, Schulman DS, Sasorda D, Farah T, Donohue BC, Reichek N. Intracoronary Doppler guide wire versus stress single-photon emission computed tomographic thallium-201 imaging in assessment of intermediate coronary stenoses. J Am Coll Cardiol 1994;24:940-947.

33. Di Mario C, Krams R, Gil R, Serruys PW. Slope of the instantaneous hyperemic diastolic coronary flow velocity-pressure relation: a new index for assessment of the physiological significance of coronary stenosis in humans. Circulation 1994;90:1215-1224.

34. Leiboff R, Bren G, Katz R, Korkegi R, Ross A. Determinants of transstenotic gradients observed during angioplasty: an experimental model. Am J Cardiol 1983;52:1311-1317.

35. Pijls NHJ, van Son AM, Kirkeeide RL, De Bruyne B, Gould KL. Experimental basis of determining maximum coronary, myocardial, and collateral blood flow by pressure measuremetns for assessing functional stenosis severity before and after percutaneous transluminal coronary angioplasty. Circulation 1993;87:1354-1367.

36. Kern MJ, Aguirre FV, Bach RG, Caracciolo EA, Donohue TJ. Translesional pressure-flow velocity assessment in patients. Cathet Cardiovasc Diagn 1994;31:49-60.

37. Kern MJ, Aguirre FV, Bach RG, Caracciolo EA, Donohue TJ, Labovitz AJ. Fundamentals of translesional pressure-flow velocity measurements. Cathet Cardiovasc Diagn 1994;31:137-143.

38. Kern MJ, Donohue TJ, Bach RG, Caracciolo EA, Flynn MS, Aguirre FV. Clinical applications of the Doppler coronary flow velocity guidewire for interventional procedures. J Interven Cardiol 1993;6:345-363.

39.   Kern MJ, Aguirre FV, Bach RG, Caracciolo EA, Donohue TJ, Flynn MS, Moore JA.
        Alterations of coronary flow velocity distal to coronary dissections before and after
        intracoronary stent placement. Cathet Cardiovasc Diagn 1994;31:309-315.

40.   Kern MJ, Aguirre FV, Donohue TJ, Bach RG, Caracciolo EA, Flynn MS. Coronary
        flow velocity monitoring after angioplasty associated wtih abrupt reocclusion. Am Heart
        J 1994;127:436-438.

41.   Kern MJ, Flynn MS, Caracciolo EA, Bach RG, Donohue TJ, Aguirre FV. Use of
        translesional coronary flow velocity for interventional decisions in a patient with multiple
        intermediately severe coronary stenoses. Cathet Cardiovasc Diagn 1993;29:148-153.

7.

ANGIOGRAPHIC STENOSIS AND ACUTE CORONARY SYNDROMES: PROGRESSION OF STENOSES TO MYOCARDIAL INFARCTION

William C. Little, M.D.
Robert J. Applegate, M.D.
Section on Cardiology
Department of Internal Medicine
Bowman Gray School of Medicine
Wake Forest University
Winston-Salem, North Carolina 27157

INTRODUCTION

Coronary angiography is used to objectively define the presence, the extent and the severity of CAD. Because of the "need to know" coronary angiography is being increasingly performed with the first suspicion of CAD (Graboys et al., 1992). The coronary angiogram is evaluated for the presence of "significant" stenoses producing more than 50-70% diameter narrowing. These stenoses limit coronary flow, may produce symptomatic ischemia (angina), and can be targeted for "revascularization". The presence of a discreet stenosis is frequently interpreted to indicate the presence of a coronary artery "lesion" and has lead to the concept of coronary artery atherosclerosis as a focal disease. Bypass of coronary arteries containing "significant" stenoses or dilation of the stenoses with angioplasty (PTCA) can relieve angina (Parisi et al., 1992). Further, it is also appealing to consider that coronary artery "lesions" are potential sites for thrombotic occlusion that will produce subsequent cardiac events. It is hoped that dilating these "lesions" will lessen the risk of future events. Recent observations reviewed here calls these assumptions into question.

CORONARY ANGIOGRAPHY - LIMITATIONS IN DETECTION OF ATHEROSCLEROSIS

Coronary angiography provides information concerning the presence and severity of obstructive coronary disease by imaging a shadow of the arterial lumen. Frequently, coronary artery disease is apparent angiographically as focal areas of luminal narrowing. Thus, based on clinical interpretation of angiograms, coronary artery disease is perceived to be a focal process. However, pathologic examination and studies employing intraoperative epicardial or intravascular ultrasound indicate that coronary artery disease is usually diffuse rather than focal (Roberts and Jones, 1979), (Roberts and Jones, 1980), (Waller, 1989), (Vlodaver et al., 1973), (Downes et al., 1991), (Dietz et al., 1992), (Mintz et al., 1995). Early in the atherosclerotic process, the coronary lumen appears to be preserved by a compensatory dilation of the external arterial diameter as the arterial wall thickens (Glagov et al., 1987), (Stiel et al., 1989), (Dietz et al., 1992), (McPherson et al., 1991). Thus, there is usually a substantial amount of atherosclerosis in the wall of the coronary artery before there is any significant narrowing of the lumen.

The presence of even a single stenosis on coronary angiography is usually a marker of diffuse atherosclerotic involvement of the coronary arteries (Mintz et al., 1995). Consistent with this concept, the endothelial function may be abnormal, indicative of atherosclerotic involvement, in angiographically normal coronary artery segments in patients with stenoses in another coronary artery (Ludmer et al., 1986), and these sites have been found by intracoronary ultrasound imaging to contain atherosclerosis not apparent angiographically (Yamagishi et al., 1994). Additionally, intravascular ultrasound demonstrates significant atherosclerosis in patients whose coronary angiograms are normal or contain only minimal luminal narrowings (Porter et al., 1993), and substantial atherosclerosis in the walls of angiographically normal segments in patients with focal stenosis elsewhere (Gayle and Braden, 1994), (Mintz et al., 1995). Thus, coronary arteriography, by detecting reductions in luminal diameter, severely underestimates the overall extent of coronary atherosclerosis which is typically a diffuse process involving the arterial wall.

CORONARY ANGIOGRAPHY BEFORE MI

Myocardial infarction (MI) is usually caused by the sudden, thrombotic occlusion of a coronary artery at the site of a fissured atherosclerotic plaque (Gorlin et al., 1986), (DeWood et al., 1980), (Constantinidines, 1989), (Falk et al., 1995). Pathologic studies indicate that the underlying atherosclerotic plaque typically reduces the luminal cross-sectional area by 80-90% (Davies, 1989), (Falk, 1983). Furthermore, the presence of a high-grade stenosis (greater than 80% or 90% angiographic diameter narrowing) is an angiographic risk factor for subsequent occlusion of a coronary artery (Moise et al., 1984), (Ellis et al., 1988). Thus, stenotic sites identified by coronary angiograms are assumed to be at risk for thrombotic occlusion, while coronary arteries that do not contain obstructive stenoses (<50%) are considered to be nearly free of the risk of occlusion (Ellis et al., 1988).

However, a growing body of literature suggests that MI's frequently develop from "non-stenotic" coronary lesions (Little et al., 1991), (Applegate et al.,

1993). For example, we analyzed 58 patients who had undergone coronary angiography both before and after suffering an MI (Little *et al.,* 1988), (Little *et al.,* 1989). On the initial angiogram, taken before MI, the location of the most severe angiographic stenosis was the site of the subsequent occlusion producing MI in 38% of patients. In 35 (60%) of our patients, the most severe luminal diameter stenosis existing in the infarct-related artery prior to the MI was less than 50% (Figure 1). Thus, an angiographically severe coronary artery stenosis was infrequently present in the infarct-related artery on the initial angiogram, while the other arteries that did contain high-grade stenoses often remained patent.

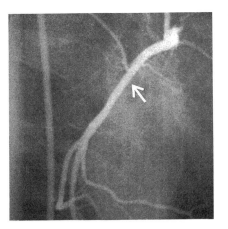 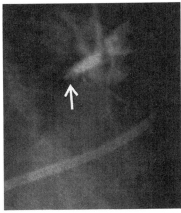

Before MI   After MI

Figure 1. A. Right coronary angiogram taken within one year of the development of acute myocardial infarction, demonstrating no stenotic areas in the right coronary artery. B. Coronary angiogram taken soon after onset of acute inferior myocardial infarction, demonstrating total obstruction of the proximal right coronary artery. From Little et al (1990)

Ambrose et al (1988) performed a analysis of 23 patients who had undergone serial coronary angiograms before and after suffering MI. Only 22% of the infarct-related arteries contained a greater than 75% diameter stenosis before MI. Similarly, Hacket et al (1989) and Giroud et al (1992) found that the overwhelming majority of patients with MI, the infarct artery contained less than 50% stenosis in an angiogram obtained prior to the MI, and that the most severely stenosed artery was the site of the subsequent occlusion in only one-third of patients. A prospective, serial angiographic study by Webster, et al (1990) at the Mayo Clinic also found that the majority of MI's occurred due to occlusion of arteries that previously contained less than a 50% stenosis. Similarly we observed that MI after coronary artery bypass surgery (CABG) or percutaneous transluminal coronary angioplasty (PTCA) frequently occurs due to occlusion of previously non-stenotic arteries (Little *et al.*, 1990), (Kerensky *et al.*, 1991). It appears that occlusion of arteries containing a preexisting severe stenosis may frequently be clinically silent presumably due to collateral formation (Webster *et al.*, 1990). These studies indicate that MI often arises from vessels that did not contain angiographically apparent stenoses, and that coronary angiography cannot adequately predict the site of a subsequent occlusion that will produce an MI.

Other investigators have reported similar findings. In a review of 313 patients who had undergone two coronary angiograms for any reason, Moise, et al (1984) found 116 newly occluded coronary vessels at the time of the second angiogram. Coronary artery segments that contained a stenosis were more likely to subsequently occlude than were segments free of stenotic lesions. However, the majority (72%) of the coronary occlusions in this study occurred in segments that were previously free of high-grade stenoses. Although stenotic segments may have a higher risk of occlusion, non-stenotic segments are not risk free and they are far more numerous (Little *et al.*, 1991).

Several lines of evidence, in addition to the serial angiographic data, indicate that MI can occur in the absence of severe atherosclerotic obstruction of the coronary lumen. First, in many patients, MI or sudden death is the initial manifestation of coronary artery disease (Alonzo *et al.*, 1975), (Turner *et al.*, 1989). The absence of exertional angina prior to the catastrophic event suggests that functionally obstructive atherosclerotic lesions may not have been present prior to the development of catastrophic coronary thrombosis. Second, serial angiographic observations in patients with unstable angina indicate that a thrombus overlying an atheroma abruptly had increased the severity of coronary artery obstruction without totally obstructing the artery (Ambrose *et al.*, 1985), (Wilson *et al.*, 1986), (Sherman *et al.*, 1986). Thus, the artery responsible for unstable ischemic syndromes frequently does not contain a high-grade stenosis prior to the onset of symptoms (Ambrose *et al.*, 1986), (Moise *et al.*, 1983). Third, after coronary flow is restored by thrombolytic therapy in patients with MI, only minor, non-stenotic lesions (<50% diameter narrowing) are present in some patients(Brown *et al.*, 1986), (Hacket *et al.*, 1989), (Serruys *et al.*, 1987), (Hacket *et al.*, 1988), (Serruys *et al.*, 1983). Finally, the highest stress in the fibrous cap overlying an atheroma, predisposing to plaque rupture and thrombus formation, occurs when the lumen is narrowed by only 40-50% (Richardson *et al.*, 1989), (Loree *et al.*, 1992).

COMPARISON WITH AUTOPSY AND NATURAL HISTORY STUDIES

The above evidence suggests that coronary angiography is relatively insensitive both in the early detection and quantitation of the extent of coronary atherosclerotic disease and that an angiographically apparent stenosis is not a prerequisite to the development of thrombus formation and

MI. How can these ideas be reconciled with: 1) the autopsy data that indicate that occlusive coronary artery thrombi frequently develop at the site of severe (80-90%) stenoses (Qiao and Fishbein, 1991), and 2) studies demonstrating that the prognosis of patients with stable angina is related to the number of angiographically stenosed coronary arteries (Mock *et al.,* 1982).

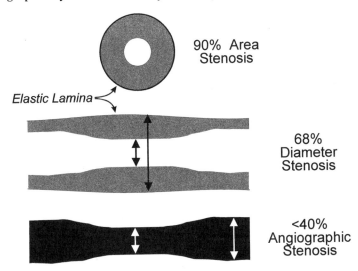

Figure 2. Illustration of the difference in the severity of stenosis quantitated as a percent area stenosis in pathologic studies and percent diameter stenosis determined angiographically. A 90% reduction in luminal cross-sectional area is equivalent to only a 68% reduction in diameter. In pathologic studies, the normal reference cross-sectional areas are defined by the internal elastic lamina. This landmark is not visible angiographically. Thus, the reference diameter is measured from an adjacent normal segment. Since coronary angiography underestimates the extent of coronary atherosclerosis, this normal segment may, in fact, be narrowed. Thus, a 90% area stenosis in an autopsy study may have produced a 40% or less diameter stenosis angiographically. Figure redrawn from Little et al 1989 (1989).

The pathologic and angiographic definition of stenosis severity differs in two ways. First, in pathologic studies, the severity of a stenosis is determined by the reduction in cross-sectional area, while angiographically the stenosis is usually quantitated as a reduction in diameter. A 68% reduction in diameter produces a 90% reduction in area. Thus, the angiographic method of quantifying stenosis severity systematically underestimates the severity as determined pathologically. The second difference is that pathologists assess the effects of atherosclerotic narrowing in the entire vessel including the wall of the artery, while angiographers examine only the effects of narrowing on the lumen of the vessel. The pathologist measures the area narrowing contained within the elastic lamina, while the angiographer quantifies the diameter narrowing of the lumen compared to an adjacent segment with a normal appearing lumen. This reference segment usually has atherosclerosis within the vessel wall (Braden and Downes, 1990). Since atherosclerosis is primarily a disease of the wall of the artery, substantially greater vessel narrowing will be observed than will be apparent by looking only at the lumen of the vessel. Because of these considerations, the culprit lesion in MI, quantitated as a 90% reduction in cross-sectional area in a pathologic study, may have been apparent only as a 40% or smaller diameter stenosis on an angiogram (Figure 2). Therefore, the observation that MI can occur in the absence of an angiographically apparent stenosis, and the autopsy data that suggest severely atherosclerotic vessels are not in conflict. Moreover, because of the limitations of coronary angiography in detecting the extent of atherosclerosis, the occlusion of an area of "angiographically insignificant" narrowing is actually thrombosis at a site of advanced atherosclerosis, albeit without narrowing of the lumen.

The prognosis of patients with stable angina is related both to the number of stenosed coronary arteries and the left ventricular ejection fraction (Mock *et al.*, 1982). However, patients with irregularities of the coronary artery walls, but without any angiographically significant stenosis (<50% diameter narrowing), have a substantially lower survival rate than patients with completely normal coronary arteries (Mock *et al.*, 1982). The impaired survival of patients with "insignificant" coronary artery disease is most likely due to the development of thrombotic coronary artery occlusion. Since patients with "insignificant" coronary artery disease usually have normal left ventricular ejection fractions, their survival should be compared to that of patients with "severe" coronary artery disease with similar left ventricular function (Epstein *et al.*, 1989). Interestingly, the survival curve of patients from the Coronary Artery Surgery Study (C.A.S.S.) registry with nonstenotic coronary artery disease is superimposable with the survival curve of patients with severe coronary artery disease with >70% diameter stenoses of all three arteries (i.e., three-vessel disease) and normal left ventricular function who were randomized to initial medical therapy in the C.A.S.S. trial (Figure 3) (Kemp *et al.*, 1986), (Alderman *et al.*, 1990), (Epstein *et al.*, 1989). This observation suggests that the presence of atherosclerosis in the coronary arterial wall, whether or not it significantly narrows the lumen, places a patient at increased risk for MI or death. It is unlikely that dilation of areas of severe coronary stenosis would make the survival of patients with CAD better than the survival of patients with angiographically "insignificant" coronary artery disease.

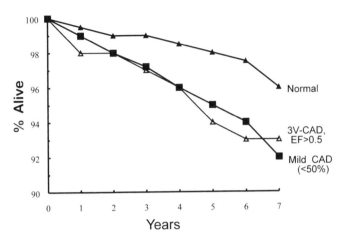

Figure 3. Diagram comparison of the survival of patients with normal coronary arteries (normal) and patients with mild coronary artery disease without any stenotic lesions (>50%) stenosis) from the CASS Registry, (Kemp *et al.*, 1986) and the survival of patients with severe three vessel coronary artery disease and normal left ventricular ejection fractions (3V-CAD, EF>0.5) (Alderman *et al.*, 1990). Note that the survival rate of patients with mild, angiographically insignificant coronary artery disease is superimposable upon the survival rate of patients with severe three vessel coronary artery disease. Figure redrawn from Little et al (1991).

ANGIOGRAPHIC PROGRESSION

As part of a clinical trial of nicardipine, coronary angiograms were performed two years apart in 335 patients (Waters *et al.*, 1990). The patients were then prospectively followed for a mean of 44±10 months after the second arteriogram. Progression of coronary artery disease was defined as a greater than 15% increase in stenosis severity at one or more sites. Much of the progression seen was relatively minor and previously would not have been considered clinically important. However, patients with progression were 7.3 times more likely to have cardiac death and 2.3 times as likely to have death or infarction during the subsequent follow-up. Although half of these patients, had been randomized to receive nicardipine during the two years between angiograms, it had no effect on progression or regression of established coronary atherosclerosis. Similar findings have also been reported from the placebo group of the Program on the Surgical Control of Hyperlipidemias (POSCH) Group (1992). In follow-up of the patients in this study, changes from a baseline angiogram, to one performed three years later, were strongly and significantly associated with subsequent overall and atherosclerotic coronary heart disease mortality. Thus, these prospective studies of the natural history of coronary artery disease, demonstrate that even minor progression of angiographic luminal narrowings is a strong predictor of future cardiac events (Applegate *et al.*, 1993).

Although it is now technically feasible to measure small changes in coronary lumen diameter (Detre *et al.*, 1975), (Sanmarco *et al.*, 1978) and the clinical studies of Waters et al (1993) and others (Buchwald *et al.*, 1992) suggest these changes are important, is it biologically plausible that the very small changes in coronary lumen dimensions seen in these serial angiography trials can lead to substantial alterations in the rate of subsequent events? Coronary angiography which images the coronary lumen severely underestimates the extent and severity of the coronary atherosclerosis present in the arterial wall. Since the initial response to coronary atherosclerosis is outward expansion, which preserves the lumen, as the wall thickens (Glagov *et al.*, 1987), even minor luminal irregularities on the coronary angiogram most likely indicate advanced atherosclerosis in the wall of the artery. All of the studies evaluating progression and/or regression of coronary artery disease have been performed in patients with angiographically demonstrable coronary artery disease. Thus, it should not be surprising that further small degrees of luminal encroachment may indicate active and advanced, although not occlusive, disease.

Q WAVE VERSUS NON-Q WAVE MI

Ambrose et al (1988) found that non-Q wave MI's were much more likely to result from the occlusion of a severely (>70%) stenotic artery than Q-wave MI's. In contrast, we found no difference in the distribution of the severity of the pre-existing stenosis in patients with Q and non-Q MI (Little *et al.*, 1989). Decanay et al (1994) in a similar study found that there are two populations of patients with non-Q MI's: patients with minimal pre-existing luminal narrowing and patients with severe pre-existing stenosis. Thus, it is clear that some non-Q MI's result from occlusion of arteries with severe pre-existing stenoses. It is likely that the stenoses stimulated the formation of collaterals that limited the extent of infarction. The lack of a severe pre-existing stenoses in patients with Q wave MI's did not provide a stimulus for protective collateral formation in these patients.

ANGIOGRAPHIC MORPHOLOGY

The endothelium of the plaque underlying the coronary thrombosis in patients with MI or unstable angina has been disrupted, exposing the thrombogenic components of the plaque to the blood stream. The fissured plaque with overlying thrombus may be angiographically apparent as a convex, intraluminal obstruction with overhanging edges, irregularities, and/or intraluminal defects (Ambrose *et al.*, 1986), (Nakagawa *et al.*, 1988). The culprit lesions frequently exhibit these angiographic characteristics after the development of MI or unstable angina (Nakagawa *et al.*, 1988), (Ambrose, 1989). The more complex the morphology of the culprit stenoses responsible for an unstable syndrome, the more likely there will be further progression (Davies *et al.*, 1991), (Chen *et al.*, 1995). It is possible that stenoses with these characteristics in patients without MI or angina may have a higher risk of subsequent occlusion (Ambrose, 1991), especially an occlusion that will produce a Q wave MI (Dacanay *et al.*, 1994). In the majority of patients before MI, the culprit plaque does not usually appear complex on angiograms performed prior to MI (Nierste and Little, 1989), (Haft and Al-Zarka, 1991). Similarly, the angiographic morphology of the culprit lesion after thrombolytic therapy does not predict subsequent reocclusion (Ellis *et al.*, 1989).

The "roughness" or degree of irregularities in the wall of the coronary artery on angiograms may indicate plaques that are at risk for rupturing. For example, prior to MI, the future infarct site may produce only minor wall irregularities or a scalloped area (Nierste and Little, 1989). Similarly, analysis of patients in the C.A.S.S. study with left anterior descending lesions suggested that lesion roughness was a predictor of subsequent occlusion (Ellis *et al.*, 1989). In contrast, Taeymans et al (1992) did not find that irregular lesion contours influenced the risk of subsequent occlusion. The extent of the angiographically apparent atherosclerosis appears to be another risk factor for subsequent occlusion (Moise *et al.*, 1988), (Mancini *et al.*, 1992).

CLINICAL IMPLICATIONS

An angiographically obstructive stenosis indicates the presence of coronary atherosclerosis and the potential for development of MI, but the coronary stenosis does not necessarily indicate the location at which the thrombotic occlusion will occur (Little *et al.*, 1988), (Little, 1990). The presence of high grade stenosis is a marker for advanced atherosclerotic coronary artery disease. It is important to recognize that localized areas of angiographic stenosis underestimate the extent of atherosclerotic involvement of the coronary arteries. In the patients whose angiogram demonstrates only non-obstructive atherosclerosis, the possibility of the future occurrence of MI cannot be ruled out, since potentially thrombogenic plaques need not be obstructive.

CABG and PTCA are appropriately directed only at the angiographically significant (i.e. stenotic or flow limiting) stenosis. Since it is difficult to predict the site of the subsequent occlusion from a coronary angiogram, these interventions may not be effective in preventing many subsequent MI's. This does not indicate that coronary arteries that do not have obstructive lesions should be dilated (Ischinger *et al.*, 1983). Instead, effective therapy to prevent MI may need to be directed at the entire coronary tree, and not just at obstructive lesions. Although mechanical treatment of high-grade coronary stenoses relieves angina and improves exercise tolerance, slowing or reversing the progression of atherosclerosis in the walls of the coronary arteries may be a more powerful intervention to prevent the catastrophic complications of coronary artery disease (unstable angina, MI, and death).

Coronary atherosclerosis is a disease of the arterial wall. The initial response to this disease process is a compensatory enlargement that preserves the lumen while potential thrombogenic plaques are developing in the wall of the artery. Thus, imaging the lumen with coronary angiography is an inaccurate means of quantitating the extent of coronary disease, and provides inadequate information to predict the site of a subsequent occlusion that will produce myocardial infarction. Restoration of a normal lumen by dilating (or even removing) a focal stenosis, does not indicate that the coronary atherosclerosis has been "fixed".

REFERENCES

ALDERMAN, E. L., BOURASSA, M. G., COHEN, L. S., DAVIS, K. B., KAISER, G. G., KILLIP, T., MOCK, M. B., PETTINGER, M., ROBERTSON, T. L. AND FOR THE CASS INVESTIGATORS: Ten-year follow-up of survival and myocardial infarction in the randomized coronary artery surgery study. Circulation 82: 1629-1646, 1990.

ALONZO, A. A., SIMON, A. B. AND FEINLEIB, M. Prodromata of myocardial infarction and sudden death. Circulation 52: 1056-1062, 1975.

AMBROSE, J. A., WINTERS, S. L., ARORA, R. R., HAFT, J. I., GOLDSTEIN, J., RENTROP, K. P., GORLIN, R. AND FUSTER, V. Coronary angiographic morphology in myocardial infarction: A link between the pathogenesis of unstable angina and myocardial infarction. J Am Coll Cardiol 6: 1233-1238, 1985.

AMBROSE, J. A., WINTERS, S. L., ARORA, R. R., ENG, A., RICCIO, A., GORLIN, R. AND FUSTER, V. Angiographic evolution of coronary artery morphology in unstable angina. J Am Coll Cardiol 7: 472-478, 1986.

AMBROSE, J. A., TANNENBAUM, M. A., ALEXOPOULOS, D., HJEMDAHL-MONSEN, C. E., LEAVY, J., WEISS, M., BORRICO, S., GORLIN, R. AND FUSTER, V. Angiographic progression of coronary artery disease and the development of myocardial infarction. J Am Coll Cardiol 12: 56-62, 1988.

AMBROSE, J. A. Coronary arteriographic analysis and angiographic morphology. J Am Coll Cardiol 13: 14921989.

AMBROSE, J. A. Prognostic implications of lesion irregularity on coronary angiography. JACC 18: 675-676, 1991.

APPLEGATE, R. J., HERRINGTON, D. M. AND LITTLE, W. C. Coronary Angiography: More than meets the eye. Circulation 87(4): 1399-1401, 1993.

BRADEN, G. A. AND DOWNES, T. R. Intravascular ultrasound detection of coronary artery "disease" rather than "lumens". Clin Res 38: 963, 1990.(Abstract)

BROWN, B. G., GALLERY, C. A., BADGER, R. S., KENNEDY, J. W., MATHEY, D., BOLSON, E. L. AND DODGE, H. T. Incomplete lysis of thrombus in the moderate underlying atherosclerotic lesion during intracoronary infusion of streptokinase for acute myocardial infarction: Quantitative angiographic observations. Circulation 73: 653-661, 1986.

BUCHWALD, H., MATTS, J. P., FITCH, L. L., CAMPOS, C. T., SANMARCO, M. E., AMPLATZ, K., CASTANEDA-ZUNIGA, W. R., HUNTER, D. W., PEARCE, M. B., BISSETT, J. K., EDMINSTON, W. A., SAWIN, H. S., WEBER, F. J., VARCO, R. L., CAMPBELL, G. S., YELLIN, A. E., SMINK, R. D., LONG, J. M., HANSEN, B. J., CHALMERS, T. C., MEIER, P., STAMLER, J. AND FOR THE SURGICAL CONTROL OF THE HYPERLIPIDEMIAS (POSCH) GROUP: Changes in sequential coronary anteriograms and subsequent coronary events. JAMA 268: 1429-1433, 1992.

CHEN, L., CHESTER, M. R., REDWOOD, S., HUANG, J., LEATHAM, E. AND KASKI, J. C. Angiographic stenosis progression and coronary events in patients with 'stabilized' unstable angina. Circulation 91: 2319-2324, 1995.

CONSTANTINIDINES, P. Plaque hemorrhages, their genesis, and their role in supra-plaque thrombosis and atherogenesis. In Pathobiology of the Human Atherosclerotic Plaque, ed. by S. Glagov, W. P. Newman and S. A. Schaeffer, pp. 393, Springer-Verlag, New York, 1989.

DACANAY, S., KENNEDY, H. L., URETZ, E., PARRILLO, J. E. AND KLEIN, L. W. Morphological and quantitative angiographic analyses of progression of coronary stenoses: A comparison of Q-wave and non-Q-wave myocardial infarction. Circulation 90: 1739-1746, 1994.

172

DAVIES, M. J. Successful and unsuccessful coronary thrombolysis. Br Heart J 61: 381-384, 1989.

DAVIES, S. W., MARCHANT, B., LYONS, J. P., TIMMIS, A. D., ROTHMAN, M. T., LAYTON, C. A. AND BALCON, R. Irregular coronary lesion morphology after thrombolysis predicts early clinical instability. J Am Coll Cardiol 18: 669-674, 1991.

DETRE, K. M., WRIGHT, E., MURPHY, M. L. AND TAKARO, T. Observer agreement in evaluating coronary angiograms. Circulation 52: 979-986, 1975.

DEWOOD, A., SPORES, J., NOTSKE, R., MOUSER, L. T., BURROUGHS, R., GOLDEN, M. S. AND LANG, H. Prevalence of total coronary occlusion during the early hours of transmural myocardial infarction. N Engl J Med 303: 897-902, 1980.

DIETZ, W. A., TOBIS, J. M. AND ISNER, J. M. Failure of angiography to accurately depict the extent of coronary artery narrowing in three fatal cases of percutaneous transluminal coronary angioplasty. J Am Coll Cardiol 19: 1261-1270, 1992.

DOWNES, T. R., BRADEN, G. A., HERRINGTON, D. M., APPLEGATE, R. J., KUTCHER, M. A. AND LITTLE, W. C. Mechanism of PTCA dilatation in coronary vessels: Intravascular ultrasound assessment. J Am Coll Cardiol 17: 126A, 1991.(Abstract)

ELLIS, S., ALDERMAN, E., CAIN, K., FISHER, L., SANDERS, W., BOURASSA, M. AND THE CASS INVESTIGATORS: Prediction of risk of anterior myocardial infarction by lesion severity and measurement method of stenoses in the left anterior descending coronary distribution: A CASS Registry Study. J Am Coll Cardiol 11: 908-916, 1988.

ELLIS, S., ALDERMAN, E. L., CAIN, K., WRIGHT, A., BOURASSA, M. AND FISHER, L. Morphology of left anterior descending coronary territory lesions as a predictor of anterior myocardial infarction: A CASS registry study. J Am Coll Cardiol 13: 1481-1491, 1989.

ELLIS, S. G., TOPOL, E. J., GEORGE, B. S., KEREIAKES, D. J., DEBOWEY, D., KRISTINA, N., SIGMON, N., PICKEL, A., LEE, K. L. AND CALIFF, R. M. Recurrent ischemia without warning. Analysis of risk factors for in-hospital ischemic events following successful thrombolysis with intravenous issue plasminogen activator. Circulation 80: 1159-1165, 1989.

EPSTEIN, S. E., QUYYUMI, A. A. AND BONOW, R. O. Sudden cardiac death without warning. N Engl J Med 321: 320-324, 1989.

FALK, E. Plaque rupture with severe pre-existing stenosis precipitating coronary thrombosis. Br Heart J 50: 127-134, 1983.

FALK, E., SHAH, P. K. AND FUSTER, V. Coronary Plaque Disruption. Circulation 92: 657-671, 1995.

GAYLE, D. D. AND BRADEN, G. A. Lack of compensatory enlargement in coronary atherosclerosis is responsible for severe stenoses: An in-vivo intracoronary ultrasound study. Clin Res 41(4): 720A, 1994.(Abstract)

GIROUD, D., LI, J. M., URBAN, P., MEIER, B. AND RUTISHAUSER, W. Relation of the site of acute myocardial infarction to the most severe coronary arterial stenosis at prior angiography. Am J Cardiol 69: 729-732, 1992.

GLAGOV, S., WEISENBERG, E., ZASINS, C. K., STANKUNAVICIUS, R. AND KOLETTIS, G. J. Compensatory enlargement of human atherosclerotic coronary arteries. E Engl J Med 316: 11371-11375, 1987.

GORLIN, R., FUSTER, V. AND AMBROSE, J. A. Anatomic physiologic links between acute coronary syndromes. Circulation 74: 6-9, 1986.

GRABOYS, T. B., BIEGELSEN, B., LAMPERT, S., BLATT, C. M. AND LOWN, B. Results of a second-opinion trial among patients recommended for coronary angiography. J Am Med Assoc **268(18)**: 2537-2540, 1992.

HACKET, D., DAVIES, G. AND MASERI, A. Pre-existing coronary stenoses in patients with first myocardial infarction are not necessarily severe. Eur Heart J **9**: 1317-1323, 1988.

HACKET, D., VERWILGHEN, J., DAVIES, G. AND MASERI, A. Coronary stenoses before and after acute myocardial infarction. Am J Cardiol **63**: 1517-1518, 1989.

HAFT, J. I. AND AL-ZARKA, A. M. The origin and fate of complex coronary lesions. Am Heart J **121**: 1050-1061, 1991.

ISCHINGER, T., GRUENTZIG, A. R., HOLLMAN, J., KING, J., DOUGLAS, J., MEIER, B., BRADFORD, J. AND TANKERSLEY, R. Should coronary arteries with less than 60% diameter stenosis be treated by angioplasty? Circulation **68**: 148-154, 1983.

KEMP, H. G., KRONMAL, R. A., VLIETSTRA, R. E., FRYE, R. I. AND & PARTICIPANTS IN THE CORONARY ARTERY SURGERY STUDY: Seven year survival of patients with normal or near normal coronary arteriograms: A CASS registry study. J Am Coll Cardiol **7**: 479-483, 1986.

KERENSKY, R. A., KUTCHER, M. A., MUMMA, M., APPLEGATE, R. AND LITTLE, W. C. Myocardial infarction late after successful PTCA: Progression of disease versus reoccurrence. J Am Coll Cardiol **17**: 304A, 1991.(Abstract)

LITTLE, W. C., CONSTANTINESCU, M., APPLEGATE, R. J., KUTCHER, M. A., BURROWS, M. T., KAHL, F. R. AND SANTAMORE, W. P. Can coronary angiography predict the site of a subsequent myocardial infarction in patients with mild to moderate coronary artery disease? Circulation **78**: 1157-1166, 1988.

LITTLE, W. C., WORKMAN, R., BURROWS, M., KAHL, F. R., KUTCHER, M. A., SANTAMORE, W. P. AND APPLEGATE, R. Coronary anatomy preceding non-Q wave myocardial infarction. J Am Coll Cardiol **13**: 6A, 1989.(Abstract)

LITTLE, W. C. Angiographic assessment of the culprit coronary artery lesion before acute myocardial infarction. Am J Cardiol **66**: 44G-47G, 1990.

LITTLE, W. C., GWINN, N. S., BURROWS, M. T., KUTCHER, M. A., KAHL, F. R. AND APPLEGATE, R. J. Cause of acute myocardial infarction late after successful coronary artery bypass grafting. Am J Cardiol **65**: 808-810, 1990.

LITTLE, W. C., DOWNES, T. R. AND APPLEGATE, R. J. The underlying coronary lesion in myocardial infarction: Implications for coronary angiography. Clin Cardiol **14**: 868-874, 1991.

LOREE, H. M., KAMM, R. D., STRINGFELLOW, R. G. AND LEE, R. T. Effects of fibrous cap thickness on peak circumferential stress in model atherosclerotic vessels. Circ Res **71**: 850-858, 1992.

LUDMER, P. L., SELWYN, A. P., SHOOK, T. L., WAYNE, R. R., MUDGE, G. H., ALEXANDER, R. W. AND GANZ, P. Paradoxical vasoconstriction induced by acetylcholine in atherosclerotic coronary arteries. N Engl J Med **315**: 1046-1051, 1986.

MANCINI, G. B. J., BOURASSA, M. G., WILLIAMSON, P. R., LECLERC, G., DEBOE, S. F., PITT, B. AND LESPERANCE, J. Prognostic importance of quantitative analysis of coronary cineangiograms. Am J Cardiol **69**: 1022-1027, 1992.

MCPHERSON, D. D., SIRNA, S. J., HIRATZKA, L. F., THORPE, L., ARMSTRONG, M. L., MARCUS, M. L. AND KERBER, R. E. Coronary arterial remodeling studied by high-frequency epicardial echocardiography: An early compensatory mechanism in patients with obstructive coronary atherosclerosis. J Am Coll Cardiol **17**: 79-86, 1991.

174

MINTZ, G. S., PAINTER, J. A., PICHARD, A. D., KENT, K. M., SATLER, L. F., POPMA, J. J., CHUANG, Y. C., BUCHER, T. A., SOKOLOWICZ, L. E. AND LEON, M. B. Atherosclerosis in angiographically "normal" coronary artery reference segments: An intravascular ultrasound study with clinical correlations. J Am Coll Cardiol **25**: 1479-1485, 1995.

MOCK, M. B., RINGQVIST, I., FISHER, L. D., DAVIS, K. B., CHAITMAN, B. R., KOUCHOUKOS, N. T., KAISER, G. C., ALDERMAN, E., RYAN, T. J., RUSSELL, R. O., MULLIN, S., FRAY, D., KILLIP III, T. AND & PARTICIPANTS IN THE CASS STUDY: Survival of medically treated patients in the coronary artery surgery study (CASS) registry. Circulation **66**: 5621982.

MOISE, A., THEROUX, P., TAYEMANS, Y., DESCOINGS, B., LESPARANCE, J., WATERS, D. D., PELLETIER, G. B. AND BOURASSA, M. G. Unstable angina and progression of coronary atherosclerosis. N Engl J Med **309**: 685-690, 1983.

MOISE, A., LESPERANCE, J., THEROUS, P., TAYEMANS, Y., GOULET, C. AND BOURASSA, M. G. Clinical and angiographic predictors of new total coronary occlusion in coronary artery disease: Analysis of 313 nonoperated patients. Am J Cardiol**54**: 1176-1181, 1984.

MOISE, A., CLEMENT, B. AND SALTIEL, J. Clinical and angiographic correlates and prognostic significance of the coronary extent score. Am J Cardiol **61**: 1255-1259, 1988.

NAKAGAWA, S., HANADA, Y., KOIWAYA, Y. AND TANAKA, K. Angiographic features in the infarct-related artery after intracoronary urokinase followed by prolonged anticoagulation. Circulation **88**: 1335-1344, 1988.

NIERSTE, D. AND LITTLE, W. C. Morphology of the culprit coronary artery lesion preceding myocardial infarction. Circulation **80**: II-349, 1989.(Abstract)

PARISI, A. F., FOLLAND, E. D. AND HARTIGAN, P. A comparison of angioplasty with medical therapy in the treatment of single vessel coronary artery disease. N Engl J Med**326**: 10-16, 1992.

PORTER, T. R., SEARS, T., FENG, X., MICHELS, A., WELSH, D. AND SHUMER, S. Intravascular ultrasound study of angiographically mildly diseased coronary arteries. J Am Coll Cardiol **22**: 1858-1865, 1993.

QIAO, J. H. AND FISHBEIN, M. C. The severity of coronary atherosclerosis at sites of plaque rupture with occlusive thrombosis. J Am Coll Cardiol **17**: 1138-1142, 1991.

RICHARDSON, P. D., DAVIES, M. J. AND BORN, G. V. R. Influence of plaque configuration and stress distribution on fissuring of coronary atherosclerotic plaques. Lancet**2**: 941-944, 1989.

ROBERTS, W. C. AND JONES, A. A. Quantitation of coronary arterial narrowing at necropsy in sudden coronary death: Analysis of 31 patients and comparison with 25 control subjects. Am J Cardiol **44**: 39-45, 1979.

ROBERTS, W. C. AND JONES, A. A. Quantification of coronary arterial narrowing at necropsy in acute myocardial infarction: Analysis and comparison of findings in 27 patients and 22 control subjects. Circulation **61**: 786-790, 1980.

SANMARCO, M. J., BROOKS, S. H. AND BLANKENHORN, D. H. Reproducibility of a consensus panel in the interpretation of coronary angiograms. Am Heart J **96**: 430-437, 1978.

SERRUYS, P. W., WIJNS, W., VAN DEN BRAND, M., RIBEIRO, V., FIORETTI, P., SIMOONS, M. L., KOOIJMAN, C. J., REIBER, J. H. AND HUGENHOLTZ, P. G. Is transluminal coronary angioplasty mandatory after successful thrombolysis? Br Heart J**50**: 257-265, 1983.

SERRUYS, P. W., ARNOLD, A. E. R., BROWER, R. W., DE BONO, D. P., BOKSLAD, M., LUBSEN, J., REIBER, J. H., RUTSCH, W. R., UEBIS, R., VAHANIAN, A., VERSRAETE, M. AND FOR THE EUROPEAN CO-OPERATIVE STUDY GROUP FOR RECOMBINANT TISSUE-TYPE PLASMINOGEN ACTIVATOR: Effect of continued rt-PA administration on the residual stenosis after initially successful recanalization in acute myocardial infarction: A quantitative coronary angiography study of a randomized trial. Eur Heart J 8: 1172-1181, 1987.

SHERMAN, C. T., LITVACK, F., GRUNDFEST, W., LEE, M., HICKEY, A., CHAUX, A., KASS, R., BLANCHE, C., MATLOFF, J., MORGENSTERN, L., GANZ, W., SAWN, H. J. C. AND FORRESTER, J. Coronary angioscopy in patients with unstable angina pectoris. N Engl J Med 315: 913-919, 1986.

STIEL, G. M., LUDMILL, L. S. G., SCHOFER, J., DONATH, K. AND MATHEY, D. G. Impact of compensatory enlargement of atherosclerotic coronary arteries on angiographic assessment of coronary artery disease. Circulation 80: 1603-1609, 1989.

TAEYMANS, Y., THEROUX, P., LESPERANCE, J. AND WATERS, D. Quantitative angiographic morphology of the coronary artery lesions at risk of thrombotic occlusion. Circulation 85: 78-85, 1992.

TURNER, S. A., RUFTY, A. J., HACKSHAW, B. T., APPLEGATE, R. AND LITTLE, W. C. Myocardial infarction as the presenting manifestation of coronary artery disease. Clin Res 37: 303A, 1989.(Abstract)

VLODAVER, Z., FRECH, R., VAN TASSEL, R. A. AND EDWARDS, J. E. Correlation of the antemortem coronary arteriogram and the postmortem specimen. Circulation 47: 162-169, 1973.

WALLER, B. F. The eccentric coronary atherosclerotic plaque: Morphologic observations and clinical relevance. Clin Cardiol 12: 14-20, 1989.

WATERS, D., LESPERANCE, J., FRANCETICH, M., CAUSEY, D., THEROUX, P., CHIANG, Y. K., HUDON, G., LEMARBRE, L., REITMAN, M., JOYAL, M., GOSSELIN, G., KYRDA, I., MACER, J. AND HAVEL, R. J. A controlled clinical trial to assess the effect of a calcium channel blocker on the progression of coronary atherosclerosis. Circulation 82: 1940-1953, 1990.

WATERS, D., CRAVEN, T. E. AND LESPERANCE, J. Prognostic significance of progression of coronary atherosclerosis. Circulation 87: 1067-1075, 1993.

WEBSTER, M., CHESEBRO, J. H., SMITH, H. C., FRYE, R. L., HOLMES, D. R., REEDER, G. S., BRESNAHAN, D. R., NISHIMURA, R. A., CLEMENTS, I. P., BARDSLEY, W. T., GRILL, D. E., BAILEY, K. R. AND FUSTER, V. Myocardial infarction and coronary artery occlusion: A prospective 5-year angiographic study. J Am Coll Cardiol 15: 218A, 1990.(Abstract)

WILSON, R. F., HOLIDA, M. D. AND WHITE, C. W. Quantitative angiographic morphology of coronary stenoses leading to myocardial infarction or unstable angina. Circulation 73: 286-293, 1986.

YAMAGISHI, M., MIYATAKE, K., TAMAI, J., NAKATANI, S., KOYAMA, J. AND NISSEN, S. E. Intravascular ultrasound detection of atherosclerosis at the site of focal vasospasm in angiographically normal or minimally narrowed coronary segments. J Am Coll Cardiol 23: 352-357, 1994.

8.

UNSTABLE ANGINA AND NON-Q WAVE MYOCARDIAL INFARCTION: PATHOGENETIC MECHANISMS AND MORPHOLOGY OF THE UNSTABLE PLAQUE

Lloyd W. Klein, M.D.
Rush-Presbyterian-St. Luke's Medical Center and
The Rush Heart Institute, Chicago, Illinois

Introduction

The acute coronary syndromes, which include unstable angina, non Q wave (NQMI), and Q wave myocardial infarction, constitute the most frequent clinical manifestations of the major disease process observed in clinical cardiology. Unstable angina and NQMI are clinically distinct syndromes of acute ischemia implying the presence of further jeopardized myocardium. Indeed, regardless of whether a small degree of myocardial necrosis has occurred (as measured by the release of creatine kinase and MB isoenzyme in the blood), both diagnoses have in common the likely potential for recurrent angina and infarct extension. Hence, these entities uniquely suggest the possibility of further hazard, rather than the necessity of accepting and managing the consequences of loss of function. The appropriate diagnostic and therapeutic approaches are governed by these characteristics[1-5].

Only during the last 15 years has coronary angiography been routinely performed in acutely unstable patients[6,7]. This has led to the subsequent development of new insights into pathogenesis[8,9]. In addition, advanced imaging modalities have been applied, permitting the direct visualization of coronary stenoses in living patients[10]. For the first time, acute events can be observed as they occur, facilitating the development of sophisticated hypotheses about their causes[11-13]. The angiographic appearance of lesions prone to cause

178

acute ischemic syndromes has been identified[14-17] and supplemented with observations made with intravascular ultrasound[18] and angioscopy[19,20], providing a complete description of the morphology and composition of the unstable
plaque and superimposed thrombus[21-25].

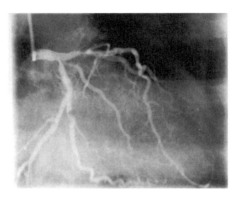

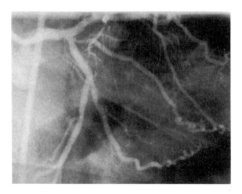

Figure 1. (top panel) A classic Ambrose eccentric type II lesion seen in the left
circumflex coronary artery in a patient with IHSS and accelerating angina.
This appearance suggests an ulcerated plaque.

(bottom panel) Following directional laser and balloon angioplasty,
no residual lesion is seen. Two years later, the patient remains asymptomatic.

Pathogenesis: Progression of Moderate Coronary Stenoses

The widespread performance of coronary angiography during acute events led to the alteration of many long held assumptions about coronary stenosis behavior and appearance. Coronary angiography performed soon after thrombolytic therapy is given for evolving ST segment elevation myocardial infarction reveals that the underlying stenosis, although irregular and ulcerated, is not usually severe[26,27]. Indeed, a 70% diameter narrowing or less is observed in 20 - 30% of cases post thrombolytic therapy, and the large majority are <90% stenoses. Nearly every angiographer active in the days of routine intracoronary streptokinase treatment for myocardial infarction has had the observation of at least one or two cases in which no angiographically evident stenosis at all was present [26]. Ambrose[15] reported that 78% of segments later the site of QMI had a <70% stenosis on angiography prior to the infarct, and 30% of segments were angiographically normal.

As discussed in the previous chapter, Little and colleagues[29] reported 42 patients undergoing angiography prior to Q wave myocardial infarction followed by repeat angiography within one month. A newly occluded artery was observed in 29 patients, 19 of these occurred at sites with ≤50% luminal diameter reduction on the first angiogram. With one exception, the remainder occurred at sites with ≤70% luminal diameter reduction. In only 34% did the occlusion occur in the artery that previously contained the most severe stenosis, which means that progression to occlusion is basically random in occurrence. It is impossible to overstate the importance this study has had in influencing thought about myocardial infarction. The basis of modern clinical practice lies in the assumption that the more severe the stenosis, the more likely that lesion is to produce a cardiac event. Consider the logic behind coronary bypass surgery or coronary angioplasty, for example: in bypass surgery, one places a conduit connecting flow from a non-obstructed zone to an area distal to a severe blockage; in angioplasty, one directly increases the luminal diameter at the site of the tightest blockage. Yet while these procedures clearly reduce chest pain and objective evidence of myocardial ischemia, neither has ever been shown to reduce the long-term incidence of sudden death, acute infarction or unstable angina. This conflicts with the hypothesis that severe stenoses lead inevitably to cardiac events, but is quite consistent with the acute progression of moderate lesions.

In fact, this is only one piece of evidence suggesting a dissociation between stenosis severity and coronary events[30]. Consider the various atherosclerosis regression trials in which lipid lowering regimens consistently reduce clinical events, but have disappointingly minimal effects on established lesions. For example, Brown et al[31] presented evidence that lipid lowering in patients with known coronary disease decreases acute coronary events despite minimal reduction in the severity of coronary stenosis. The Posch Trial[32] showed similar outcomes, which we pointed out[33] could be explainable by several pathophysiologic pathways.

Studies like these show that angiographically severe coronary disease merely represents a marker for the likelihood of non-critical plaques to be prone to acute ulceration and coronary thrombosis, rather than predicting the site. Indeed, it appears that the less severely stenosed segments may be more prone to disruption and subsequent thrombotic occlusion[29,34].

Moise et al[35] reported a somewhat different finding that further explicates this matter. They found that both the extent of coronary disease and the severity of the most severely stenotic lesion were predictive of future progression. The more severely stenotic vessel occluded somewhat more frequently, usually without clinical consequences, whereas occlusion of less severe stenoses led to acute infarction or unstable angina. In part, this is the result of myocardial protection by collaterals; ischemic preconditioning may also play a role. However, the clear indication and direction of these findings is that clinicians have been attentive to the wrong lesions. The most severe lesions produce symptoms - but not necessarily heart attacks!

Thrombosis and Vasospasm - Causes of Rapid Progression

The pattern of plaque progression is not linear over time, but rather is occasionally rapid at times and slow at other times[8,9]. Rapid progression is produced by thrombus formation, while slow progression is accompanied by lipid deposition within the arterial wall.

How and why do some moderate stenoses progress rapidly[36]? Certain plaques are prone to ulceration, damaging the overlying endothelium. This exposes the collagen and other procoagulant material within the atheroma (see below) to the circulating blood, including platelets and hemostatic factors. This leads to acute thrombus formation and increased vascular tone[37].

The precise sequence of events causing a previously stable atherosclerotic plaque to rupture, fissure or ulcerate remains unclear, but the etiology of plaque disruption includes: (1) vasospasm, (2) stress fracture of the plaque due to increased wall stress, (3) injury to coronary arterial vaso-vasorum, resulting in intramural hemorrhage and (4) platelet aggregation with release of thromboxanes and other vasoactive substances. A combination of all or some or these processes may be operative, either sequentially or simultaneously, in an individual patient[38].

182

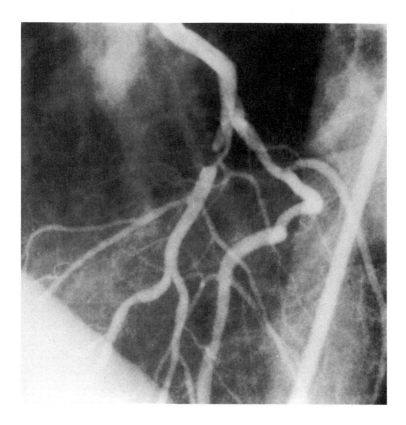

Figure 2. An unusually vivid eccentric lesion with smooth luminal contour but scalloped edges. This appearance is said to represent intraplaque hemorrhage. This patient presented with rest angina, and chose single vessel internal mammary artery bypass surgery.

The progression of early atherosclerotic plaques to clinically manifest, flow limiting stenosis causing exertional angina clearly is a separate pathway of growth. This process is accelerated in people with risk factors, but in all cases is a process initiated by chronic endothelial damage. Activated platelets are known to provide cholesterol for esterification by evolving foam cells, and there are observations of thrombophagocytosis by macrophages. Fibrin deposited in the vessel wall also promotes atheroma growth. Coronary mural thrombi and its subsequent fibrotic organization may cause episodes of rapid plaque growth followed by long dormant periods. This is consistent with pathologic studies showing a morphology suggesting numerous previously healed fissures with various stages of thrombus and its organization: the plaques appear to be composed of layers of thrombus overlying fissured plaques[9]. Thus, thrombotic events are also a critical element in the formation of atheroma.

Platelet aggregates in the environment of a severe coronary stenosis abets thrombus formation and propagation. The turbulent flow and regions of stasis produced are capable of activating the platelet release reaction. When platelet aggregates develop beyond critical stenoses, a periodic, cyclic reduction in coronary blood flow follows. These are associated with elevated levels of thromboxane B2, a stable metabolite of thromboxane A2. Leukocytes may also participate in the genesis of acute thrombosis via release of leukotrienes and/or superoxides. Granulocyte and monocyte adhesion receptors are also increased. Such substances are also vasoactive, and thus may initiate or contribute to vasospasm. A potential for a spiral between vasospasm and thrombosis caused by these humoral factors is thus created[38].

Coronary vasospasm clearly plays an important role in the genesis of coronary thrombosis. The presence of smooth muscle contraction bands have been identified in the medial layer of coronary arteries in patients with fatal MI. Angiographic studies of patients who developed acute MI during coronary angiography also document the role of vasospasm. Arterial vasospasm also likely is an important element in plaque rupture.

Stenosis Severity, Thrombus Burden and Time Course

DeWood and colleagues, in two classic studies, performed coronary angiography in the early hours after Q wave[6] and NQMI[7]. In the latter study, 341 patients with NQMI were studied within 1 week after acute presentation. The patients were subdivided into 3 groups: 192 patients who underwent angiography within 24 hours of peak symptoms, 94 patients evaluated within a 24-72 hour period, and a third group of 55 patients studied 3-7 days after peak symptoms. In contrast to the QMI study, in which the infarct related artery was totally occluded in the first 24 hours, only 26% of the comparable NQMI group had total occlusions. Additionally, while the trend in QMI patients suggested that the infarct artery was more likely to be patent over time, the opposite was seen with NQMI: 37% of the second group and 42% of the third group had total occlusions (p <.05). Importantly, stenoses of 90% - 99% were observed in 34% of group 1, 26% of group 2 and 18% of group 3 (p <.05); whereas stenoses of 70 -90% were distributed equally among the three groups. Also, collaterals were present in 85% of NQMI patients with total occlusions; this was much less common in the QMI patients. Finally, in contrast to the prevalence of angiographically evident thrombus in QMI, NQMI only occasionally demonstrated intraluminal filling defects. When present, these were not usually associated with total occlusion.

Consequently, the patient with NQMI is less likely to have a totally occlusive thrombus, but more likely to have a high grade stenosis in the infarct related vessel than QMI patients. This indicates that NQMI represents a severe imbalance between supply and demand in the presence of a patent but severely narrowed coronary artery. This situation may produce just severe enough blood flow reduction to cause necrosis of a limited extent of myocardium.

The severity of the underlying stenosis in the setting of acute myocardial infarction can not be appreciated until the occluding thrombus has completely resolved. Brown et al[39] used magnified angiograms and computerized quantitative measurements to distinguish the coronary atheroma from the underlying thrombus in 33 patients treated with intravenous streptokinase. In this report, the average atherosclerotic lesion was only 56% stenosis. In the TIMI IIA trial, patients underwent angiography within 90 minutes after receiving t-PA and again at the time of hospital discharge. Between the time of initial thrombolysis and follow-up angiography, there was a reduction in the degree of narrowing from a mean of 80.5% to 34%. In the majority of patients the final lumen was less than 50% narrowed[40].

Many retrospective studies have shown that the "culprit lesion" responsible for coronary occlusion in patients with acute MI characterized by ST segment elevation is not necessarily as severe as would be suggested by coronary angiography performed in the immediate post-reperfusion phase. Giroud et al[34] found that in 92 patients who presented with acute MI, 78% of lesions responsible for the infarct occurred in patients with a previously significantly diseased vessel, as determined by angiograms obtained at a median of 26 months (range 1 to 144)before the index myocardial infarction.

We have demonstrated that acute changes in the morphology of a non-obstructive plaque are associated with the conversion of stable atherosclerosis to an acute coronary syndrome. Dacanay et al[4] documented substantial differences between the angiographic appearance of stenoses that progress to QMI versus NQMI. There was significantly more severe luminal diameter narrowing at the site of stenoses that progressed to QMI than to NQMI. Many of the coronary arterial segments that later become the site of NQMI have either minimal plaques with little or no angiographic evidence of atherosclerotic disease or else are severe stenoses of variable angiographic morphology. QMI are associated with an intermediate stenosis with complex stenosis morphology that progresses to acute thrombotic occlusion within 18 months; if a QMI occurs after this time period, an intermediate-severity, simple morphology (i.e, not eccentric type II) stenosis is often demonstrated on the earlier angiogram. Taken together, these findings suggest that the plaque substrate differs between QMI and NQMI, at least at some point in time before the acute event, and persisting up to the time of plaque rupture. This study demonstrates that either of two processes may lead to NQMI: a relatively rapid progression at a minimally diseased site or occlusion at the site of a severe stenosis with collateral recruitment. The existence of such apparently rapid growth is well known to clinicians who have had occasion to repeat angiograms at frequent intervals in anecdotal cases.

Clinically, it is very difficult to distinguish between unstable angina and NQMI until enzymatic testing for myocardial infarction has been completed. Angiographic distinction between the two is impossible, although filling defects consistent with thrombus are more commonly seen in patients with NQMI. Unlike QMI, which is characterized by complete occlusion of the culprit vessel, these syndromes are characterized by incomplete occlusion. Since contrast material fills the lumen of the vessel at least partially, morphologic characteristics of the lesion are more apparent in these patients than those with QMI. Although intense activation of platelets and the coagulation system occur in patients with rest angina and angioscopic findings of patients undergoing emergency bypass indicate intraluminal red thrombus in nearly all cases,

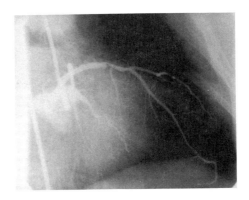

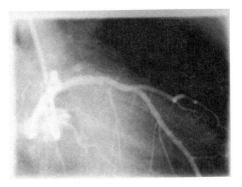

Figure 3. A 37 year old woman presenting with NQMI: Angiography 1-1/2 years previously for atypical chest pain showed completely normal vessels.

(top panel) Eccentric, irregular lesion with overhanging edges in the anterior descending artery.

(bottom panel) Result after directional atherectomy. This patient remained asymptomatic for 2 years until another NQMI occurred, this time involving the previously normal right coronary artery.

188

the angiographic detection of thrombosis is considerably less sensitive. The frequency with which filling defects are reported ranges from 56% in patients studied during an episode of unstable angina to 35% in patients within 24 hours of an episode of rest angina to 1% in patients studied after one month. These differences reflect both the effects of endogenous fibrinolytic mechanisms and the exclusion of patients in whom continued instability necessitates an emergent revascularization procedure. In the latter group of patients, the frequency of angiographically visible thrombus is higher.

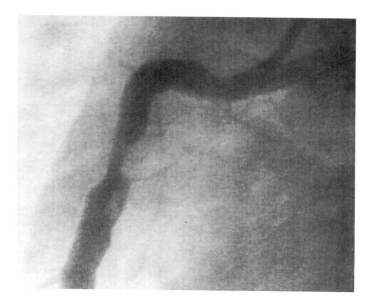

Figure 4. A 30 year old man under severe personal stress presenting with NQMI. A huge thrombus beyond only a 40% atherosclerotic lesion in the right coronary artery is seen. Stress testing was negative. The patient has done well for 1 year on antiplatelet therapy. No medical risk factor (including homocysteine and anti-thrombin III levels) has been established.

Pathogenesis and Morphologic Correlates

There is compelling data indicating that the initiating patho-physiologic event in the acute coronary syndromes is due to a change in the coronary endothelial surface.

Rupture of an atherosclerotic plaque is the most important mechanism underlying sudden and rapid plaque progression. In patients presenting with unstable angina or NQMI in whom extensive plaque rupture has occurred, even though the coronary arterial lumen is compromised, the plaque can be visualized easily. Comparison of angiograms performed remotely preceding an acute ischemic event with those performed in the same patient during an ischemic presentation usually indicates that the "culprit" lesion was not the most severe narrowing at the time of the initial angiogram and that a relatively "insignificant" plaque has undergone an abrupt change to produce the acute syndrome[29,40,41]. Nevertheless, as reported by us many years ago[42], it is not possible to state with great reliability, based on angiographic appearance, which plaques will become unstable and undergo rupture. One can not predict what subsequent behavior any stenosis may exhibit, other than to infer a likelihood, based on morphology.

It is now widely accepted that all of the acute coronary syndromes share a common pathogenetic mechanism involving plaque disruption and superimposed thrombus[43,44]. Ambrose and associates[14-17] have demonstrated in a remarkable series of papers that these acutely ruptured plaques have a characteristic angiographic appearance, referred to as "complex plaques" or "eccentric type II" lesions. The morphologic appearance is that of an asymmetric convex obstruction with a narrow neck or base containing sharp, overhanging edges, irregular or scalloped borders, and sometimes intraluminal lucency. These morphologic patterns represent ruptured plaques, intracoronary thrombus, or both. This appearance, based on the post mortem studies of Levin and Fallon[45], have revolutionized the manner in which angiograms are interpreted and used in clinical practice. Such lesions occur in about 70% of patients with unstable angina, NQMI and QMI after thrombolysis versus only 10 - 20% of patients with stable angina[14-17]. The similarities in stenosis morphology in all three syndromes strongly lend credence to a common pathogenesis.

Many studies[21-25] have angiographically documented the presence of intracoronary thrombus during unstable angina. The presence of a hazy, fuzzy intraluminal appearance is suggestive, but a well delineated, ovoid filling defect surrounded on at least 3 sides by contrast is diagnostic when distal flow is present. A total occlusion precludes this observation during acute MI, but instead a concave cut-off with contrast staining is commonly seen.

One of the difficulties in assessing the value of morphologic analysis is that the presence of eccentric, irregular stenoses, although statistically associated with unstable angina, can also be present in stable angina[16,42]. Furthermore, the natural history of such lesions is incompletely described[16,46]. Despite their propensity to rapidly progress to total occlusion, we do not really know how often they may heal without acute thrombosis. How rapidly can stenoses alter activity/growth levels, and hence change morphology? Do stenoses exhibit different morphological features at various stages of activity? How closely does the angiographic appearance represent acute rupture and healing of plaque fissuring?

Chen et al[47] prospectively studied 85 consecutive patients with unstable angina who stabilized with medical therapy, but were found to require angioplasty for treatment of their coronary disease. Angiography was carried out 8 ± 4 months after the first angiogram. Stenosis morphology and severity was assessed at both times. At restudy, 25% of the complex

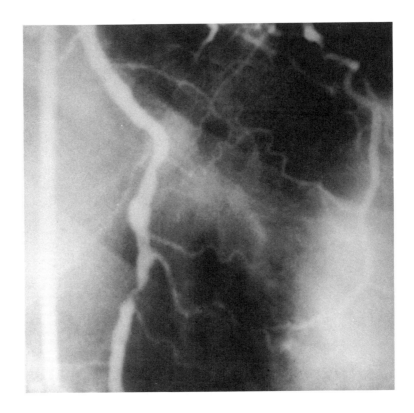

Figure 5. Classic irregular, eccentric stenosis with the vague suggestion of an ovoid filling defect centrally. Such difficulties in morphologic assessment of angiograms illustrate the limitations of this technique. Furthermore, this lesion was the only stenosis found in a patient with stable, exertional anginal correlating with a thallium defect, underscoring the non-specificity of the Ambrose criteria.

lesions progressed vs. 7% of the non complex lesions (p = .001). 17 of the complex stenoses that progressed developed into total occlusion compared to 3 of the 8 non complex lesions (p = .02). Changes in stenosis severity was significantly larger in the complex lesions (p = .03). 34% of the complex lesions progressed compared with 10% of the non complex lesions. Thus, in unstable angina patients who stabilize medically, the unstable coronary lesion will commonly progress over the short-term. This is consistent with the hypothesis of stenosis progression described earlier[9].

Another issue is whether stenosis location at certain places in the coronary tree could predispose to rupture. Taeymans et al[48] analyzed 38 coronary lesions in patients who had undergone thrombolysis for myocardial infarction and compared them to 64 control (non-infarct related) lesions in the same patients. Infarct-related lesions shared characteristics that would be expected to increase shear stress and flow separation, such as branch division (76% vs. 52%) and steeper inflow or outflow angles of stenosis (21 ± 10 vs.16 ± 7, $p<0.05$ and 20 ± 10 vs. 16 ± 8, $p<0.05$, respectively). These authors concluded that such conditions seemed to enhance plaque fissuring and rupture and thus enhancing the risk of thrombotic occlusion. Other reported predictors of progression include lesions found in larger arteries, and stenoses found in a proximal or mid artery position[49].

Recent angioscopic studies in unstable angina[10,20] and myocardial infarction[19] clearly suggest that the acutely injured plaque has undergone a transformation beyond the ulceration itself. Stable atheroma appear white or light grayish, with a glistening, smooth appearance. In contrast, the acute atheroma in its earliest stage is yellowish and friable with a divided surface and ragged edges. There is often a darkened, purplish area consistent with a subintimal hemorrhage at the surface radiating into the subendothelium. When a

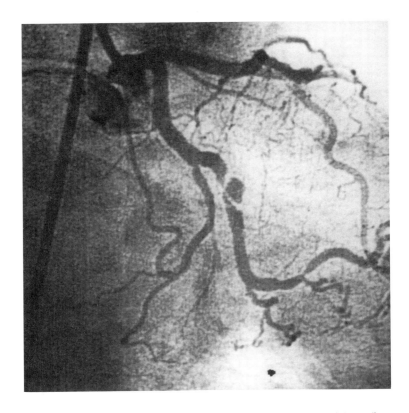

Figure 6. Although this lesion appears to be a partially healed, intervention-related dissection, this was the spontaneous angiographic presentation in a patient with progressive, but not "not", unstable angina. A colleague observed that "it looks like a bomb went off inside this artery". Again, the inability to correlate the acuity of the clinical syndrome with stenosis morphology is emphasized. Directional atherectomy was initially successful, but the development of stenoses in other locations over a 2 year period led to bypass surgery ultimately. This scenario (also present in the case in figure 3) shows how high grade, "ugly" stenoses may develop rapidly in previously angiographically normal segments.

coronary thrombus is present in unstable angina, it is grayish-white, whereas thrombus seen in acute MI is red. Such macroscopic morphology may be descriptive in nature, but there is demonstrably an underlying mechanism of infinite complexity[50]. The mere fact of these observations is an important step in the comprehension of how lesion appearance is related to their composition, activity and propensity to cause acute cardiac events.

Intravascular ultrasound studies in our laboratory[18] have shown that the underlying stenosis in unstable angina may exhibit marked ulceration and dissection approaching that seen after balloon angioplasty of stable lesions. Thrombus may be present on ultrasound even when it is not angiographically evident.

What Determines Which Coronary Syndrome Develops?

Although plaque disruption with thrombus formation is clearly the major pathogenetic mechanism for acute coronary syndromes, the determinants of which syndrome a patient develops after disruption is not understood. Further, most plaque fissures are probably asymptomatic, resulting only in slow progression of lesions. Thus, what factors influence whether plaque disruption leads to an acute clinical syndrome, and to which one, requires further study[51].

Clearly, the syndrome experienced by the patient after plaque rupture could depend on many factors, including the degree and acuteness of the ulceration, the duration of decreased perfusion, the volume of myocardium that is ischemic, the changes produced in myocardial oxygen demand and the degree of collateralization which develops. The presence of ischemic pre-conditioning, amount and perhaps the composition of the intracoronary thrombus may also be a significant determinant; in MI the thrombus is larger and more fibrin rich than the thrombus observed in unstable angina[52]. Thrombus at the site of coronary artery disruption is platelet rich, whereas that extending distal to the site of the disruption at the total occlusion is fibrin and red cell rich.

The central role of thrombus burden and avidity in patients presenting with NQMI is well shown in two important therapeutic trials. In the TIMI 3A Trial[53], thrombolytic therapy was administrated to patients presenting with either NQMI or unstable angina. In most cases, a clinical diagnosis of NQMI was associated with angiographic evidence of thrombus. In addition, NQMI was associated with angiographic improvement after tPA. Unstable angina more commonly had complex lesions and were less likely to exhibit intracoronary filling defects: there was little angiographic or clinical improvement with tPA administration. The TAUSA Trial[54] showed that intracoronary urokinase treatment was ineffective as a therapeutic strategy in unstable coronary angina. This trial also showed that prophylactic thrombolysis with intracoronary urokinase was actually detrimental as adjunctive therapy to balloon angioplasty. Conventional therapy with heparin and aspirin was superior to the use of urokinase.

One of the difficult aspects in describing the intravascular events leading to unstable angina relates to its wide clinical spectrum: the diagnosis of unstable angina includes patients with many different types of clinical syndromes. In patients with new onset angina, angina at low workload, or recent change in angina that has been previously stable, the incidence of complex plaque and thrombus is about 70%. In patients with an abrupt change in anginal pattern or very recent onset of rest pain, the incidence of thrombus is higher.

There are important therapeutic considerations inherent in these observations. Balloon angioplasty is known to have a somewhat increased risk of abrupt closure and restenosis in unstable angina generally, but this is not, in itself, a contraindication to proceeding with intervention. However, when a thrombus is evident angiographically, further increased risk is involved. The decision to proceed in this circumstance requires a judgment balancing risks and benefits. Thus, the presence of an ovoid filling-defect suggests a higher degree of risk, even though the likely presence of thrombus can be inferred on clinical grounds even if not visualized by angiography, perhaps because this finding implies a relatively large thrombus.

In possibly the seminal study of the past decade, Sherman and colleagues[10] performed coronary angioscopy during coronary bypass surgery to directly visualize lesions. A total of 32 vessels were examined in 10 patients with unstable angina and in 10 patients with stable angina. The findings at coronnary angiography were compared to the angioscopic observations. On angioscopy, 0/17 arteries in patients with stable coronary disease had either complex plaque or thrombus. In the culprit arteries of the unstable angina patients, all 3/3 patients with accelerated angina had complex palques and all 7/7 with angina at rest had thrombus. Angiography correctly identified the absence of acute lesions in all 22 "quiescent" arteries, but detected only 1/4 complex plaques and 1/7 thrombi. This difference could not be explained by treatment modalities or spontaneous changes in clinical status. Two crucial conclusions arise from these findings. First, angiography fails to detect acute lesions in a substantial number of patients - therefore, when the morphologic findings of thrombus or ulcerated plaque are present, this should be regarded as relatively specific, but their absence should not be considered particularly sensitive. Second, the wide spectrum of unstable angina can be categorized into at least two entities (rest vs. accelerated angina) with a pathophysiologic rationale. Specifically, partially occlusive thrombus is commonly present in unstable rest angina.

While these angiographic, angioscopic and clinical distinctions between NQMI and unstable angina are descriptive, precisely what determines these differences remains controversial. An important observation is the progressive increase of the incidence of total occlusion from about 10% in patients with unstable angina to 80 or 90% in those with acute infarction with ST elevation. In patients with NQMI, the incidence of total occlusion is between 20 and 40%. The higher incidence of total occlusion in QMI suggested to Ambrose[51] a more acute event within the coronary arteries, because "the clinical presentation of myocardial infarction is more profound than that of unstable angina. One might expect a more sudden decrease in coronary perfusion after infarction as might occur with an occlusive thrombus".

This teleological argument not only defies common sense, but also can not fully explain "why" certain events happen in one case but not another. Clearly, the amount of thrombus developing after coronary plaque rupture is an important determinant of the acute clinical syndrome. Additionally, the thrombus in QMI contains more fibrin, enhancing its adhesive properties, whereas in unstable angina it is more rich in platelets. These differences undoubtedly explain in part the variable angiographic incidence of occlusion and response of thrombolytic agents in the two syndromes, but represents phenomenology. The real question is why this differential thrombus adherence and burden occurs. The incidence of angiographic total occlusion of the culprit lesion may suggest possible differences in pathologic coronary lesion substrate. As reviewed earlier in this chapter, we[41] have presented evidence that one underlying factor is the size and speed of growth of the underlying atherosclerotic plaque that ruptures. The data supports the opposite view to that of Ambrose. NQMI probably occurs on an even more minimal plaque than QMI: because less underlying collagen is exposed, or because the size of the rupture is less, the thrombus is smaller and less avid. Other variables which could be involved include differences in local mediator release, platelet activation, and the local activity of the thrombotic and fibrinolytic systems. Such factors are themselves influenced by atheromatous injury and severity.

DiSciascio[55] used the benefit of tissue retrieval during directional coronary atherectomy to study the histopathologic correlates of unstable ischemic syndromes. They demonstrated the presence of thrombus in 50% of the patients with rest angina, 41% of patients with crescendo angina in 69% of patients with recent MI. In addition, 25% of patients with recent MI had ulceration compared to 12% with rest angina and 7% with cresecendo angina. Chronic inflammation (as observed by the presence of inflammatory cells) was observed in 67% of patients with recent MI, 47% of patients with rest angina and 41% with crescendo angina. Thus, the degree of inflammation (and its cause) may well be a marker, as well as an etiologic factor, as to which acute coronary syndrome develops.

The Rupture Prone Plaque

Atherosclerotic plaques consist of a lipid rich core in a central portion of an eccentricity thickened intimal. This central core contains many lipid rich macrophages, called foam cells. The lipid is composed of oxidized LDL cholesterol. The lipid core boundary on the luminal aspect is formed by a thin fibrous cap. During coronary arterial stress, vigorous bending and twisting of these plaques may lead to their rupture, releasing large amounts of tissue factor from the foam cells, which is strongly procoagulant. Consequently, the integrity of the fibrous cap determines the stability of the plaque. Rupture prone plaques are composed of thin, friable fibrous caps. Those which are stable and not likely to precipitate events have thicker caps that protect the blood from contact with the thrombogenic lipid core[56,57].

The fibrous plaque is composed of extracellular matrix, a primary component of which is collagen. Collagen types 1 and 3 are the main constituents of the fibrous plaque[58]. The smooth muscle cells which produce this collagen are found in significant amounts, but usually in a non-activated state in the lipid core. However, the vulnerable plaque contains many activated smooth muscle cells which produce cytokines[38].

The cause of cap rupture thus becomes the key to understanding the proximate causes of acute ischemic events. Mechanical stresses, such as those due to hypertension, smoking or other vasoreactive influences, concentrate on the fibrous cap and are certainly involved. These may include shear stress, incessant bending with each cardiac cycle, and the impact of velocity and acceleration changes in blood flow predicted by Bernoulli's principle once a focal atheroma has developed. Also clearly incriminated as an initiating factor is catecholamine release, which not only vasoconstrict coronary vessels, raise blood pressure and myocardial oxygen demand, but also render platelets more prone to aggregation[9]. The fibrous cap must be resistant towards these high stresses to avoid rupture and thus, precipitation of a coronary event[59].

Inflammation, perhaps the result of a latent viral infection, has also been implicated. Vulnerable plaques are abundant in macrophages and t-lymphocytes. Cytokines also play an important modulating role in this process: whereas TGF-beta and PDGF increase RNA and the synthesis of collagen, interferon-gamma diminishes its production; t-lymphocytes produce interferon-gamma. Consequently, in the unstable plaque, t-lymphocytes inhibit collagen synthesis. Additionally, macrophages produce proteases which enhance the breakdown of collagen. Thus, many characteristics of a chronic inflammatory process in the unstable plaque are present; the end-pathway involves both decreased production and increased metabolism of extracellular matrix, rendering the plaque vulnerable[38].

van der Wal[60] showed in a study of 20 patients at necropsy who died of myocardial infarction that the immediate site of plaque rupture was always marked by a inflammatory process suggesting a causative role in destabilizing the fibrous tissue.   Fibrin deposition in the vessel wall promotes atheroma formation, and several serological links between inflammation and fibrin exist. Fibrinogen, an independent risk factor for coronary disease, is an acute phase reactant. Both by increasing serum viscosity and by promoting platelet deposition, fibrinogen creates further hemodynamic stress as well as initiating a cascade of events[61] .

Stabilization of Vulnerable Plaques

The title of the final section of this chapter suggests one observer's view of the future of clinical cardiology. Before it can be written, however, progress is necessary both in regard to pharmacologic and mechanical therapeutic approaches as well as to better diagnostic procedures to assess the effectiveness of the treatment.

Topol and colleagues[62] discussed the mechanisms by which currently employed anti-ischemic and anti-thrombotic drugs alter the activity of plaques, rendering them quiescent. Certainly, effective pharmacologic agents act partially in this manner, but the underlying strategies dictating their use and dosage are based on their traditional actions. Clinical medicine has not progressed to the point where therapy is consciously applied to stablilize vulnerable plaques, even if some do work in this manner. The development of new agents aimed at unique sites involved in the process (such as the recent introduction of glycoprotein IIb/IIIa receptor inhibition) and a better comprehension of gene therapy as a therapeutic method are clear first steps before this goal can be achieved.

The futher investigation of pathophysiologic factors is an important facet of therapy. It would be easy to be mesmerized by how much more is now known than before into believing that all the pieces have been identified; this is not likely so. The potential role of viral (or other infectious) vectors in initiating inflammation and the humoral factors responsible for differential fibrous plaque growth are just two of the obvious issues that need further exploration. Indeed, many of the factors which are thought to be understood require yet another layer of understanding. The interplay of circumferential shear stress, mediators of vascular tone, viscosity (and its relationship to fibrinogen and low density lipoprotein levels) and endothelial damage is just beginning to be understood, for example.

Finally, before the potential role of any new therapeutic agent can be tested, better "gold standards" to measure its effects on thrombus, atheroma, platelet activation and/or endothelial function are needed. Although stenosis morphology has been a crucial first step on the pathway to understanding pathophysiology and designing treatment, it is not a truly definitive test. For example, morphology is not even a predictor of clinical outcome in unstable angina[64]. The angiogram, and its interpretation for morphologic analysis, should be recognized as an effective, but crude, tool. The additional information gathered with any new diagnostic technique will be weighed against the ease of performance of the angiogram; to be useful as more than a research tool, it must achieve widespread applicability. Only when it can be accepted as the "better reference standard" available in all clinical settings, will medicine finally be able to move in the direction of stabilizing vulnerable plaques - and preventing their transformation to active plaques.

Bibliography

1. Braunwald E. Unstable angina: a classification. Circulation 1989; 80:410-414.

2. Braunwald E, Mark DB, Jones RH, et al. Unstable angina: Diagnosis and management. In: Clinical Practice Guidelines, Number 10. Rockville, MD: US Dept. of Health and Human Services, 1994. Agency for Health Care Policy and Research, Publication 94-0602.

3. Calvin JE, Klein LW, VandenBerg BJ, et al. Risk stratification in unstable angina. Prospective validation of the Braunwald classification. J Am Med Assoc 1995; 273:136-141.

4. Gibson RS. Non Q wave myocardial infarction. Diagnosis, prognosis and management. Curr Probl Cardiol 1988; 13:1-72.

5. Klein LW, Helfant RH. The Q wave and non-Q wave myocardial infarction: Differences and similarities. Prog Cardiovasc Dis 1986; 29:205-220.

6. DeWood MA, Spores J, Notske R, et al. Prevalence of total coronary occlusion during the early hours of transmural myocardial infarction. N Engl J Med 1980; 303:897-902.

7. DeWood MA, Stiffer WF, Simpson CS, et al. Coronary angiographic findings soon after non-Q wave myocardial infarction. N Engl J Med 1986; 315:417-423.

8. Fuster V, Badimon L, Cohen M, Ambrose JA, Badimon JJ, Cheseboro J. Insights into the pathogenesis of acute coronary syndromes. Circulation 1988; 77:1213-1220.

9. Fuster V, Badimon L, Badimon JJ, Chesebro J. The pathogenesis of coronary artery disease and the acute coronary syndromes. Parts 1 & 2. N Engl J Med 1992; 326:242-250, 310-318.

10. Sherman CT, Litvack F, Grundfest W, et al. Coronary angioscopy in patients with unstable angina pectoris. N Engl J Med 1986: 315:913-919.

11. Davies MJ, Thomas AC. Plaque fissuring - the cause of acute myocardial infarction, sudden ischemic death, and crescendo angina. Br Heart J 1985; 53:363-373.

12. Falk E. Plaque rupture with severe pre-existing stenosis precipitating coronary thrombosis. Characteristics of coronary atherosclerotic plaques underlying fatal occlusive thrombi. Br Heart J 1983; 50:127-134.

13. Falk E. Unstable angina with fatal outcome. Dynamic coronary thrombosis leading to infarction and/or sudden death. Autopsy evidence of recurrent mural thrombosis with peripheral embolization culminating in total vascular occlusion. Br Heart J 1985; 71:699-708.

14. Ambrose JA, Winters SL, Stern A, Eng A, Teichholz LE, Gorlin R, Fuster V. Angiographic morphology and the pathogenesis of unstable angina pectoris. J Am Coll Card 1985; 5:609-616.

15. Ambrose JA, Winters SL, Arora R, Haft JI, Goldstein J, Rntrop KP, Gorlin R, Fuster V. Coronary angiographic morphology in myocardial infarction: A link between the pathogenesis of unstable angina pectoris and myocardial infarction. J Am Coll Card 1985; 6:1233-1238.

16. Ambrose JA, Winters SL, Arora R, Eng A, Riccio A, Gorlin R, Fuster V. Angiographic evolution of coronary artery morphology in unstable angina. J Am Coll Card 1985; 5:609-616.

17. Ambrose JA, Hjemdahl-Monsen CE, Borrico S, Gorlin R, Fuster V. Angiographic demonstration of a common link between unstable angina pectoris and non-Q wave acute myocardial infarction. Am J Cardiol 1988; 61:244-247.

18. Liebson PR, Klein LW. Intravascular ultrasound in coronary atherosclerosis: A new approach to clinical assessment. Am Heart J 1992; 123:1643-1660.

19. Mizuno K, Satomura K, Miyamoto A, et al. Angioscopic evaluation of coronary artery thrombi in acute coronary syndromes. N Engl J Med 1992; 326:287-291.

20. Ramee SR, White CJ, Collins TJ, Mesa JE, Murgo JP. Percutaneous angioscopy during coronary angioplasty using a steerable microangioscope. J Am Coll Cardiol 1989; 13:363-368.

21. Holmes DR Jr, Hartzler GB, Smith HC, Fuster V. Coronary artery thrombosis in patients with unstable angina. Br Heart J 1981; 45:411-416.

22. Vetrovec GW, Cowley MJ, Overton H, Richardson DW. Intracoronary thrombus in syndromes of unstable myocardial ischemia. Am Heart J 1981; 102:1201-1208.

23. Capone G, Wolf NM, Meyer B, Meister SG. Frequency of intracoronary filling defects by angiography in angina pectoris at rest. Am J Cardiol 1985; 56:403-406.

24. Rehr R, DiSciascio G, Vetrovec G, Cowley M. Angiographic morphology of coronary artery stenoses in prolonged rest angina: evidence of intracoronary thrombus. J Am Coll Cardiol 1989; 14:1429-1437.

25. Freeman MR, Williams AE, Chisholm RT, Armstrong PW. Intracoronary thrombus and complex morphology in unstable angina relation to timing of angiography and in-hospital cardiac events. Circulation 1989; 80:17-23.

26. Kereiakes DJ, Topol EJ, George BS, et al. Myocardial infarction with minimal coronary atherosclerosis in the area of thrombolytic reperfusion. J Am Coll Cardiol 1991; 17:304-312.

27. Nakogawa S, Hanada Y, Kaiwaya Y, Tanaka K. Angiographic features in the infarct-related artery after intracoronary urokinase followed by prolonged anticoagulation. Circulation 1988; 78:1335-1344.

28. Davies SW, Marchant B, Lyons JP, et al. Coronary lesion morphology in acute myocardial infarction: demonstration of early remodeling after streptokinase treatment. J Am Coll Cardiol 1990; 16:1079-1086.

29. Little WC, Constantinescu M, Applegate RJ, et al. Can coronary angiography predict the site of a subsequent myocardial infarction in patients with mild to moderate coronary artery disease? Circulation 1988; 78:1157-1166.

30. Matsuda Y, Kramer JR, Matsuda M. Progression and regression of coronary artery disease - Linkage of clinical pathologic and angiographic findings. Clin Cardiol 1995; 18:412-417.

31. Brown BG, Zhoo XQ, Sacco DE, Albers JJ. Lipid lowering and plaque regression: new insights into prevention of plaque disruption and clinical events in coronary disease. Circulation 1993; 87:1781-1791.

32. Karnegis JN, Matts JP, Tuna N, Amplatz K, (POSCH Group). Relation between changes in severity coronary artery stenosis and anginal patterns. Cath Cardiovasc Diagn 1994; 32:324-329.

33. Klein LW, Liebson PR. Coronary angiography in patients with established coronary artery disease: how much does the angiogram help in assessing changes in symptoms? Cath Cardiovasc Diagn 1994; 32:330-331.

34. Giroud D, Li JM, Urban P, Meier B, Rutishauser W. Relation of the site of acute myocardial infarction to the most severe coronary arterial stenosis at prior angiography. Am J Cardiol 1992; 69:729-732.

35. Moise A, Lesperance J, Theroux P, Taeymans Y, Goulet C, Bourassa MG. Clinical and angiographic predictors of new total coronary occlusion in coronary artery disease: analysis of 313 nonoperated patients. Am J Cardiol 1984; 54:1176-1181.

36. Conti CR. Identifying coronary stenoses prone to thrombus. Clin Cardiol 1995; 18:491-492.

37. Levin RI. The biology of unstable atherosclerosis. Primary Cardiology 1990; 16:16-27.

38. Libby P. Molecular bases of the acute coronary syndromes. Circulation 1995; 91:2844-2850.

39. Brown BG, Gallery CA, Badger RS, et al. Incomplete lysis of thrombus in the moderate underlying atherosclerotic lesion during intracoronary infusion of streptokinase for acute myocardial infarction: quantitative angiographic information. Circulation 1986; 73:653-661.

40. The TIMI Research Group. Immediate vs. delayed catheterization and angioplasty following thrombolytic therapy for acute myocardial infarction: TIMI IIA results. J Am Med Assoc 1988; 260:2849-2858.

41. Dacanay S, Kennedy HL, Uretz E, Parrillo JE, Klein LW. Morphologic and quantitative angiographic analysis of progression of coronary stenoses: A comparison of Q wave and non-Q wave myocardial infarction. Circulation 1994; 90:1739-1746.

42. Rubinstein RI, Herlich MB, Agarwal JB, Klein LW, Helfant RH. Predictive value and prognosis of coronary angiographic morphology. Circulation 1986; 74:II-305.

43. Gorlin R, Fuster V, Ambrose J. Anatomic - physiologic links between acute coronary syndromes. Circulation 1986; 74:6-9.

44. Willerson JT, Hillis LD, Winnford M, Buja LM. Speculation regarding mechanisms responsible for acute ischemic heart disease syndromes. J Am Coll Cardial 1986; 8:245-250.

45. Levin DC, Fallon JT. Significance of the angiographic morphology of localized coronary stenoses. Circulation 1982; 66:316-320.

46. Haft JI, Al-Zarka AM. Comparison of the natural history of irregular and smooth coronary lesions: Insights into the pathogenesis, progression and prognosis of coronary atherosclerosis. Am Heart J 1993; 126:551-561.

47. Chen L, Chester MR, Redwood S, Huang J, Leatham E, Kaski JC. Angiographic stenosis progression and coronary events in patients with "stabilized" unstable angina. Circulation 1995; 91:2319-2324.

48. Taeymans Y, Theroux P, Lesperance J, Waters D. Quantitative angiographic morphology of coronary artery lesions at risk for thrombotic occlusion. Circulation 1992; 85:78-85.

49. Jost S, Deckers JW, Nikatta P, et al. Progression of coronary artery disease is dependent on anatomic location and diameter. J Am Coll Cardiol 1993; 21:1339-1346.

50. Forrester JF. Intimal disruption and coronary thrombosis: Its role in the pathogenesis of human coronary disease. Am J Cardiol 1991; 68:69B-76B.

51. Ambrose JA. Plaque disruption and the acute coronary syndromes of unstable angina and myocardial infarction: If the substrate is similar, why is the clinical presentation different? J Am Coll Cardiol 1992; 19:1653-1658.

52. Chesebro JH, Zoldhelyi P, Fuster V. Pathogenesis thrombosis in unstable angina. Am J Cardiol 1991; 68:2B-10B.

53. TIMI 3A Investigators. Early effects of tissue-type plasminogen activator added to conventional therapy on the culprit coronary lesion in patients presenting with ischemic cardiac pain at rest. Circultion 1993; 87:38-52.

54. Ambrose JA, Almeida OD, Sharma S, et al. Adjunctive thrombolytic therapy during angioplasty for ischemic rest angina - Results of the TAUSA Trial. Circulation 1994; 90:69-77.

55. Di Sciascio G, Cowley MJ, Goudreau E, Vetrovec GW, Johnson DE. Histopathologic correlates of unstable ischemic syndromes in patients undergoing directional atherectomy: In vivo evidence of thrombosis, ulceration and inflammation. Am Heart J 1994; 128:419-426.

56. Falk E. Why do plaques rupture? Circulation 1992; 86(suppl III):III-30-42.

57. Cheng GC, Loree HM, Kamm RD, Fishbein MC, Lee RT. Distribution of circumferential stress in ruptured and stable atherosclerotic lesions. Circulation 1993; 87:1179-1187.

58. Moore JA, Bach RG, Kern MJ. Application of translesional pressure and flow velocity assessment in a severely calcified coronary narrowing in a patient with unstable angina. Cath Cardiovasc Diagn 1995; 35:270-276.

59. Falk E, Shah PK, Fuster V. Coronary plaque disruption. Circulation 1995; 92:657-671.

60. van der Wal AC, Becker AE, van der Loos CM, Das PK. Site of intimal rupture or erosion of thrombosed coronary atherosclerotic plaques characterized by an inflammatory process unrespective of the dominant plaque morphology. Circulation 1994; 89:36-44.

61. Loscalzo J. Thrombotic mechanisms in atherogenesis. Am J Cardiol (supplement), Mechanisms of Coronary Disease; Part I: Development of Atherosclerosis and Thrombosis, pages 23-27.

62. Mac Isacc AI, Thomas JD, Topol EJ. Toward the quiescent coronary plaque. J Am Coll Cardiol 1993; 22:1228-1241.

63. Kragel AH, Reddy SG, Wittes JT, Roberts WC. Morphometric analysis of the composition of coronary arterial plaques in isolated unstable angina pectoris with pain at rest. Am J Cardiol 1990; 66:562-567.

64. Bar FW, Raymond P, Renkin JP, Vermeer F, de Zwaan C, Wellens HJ. Coronary angiographic findings do not predict clinical outcome in patients with unstable angina. J Am Coll Cardiol 1994; 24:1453-1459.

9.

DEFINING CORONARY PATHOLOGY AND CLINICAL SYNDROMES BY CORONARY ANGIOSCOPY

James S. Forrester, M.D., Frank Litvack, M.D., Neal Eigler, M.D., Robert J. Siegel, M.D., Cedars-Sinai Medical Center, Los Angeles, California

Introduction

In the mid 80's, Spears et al and Litvack et al[2] reported the use of large diameter (1.8-3.3 mm) endoscopes to visualize the surface of peripheral and coronary blood vessels during surgery. In the last five years, major improvements in fiberoptic technology have made it possible to perform percutaneous coronary and peripheral vascular imaging in the catheterization laboratory. Angioscopy provides unique intravascular information. The interventional cardiologist can determine the etiology of unstable coronary chest pain syndromes, assess the trauma created by angioplasty, determine the appropriateness of stent placement, and evaluate the completeness of thrombolysis. Vascular surgeons can inspect anastomoses and determine the completeness of thrombectomy. Despite the unique vascular detail provided to coronary interventionalists by angioscopy, it probably will not evolve into routine use, because catheterization laboratory decisions rarely depend on such information. Conversely angioscopy continues to have great value in clinical coronary research, and is widely used by peripheral vascular surgeons for intraoperative decision-making.

The New Angioscopic Technology

Each fiber in a fiberoptic bundle is composed of an inner core which conveys light, and a surrounding cladding which traps the light within the inner core. When the ratio between the refractive indices of the core and cladding material is appropriately chosen, light is completely reflected within the core, resulting in transmission of light around bends with minimal loss of intensity. Individual fibers are assembled into a bundle, such that each fiber forms one pixel of the intravascular image. A lens attached to the distal end of the bundle to focus the output.

In the past several years, there have been major advances in flexibility, lens attachment, and guidance systems for angioscopes[3-5]. One way to increase flexibility is to decrease the outer diameter of the fiberoptic. A fused imaging bundle becomes flexible when its diameter is less than 0.5 mm. This diameter has been achieved by decreasing the thickness of the cladding. An alternative is to use individual fibers that are free to slide over each other throughout the body of the fiberoptic, and are bound together at each end. Although this technology offers flexibility, the individual fibers are more prone to damage. Another advance involves attachment of the distal lens assembly that gathers the light from within the artery and focuses it into the fiberoptic bundle. Until recently, it was not possible to attach lenses to very small diameter fiberoptic bundles. Through the use of special epoxies, gradient index lenses, and new attachment techniques, it has become feasible to attach a lens measuring 0.35 mm in diameter. For such small lenses, however, there is a trade-off: The wider the viewing angle, the more the required illumination. The ideal distal objective has an absolute minimum focal length and a wide angle. Lenses with a minimum focal length, e.g., 0.5 mm, and relatively wide angle lens, e.g., 90 degrees, are now available.

To steer the angioscope through tortuous vessels, and to center the lens in the vessel during imaging, guidance systems have been markedly improved. New guidewire systems[5] provide 20% increase in successful intracoronary image acquisition (80% vs 60%). For centering the angioscope, a balloons are now used. The balloon also obstructs antegrade blood flow, allowing more prolonged imaging during flushing of blood from the imaging site. These technologic advances allow performance of percutaneous intracoronary angioscopy with relative ease in the catheterization laboratory.

Classification of Angioscopic Images

Angioscopic images are classified using color, mass and the surface characteristics of the vessel (Table 1). We use four categories [7,8]: normal, stable atheroma, intimal disruption and thrombus. Post-intervention, we also identify intimal flaps and dissections. In our classification, normal is defined as smooth, white, and without masses (Figure 1). Stable atheromas are white or yellow masses with a smooth surface (Figure 2). Intimal disruption is defined as a torn surface without thrombus (Figure 3). Thrombus is a red or which mass (Figure 4). Recently the European Working Group on Coronary Angioscopy has proposed a similar angioscopic image classification system[8]. The group is currently evaluating intraobserver and interobserver variability for this system.

The accuracy of these classification systems have been determined by independent histopathologic correlation. We studied current 70 postmortem human arterial segments in vitro[9]. Three observers categorized each angioscopy image, and the pathologist independently classified each lesion. For stable atheroma the sensitivity, specificity, and accuracy of angioscopic classification all were greater than 90%. For intimal disruption, the angioscopic sensitivity was 73%, and for thrombus detection it was 100%. In an analogous study, Schwartz et al reported independent angioscopic-histopathologic correlation studies in carotid arteries at autopsy[10]. The angiographic images and pathologic sections were classified as normal, fibrous ridges, fatty streaks, atheromas, or complicated lesions, which included ulceration, thrombosis and hemorrhage. The angioscopic and histologic classification agreed in 43/48 cases. Angioscopic misclassification of 5 vessels as "normal" was due to inability to reach a lesion; in no case was an ulceration visualized and misclassified. From these studies we can conclude that although angioscopic image interpretation is subjective, the accuracy and reproducibility of interpretation is adequate for clinical use.

The Relative Value of Angioscopy and Angiography

Angioscopy and angiography are complementary[11-15]. Angioscopy is far superior for detecting localized damage to the vessel surface; angiography is best for defining the magnitude of coronary disease throughout the length of a vessel. The superiority of angioscopy for detecting local abnormalities is quite striking. Van Stiegman et al found thrombus in 30 angioscopic images, only 11 of which were detected by angiography[11]. Further, angioscopy revealed free-floating clots, atherosclerotic debris and membrane-like obstructions which were undetectable by angiography. Johnson et al found 26 subintimal dissections by angioscopy, none of which were detected by cineangiography[12], and 6 distal emboli detected by angioscopy were identified in only two cases by angiography. More recently, den Heijer et al reported that "no fewer than 48% of angioscopically observed thrombi remained undetected at angiography", and that the frequency of angioscopically detected dissection (77%) greatly exceeded that of angiography (29%)[13]. This distinction holds for every clinical subset, including infarction, unstable angina, old infarction and stable angina[14]. The differences between angioscopic and angiographic detection of thrombus is clearly related to the size of the lesion. Whereas angiography detects 100% of large angioscopic thrombi, it detects only 30% of small ones[15]. We can conclude that the unique value of angioscopy is its superiority for detecting small to medium sized intracoronary thrombi and intimal disruptions that are undetectable by angiography.

In contrast, angiography is superior for quantitative measurements, and for visualizing the entire coronary tree. In principle, angioscopy can be used to assess the magnitude diameter stenosis[16-18] but the methodology is impractical (Table 2). Quantitation has been performed using a transverse circle of light emitted from a guidewire passed a known distance beyond the tip of the angioscope. In phantoms, the mean difference between measured and known areas has been small (6.5%)[16]. In intraoperative application, quantitative cross-sectional luminal areas obtained by intraoperative coronary angioscopy and luminal areas calculated from angiographic findings also are closely correlated[17]. In these intraoperative studies, however, it is possible to measure the distance from the angioscope tip to the object being imaged. In percutaneous angioscopy, as performed in the catheterization laboratory, this crucial measurement is not available. With the inability to calibrate the lens-to-object distance, pincushion distortion makes quantitation subject to gross errors. Further the angioscopic quantitation system is ineffective in tortuous segments and for segments with complex morphology[18]. Thus, angiography is far superior to angioscopy for assessing diameter stenosis.

Use of Angioscopy for Defining Acute Coronary Syndromes

Angioscopy has played a central role in defining the pathogenesis of acute ischemic syndromes (Figure 5). We reported on intraoperative angioscopy in 71 patients with chronic stable angina, unstable angina, myocardial infraction and acute closure during failed balloon angioplasty[7]. Of the patients with stable angina, all but one had smooth, yellow-white atheromatous coronary arteries, whereas 86% of patients with unstable angina had intimal disruption or thrombus. In (post infarction) patients the culprit lesion revealed ulceration or thrombi as well as strands of intima floating within the lumen. In an analoguous study of 63 patients studied by percutaneous angioscopy in the catheterization laboratory, Mizuno et al found the frequency of thrombus and intimal disruption in unstable angina was somewhat lower than in our intraoperative study -- presumably related to the difference in population studied --but the results generally corresponded[19]. In patients with unstable angina in which saphenous vein grafts were the culprit vessel, thrombi were found in 71% by angioscopy[20]. The majority of grafts also had dissection and friable plaques, which were undetected by angiography. There was no correlation between age of the graft and the presence of friable plaque. Taken together these data indicate that intimal disruption, with platelet aggregation and thrombus formation, play a central causative role in acute coronary syndromes.

Angioscopy also has provided a fascinating, previously unrecognized insight about unstable angina, compared to acute myocardial infarction[21]. Seventy one percent of those with unstable angina had gray-white thrombi; whereas all of the acute infarction patients had red thrombi. This angioscopic observation suggests that the thrombi in unstable angina are older and more platelet-rich. We may speculate, therefore, that the relative ineffectiveness of thrombolytic agents in unstable angina, compared to its established efficacy in acute myocardial infarction, reflects an unrecognized difference in the composition of the thrombus which causes the syndrome.

Angioscopy During Coronary Interventions

In the catheterization laboratory, the interventionist deals with acute closure, due to arterial dissection and/or thrombosis (Figure 6). Angioscopy has provided insight about how it disappears during thrombolysis.

In dogs, a friable gray mesh develops a few minutes after insertion of a copper coil. Over a period of 1 to 3 hours, a red thrombus develops and becomes progressively occlusive. During subsequent thrombolysis, residual thrombus undetectable by angiography, is usually present by angioscopy[22]. The presence of residual intimal disruption (Figure 7) and thrombus after successful thrombolysis is also common in man. For this reason, angioscopy can be used to assess the completeness of thrombolysis, e.g., when intra-arterial urokinase infusion is used as therapy of subacute thrombosis.

Several groups have described angioscopy before and after coronary interventions. Angioplasty damages the blood vessel surface in ways that are largely undetectable by angiography. Since some of this damage (e.g., undetected partial thrombosis) may be correctable, angioscopy could provide a means for reducing the rate of both acute complications and late restenosis. Uchida found that before angioplasty, the stable angina patients had yellow-white atheroma with smooth surfaces. Immediately after angioplasty, there was intimal denudation with scattered thrombi in 10 of 11 segments examined. In 7 of these segments, the post-procedure abnormalities including fissures and dissections, could not be identified by angiography[23]. den Heijer et al studied dilated segments at 15 minute intervals for up to one hour post PTCA[24]. Significant progression of intimal dissection and thrombus formation was seen, which was entirely undetected by angiography. Angioscopy also has been used to evaluate the effect of new interventional devices, including excimer and holmium YAG lasers[25-27], and extraction atherectomy[28]. These studies reveal that the magnitude of procedure-induced injury is comparable to that created by balloon angioplasty. Flaps, fractures and abundant tissue remnants are common.

Angioscopy also has provided some provocative new information about restenosis. Itoh et al [29] found that there is a major difference in the risk of restenosis based on plaque color. Yellow plaques had an 18% restenosis rate, compared to a 58% rate in white plaques. It is possible that this difference relates to plaque compliance and risk of dissection, since fatty yellow plaques are more compliant than fibrous white plaques. At restudy of patients who developed restenosis, White et al compared the surface morphology of these lesions to primary atherosclerotic lesions[30]. Restenotic lesions typically were smooth and white, as opposed to native lesions, many of which were yellow or yellow-brown. These findings are consistent with the hypothesis that restenosis results from smooth muscle cell proliferation with abundant formation of collagenous extracellular matrix, and may explain why restenotic lesions rarely are the culprit lesion of an acute coronary syndrome.

We can conclude from the pre and post angioplasty studies that all types of angioplasty cause severe angiographically undetected damage in most cases. As more experience is accumulated, such data could provide insight into the mechanisms responsible for acute closure and restenosis following coronary and saphenous vein graft angioplasty, analogous to the contribution of angioscopy to the understanding of the pathogenesis of acute coronary syndromes.

Angioscopy During Placement of Intracoronary Stents

Angioscopy has also been used during and after coronary stent placement. Investigators have reported that angioscopy influenced their clinical management in 30 50% of their cases[31-32]. The great majority of these cases involved detection of unsuspected thrombus, or withholding thrombolytic therapy in patients with suspected thrombus. In addition there are case reports of unexpected incidental observations. Early stent obstruction, assumed to the caused by thrombus, was found to be due to an intimal dissection[33] and to intimal hyperplasia[34], in both cases obviating the need for thrombolytic therapy and prolonged anticoagulation. We also have insight about reendothelialization after stent placement. Serial angioscopy reveals absence of a neointimal layer at 8-18 days, and its uniform presence at 65-142 days[35]. Although it now seems likely that both intravascular ultrasound and angioscopy will not be required for routine stent placement, angioscopy may find a role in choice of interventional devices in some clinical subsets (e.g., vein graft stenosis) or when stent placement is difficult.

Angioscopy During Coronary and Peripheral Vascular
Surgery

Angioscopy has been used sparingly during coronary
vascular surgery and extensively in peripheral vascular
surgery. Bessou et al reported the use of coronary and
internal thoracic artery angioscopy in 38 patients over an
11 month period[36]. Of 13 internal mammary arteries examined, one was rejected on the basis of the angioscopic
detection of an intimal fracture. The authors also found
angioscopy useful for examining distal graft anastomoses. While at al found abnormalities in 110/48 (23%) of
coronary bypass anastomoses[37]. Nevertheless the value
of angioscopy during cardiac surgery remains undefined -
- on the one hand, unexpected pathology can be detected, albeit in low prevalence. On the other, the added
time and minimal risk associated with intraoperative angioscopy suggest it is unlikely to be used routinely.

In contrast, angioscopy has clear value in peripheral vascular surgery. We performed angioscopic inspection
during 85 peripheral vascular procedures, predominantly
femoral-popliteal and aortofemoral bypasses[38]. Changes
in intraoperative management based on angioscopic
findings included revision of 47% in situ venous valves,
and repeat thrombectomy in 85% (Figure 8). In 22 of 73
graft angioscopies, a potential cause of graft occlusion
was recognized. Others have used angioscopy for pre-
treatment assessment. In 23 patients with symptomatic
peripheral vascular disease, lesions best treated by atherectomy were identified in 12 patients, and 7 occlusions
were successfully treated with laser angioplasty. Angioscopy also identified 4 cases of incomplete recanalization despite a satisfactory angiographic image. Hofling
et al performed percutaneous peripheral vascular angioscopy in patients with superficial femoral or popliteal
artery stenoses before, during and after atherectomy[40].

Although angiographically acceptable results were obtained in all patients, angiocopy revealed flaps or obstructing residual material at 4 of the 15 sites. Based on this information additional passages of the atherectomy catheter were used to improve the therapeutic outcome.

These data suggest that angioscopy may be a valuable tool in peripheral vascular surgery. This possibility is further supported by a follow-up study which suggests that angioscopic evaluation may significantly alter long term outcomes[41]. In a cohort of 135 in situ femorodistal bypasses, 96 patients were studied by angioscopy, whereas in 39 patients the scope was not available. Using lifetable analysis, patency rates for the two groups were 76% and 76% at 30 days, 62% and 44% at 1 year, and 43% and 27% at 4 years. We can conclude that the use of angioscopy causes peripheral vascular surgeons to change their decisions in about 25% of cases. Because it alters both intraoperative decisions and probably alters long term outcomes, angioscopy probably will have an expanding role in peripheral vascular surgery.

Summary

Flexible, steerable angioscopes with diameters suitable for coronary use provide unique information about the coronary vessel surface. Although interpretation of images is subjective, angioscopic image analysis is reasonably accurate and reproducible when compared to histopathologic data. Angioscopy consistently detects clinically important intimal disruption and partially occlusive thrombosis that is undetectable by angiography. Images before and after atherectomy, balloon and laser angioplasty indicate that angioplasty causes severe trauma which is not detected by angiography. These data provide insight into the mechanisms responsible for angioplasty-induced acute closure and restenosis. Finally, although the value of angioscopy continues to come from its ability to clarify the pathogenesis of a broad spectrum of vascular syndromes, its use in selected clinical subsets, such as stent placement and thrombectomy, has direct relevance to clinical decision-making.

REFERENCES

1. Surg 1994; Spears JR, Spokojny AM, Marais HJ. Coronary angioscopy during cardiac catheterization. JACC 1985; 6:93-7.

2. Litvack IF, Grundfest W, Lee ME, Carroll RN, Foran R, Chaux A, Berci G, Rose HB, Matloff JM, Forrester JS. Angioscopic examination of blood vessel interior in animals and humans. Clin Card 1985; 8:65-70.

3. Katzir A. Optical Fibers in Medicine. Sci Am 1989; 120-125.

4. Auth D, Physical principles and limitations of fiberoptic angioscopy in Endovascular Surgery 1989; W. B. Saunders and Co., ed Moore WS and Ahn SS, 31-38.

5. Franzen D, Hopp HW, Korsten J, Hilger HH. A prospective study on percutaneous coronary angioscopy with different guiding techniques in patients with coronary heart disease. Eur Heart J 1992; 13:655-660.

6. Sherman CT, Litvack F, Grundfest W, Lee M, Hickey A, Chaux A, Kass R, Blanche C, Matloff J, Morgenstern L, Ganz W, Swan HJC, Forrester J: Demonstration of thrombus and complex atheroma by in-vivo angioscopy in patients with unstable angina pectoris. NEJM 315:913-919, 1986.

7. Forrester J, Litvack F, Grundfest W, Segalowitz J, Hickey A. Symposium: intravascular imaging and flow: Cardiac angioscopy in acute ischemic syndromes. Amer J of Cardiac Imaging 1988; 2:178-184.

8. den Heijer P, Foley DP, Hillege HL, Lablanche JM. The 'Ermonville classification of observations at coronary angioscopy--evaluation of intra- and inter-observer agreement. European Working Group on Coronary Angioscopy. Eur Heart J 1994; 15:815-22.

9. Siegel RJ, Ariani M, Fishbein MC, Chae JS et al. Histopathologic validation of angioscopy and intravascular ultrasound. Circulation 1991; 84:109-17.

10. Schwartz A, Burrig KF, Aulich A. Usefulness of angioscopy in stenotic processes of the carotid - a comparison with morphological findings. Endoscopy 1988; 20:107-110.

11. Van Stiegman G, Perace W, Bartle E et al. Flexible angiscopy seems faster and more specific than arteriography. Arch Surg 1987; 122:279-283.

12. Johnson C, Hansen D, Vracko R, Ritchie J. Angiscopy-more sensitive for identifying thrombus, distal emboli, and subintimal dissection. J Am Coll Cardiol 1989; 13:146A.

13. den Heijer P, Foley DR, Escaned J, Hillege HL. Angioscopic versus angiographic detection of intimal dissection and intracoronary thrombus. JACC 1994; 24:649-54.

14. Mizuno K, Yanagida T, Shibuya T, Arakawa K. The effectiveness of coronary angioscopy in detecting intraluminal pathologic changes. Jpn Circ J 1992; 56:586-91.

15. Uretsky BF, Denys BG, Counihan PC, Ragosta M. Angioscopic evaluation of incompletely obstructing coronary intraluminal filling defects; comparison of angiography. Cathet Cardiovasc Diagn 1994; 33:323-9.

16. Spears JR, Ati M, Raza SJ, Iyer GS. Quantitative angioscopy: A novel method of measurement of luminal dimensions during angioscopy with the use of a lightwire. Cardiovasc Intervent Radiol 1994; 17:197-203.

17. Lee G, Garcia J, Corso P, Chan M, Rink J, Pichard A, Lee K, Reis R, Mason D. Correlation of coronary angioscopic to angiographic findings in coronary artery disease. ACC 1986; 57:238-241.

18. Schuurbiers JC, Slager CJ, Serruys PW. Luminal volume reconstruction from angiscopic video images of casts from human coronary arteries. Am J Cardiol 1994; 78:764-8.

19. Mizuno K, Miyamoto A, Satomura K, Kurita A et al. Angioscopic coronary macromorphology in patients with acute coronary disorders. Lancet 1991; 337:809-12.

20. White CJ, Ramee SR, Collins TJ, Mesa JE, Jain A. Percutaneous angioscopy of saphenous vein coronary bypass grafts. J Am Coll Cardiol 1993; 21:1181-5.

21. Mizuno K, Satomura K, Miyamoto A, Arakawa K et al. Angioscopic evaluation of coronary artery thrombi in acute coronary syndromes. New Engl Journal of Medicine 1992;326:287-91.

22. Uchida Y, Nakamura F, Tomaru T, Sonoki H, Sumino S, Sugimoto T. Angiographic and angioscopic observations of the arterial luminal changes induced by vasospasm. Am Heart J 1987; 114:1096-1101.

23. Uchida Y, Hasegawa K, Kawamura K, Shibuya I. Angiocopic observation of the coronary luminal changes induced by percutaneous transluminal coronary angioplasty. Am Heart J 1989; 117:769-776.

24. den Heijer P, van Dijk RB, Hillege HL, Pentinga ML. Serial angioscopic and angiographic observations during the first hour after successful coronary angioplasty: a preamble to a multicenter trial adressing angioscopic markers for restenosis. Am Heart J 1994; 128:656-63.

25. Barrazet FS, Dupouy PJ, Rande JL, Hirosaka A. Angioscopy after laser and balloon coronary angioplasty. J Am Coll Cardiol 1994; 23:1321-6.

26. Nakamura F, Kvasnicka J, Uchida Y, Geschwind HJ. Percutaneous angioscopic evaluation of luminal changes induced by excimer laser angioplasty, Am Heart J 1992; 124:1467-72.

27. Ito A, Miyazaki S, Nonogi H, Ozono K, et al. Angioscopic and intravascular ultrasound imagings before and after percutaneous holmium-YAG laser coronary angioplasty. Am Heart J 1993; 125:556-8.

28. Annex BH, Sketch MH Jr, Stack RS, Phillips HR. Transluminal extraction coronary atherectomy. Cardiol Clin 1994; 12:611-22.

226

29. Itoh A, Miyazaki S, Nonogi H, Daikoku S, Haze K. Angioscopic prediction of successful dilatation and of restenosis in percutaneous transluminal coronary angioplasty. Significance of yellow plaque. Circ 1995; 81:1389-96.

30. White CJ, Ramee SR, Mesa JE, Collins TJ. Percutaneous coronary angioscopy in patients with restenosis after coronary angioplasty. J Am Coll Cardiol 1991; 17:46b-49b.

31. Teirstein PS, Schatz RA, Wong SC, Rocha-Singh KJ. Coronary stenting with angioscopic guidance. Am J Cardiol 1995; 75:344-7.

32. Strumpf RK, Heuser RR, Eagan JT Jr. Angioscopy: a valuable tool in the deployment and evaluation of intracoronary stents. Am Heart J 1993; 126:1204-10.

33. den Heijer P, van Dijk RB, Twisk SP, Lie K. Early stent occlusion is not always caused by thrombosis. Cathet Cardiovasc Diagn 1993; 29:136-40.

34. Resar JR, Brinker J. Early coronary artery stent restenosisl utility of percutaneous coronary angioscopy. Cathet Cadiovasc Diag 1992; 27:276-9.

35. Ueda Y, Nanto S, Komamura K, Kodama K. Neointimal coverage of stents in human coronary arteries observed by angioscopy. J Am Coll Cardiol 1994; 23:341-6.

36. Bessou JP, Melki J, Bouchart F, Mouton-Schleifer D, et al. Intraoperative coronary angioscopy-technique and results: a study of 38 patients. J Card Surg 1993; 8:483-7.

37. White GH, Siegel SB, Colman PD, Kopchok GE, White RA. Intraoperative coronary angioscopy: development of practical techniques. Angiology 1990; 41:793-800.

38. Grundfest W, Litvack F, Glick D, Segalowitz J, Treiman R, Cohen L, Foran R, Levin P, Cossman D, Carroll R, Spigelman A, Forrester J, Circ 1988; 78:3.

39. Dietrich EB, Yoffe B, Kiessling JJ, Santiago O, et al. Angioscopy in endovascular surgery: recent technical advances to ehance intervention selection and failure analysis. Angiology 1992; 43:1-10.

40. Hofling G, Polnita A, Bauriedel G, Backa D, Lauterjung L, Simpson J. Use of angioscopy to assess the results of percutaneous atherectomy. Am J Cardiac Imaging 1989; 3:20-26.

41. Trubel W, Magoometschnigg H, al-Hachich Y, Staudacher M. Intraoperative control following femorodistal revascularization: angioscopy is superior to angiography. Thorac Cardiovasc 42:199-207.

228

ACKNOWLEDGEMENTS

The authors would like to express their appreciation to the Grand Foundation, Helga and irving Cooper and Miriam and Al Winner for their financial support, and to Ms. Dwana L. Williams for her editorial support.

TABLE 1:

CLASSIFICATION OF NATIVE LESIONS IN
CORONARY ARTERIES

	Normal	Stable Atheroma	Disrupted	Thrombus
Surface	Smooth	Smotoh	Torn	Smooth
Color	White yellow	White Yellow*	White/or	Red
Mass	None lumen	Obstructs	Usually	Obstructs or occludes

*Some disrupted surfaces have subintimal hemorrhage

TABLE 2

LIMITATIONS OF ANGIOSCOPY AND ANGIOGRAPHY

<u>Angioscopy</u>

Length of vessel examined is limited
Quantitative measurements are impractical
Interpretation is subjective
Difficult to perform in tortuous vessels

<u>Angiography</u>

Major damage is often undetectable
Underestimates complex lesion morphology
Does not detect small thrombi
Does not identify plaque composition

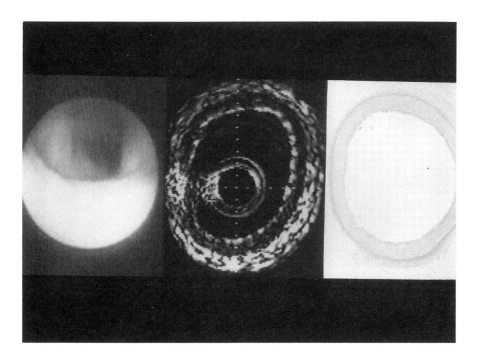

Figure 1. A Normal blood vessels as seen by angioscopy, intravascular ultrasound (IVUS) and microscopy. The angioscopic image (top) has a white, smooth, and flat surface. Intravascular ultrasound image reveals circular vessel with a smooth luminal surface, and the typical "three-ringed" appearance representing internal elastic lamina media and adventita. The circular structure in the center of the image is the IVUS catheter artifact. Microscopy demonstrates a normal musclular artery. The vessel was classified as a normal artery by angioscopy, ultrasound, and microscopy. Hematoxylin and eosin stain, original magnification X2.

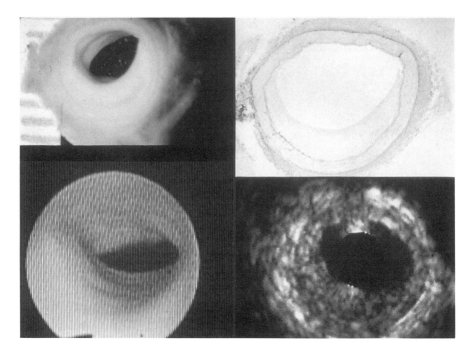

Figure 2. A stable atheroma as seen by angioscopy, IVUS, gross inspection and microscopy. The angioscopic image is a yellow mass with a smooth surface; the lumen is elliptical. The intravascular ultrasound image reveals increase in an wall thickness from 3 to 9 o'clock and a smooth luminal surface. Gross pathology and histology demonstrate eccentric fibrous plaque in the area of increased wall thickness by ultrasound. This vessel was classified as stable atheroma by angioscopy, ultrasound and histopathology. Hematoxylin and eosin stain, original magnification X2.

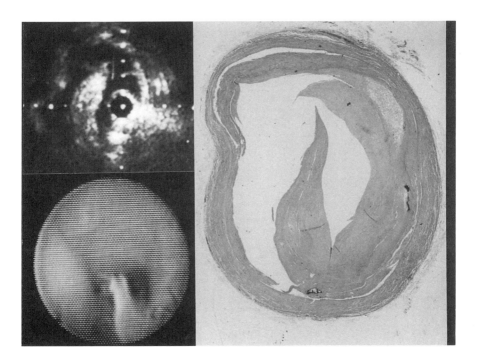

Figure 3. A typical intimal disruption. The images angioscopic and IVUS images demonstrate separation of
plaque (arrow) from the arterial wall. These findings are
confirmed bymicroscopy (C). This artery was classified
as disrupted by all three methods. Hematoxylin and eosin stain, original magnification X2.

234

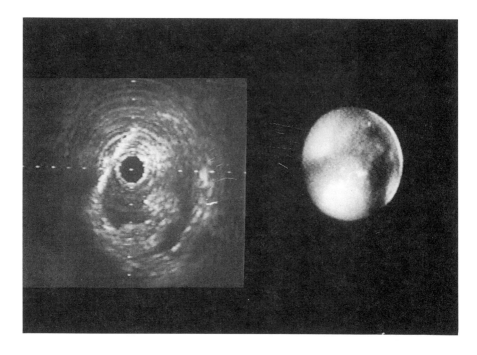

Figure 4. A thrombus is imaged by angioscopy and IVUS. Angioscopic image reveals elevated red tubular intraluminal mass (*). The IVUS image reveals a pedunculated smooth intraluminal mass (*). Both images were classified as thrombus.

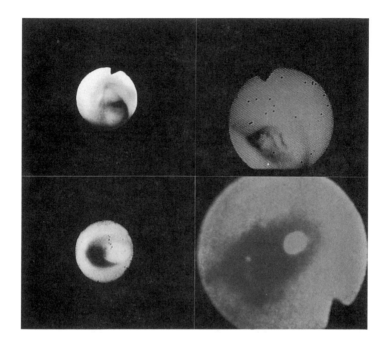

Figure 5. The four stages of atheroma evolution, top left, stable atheroma in vivo as seen by angioscopy. This lesion is smooth, yellow and partially occludes the coronary lumen. Top left, a disrupted attheroma in the left anterior descending coronary artery of a patient with unstable angina who was referred to bypass surgery. Bottom right, a crescent-shaped fresh, partially occlusive coronary thrombosis in a patient with acute unstable rest angina pectoris unresponsive to medical therapy. The surface of the clot undulated during routine flushing to clear blood from the imaging field. Coronary thrombi are typically adherent and do not dislodge during flushing. Bottom right, a completely occlusive coronary thrombosis in the left anterior descending coronary artery of a patient having an acurte myocardial infarction. The angioscope is very close to the thrombus, and the vessel walls are outside the field of view. The central white spot is the angioscope's imaging lightr reflected back off the glistening thrombus.

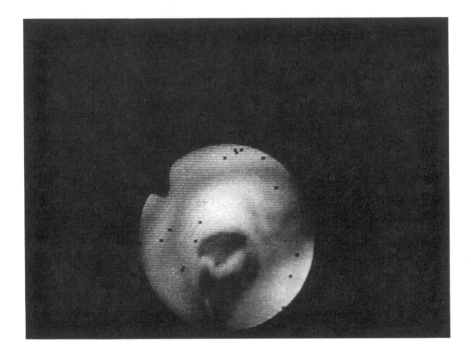

Figure 6. Angioscopic evidence of severe intimal change caused by balloon angioplasty. The angiogram revealed a subtle linear dissection. The angioscopic image shows the double lumen created by the dissection, and subintimal hemorrhage.

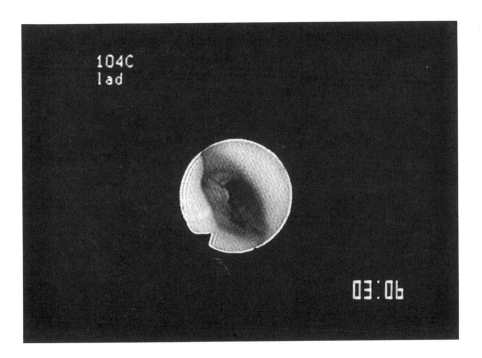

Figure 7. Atheroma with residual disruption, but without thrombosis two weeks after transmural infarction. The patient had not been treated with a thrombolytic agent. Thus, this is an example of spontaneous endogenous thrombolysis after presumed coronary occlusion.

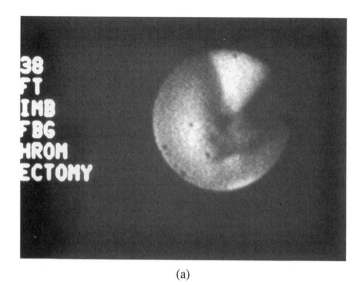

(a)

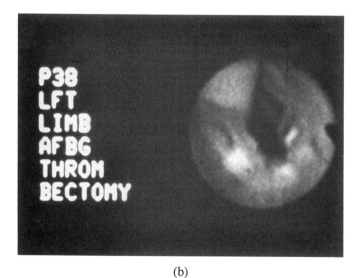

(b)

Figure 8a, 8b. Top, retained intimal debris is seen after thrombectomy in this 59 year old male with an acutely failed limb of his aorta femoral bypass graft after arteriography. Bottom, the same area as in figure 4, after repeat thrombectomy.

10.

USEFULNESS OF INTRAVASCULAR ULTRASOUND FOR
DETECTING ATHEROSCLEROSIS PROGRESSION OR
REGRESSION.

Mun K. Hong, MD, Martin B. Leon, MD, and
Gary S. Mintz, MD

from the Intravascular Ultrasound Imaging and Cardiac
Catheterization Laboratories, Washington Hospital Center,
Washington, DC.

Author for correspondence and reprint request:

Gary S. Mintz, MD
Director, Intravascular Ultrasound Program
Washington Cardiology Center
110 Irving St., NW, 4B-1
Washington, DC 20010
(202)877-5975
(202)877-3339 (FAX)

INTRODUCTION

Atherosclerosis as the major contributor to coronary artery disease and mortality:

Atherosclerosis is the major cause of death in the United States, despite recent evidence suggesting an overall reduction in cardiovascular mortality (1-6). Findings of the International Atherosclerosis Project (7) and others (8) indicate that cardiovascular morbidity and mortality are related to the overall extent of atherosclerosis. The ubiquitous nature of atherosclerosis, even in young subjects, is well established (9). Likewise, the contribution of dyslipidemia as the most powerful predictor of coronary artery disease, with the exception of age, is well understood (10,11). Therefore, reduction (ideally, prevention) of atherosclerosis should have a major impact on cardiovascular morbidity and mortality. In this regard, both the treatment options to reduce atherosclerosis and the imaging modalities to document the progression or regression of atherosclerosis are important.

The relationship between the plaque burden and luminal narrowing:

One may speculate that there would be a linear relationship between the amount of atherosclerosis and luminal encroachment with adverse clinical consequence. However, there have been pathologic, angiographic, and clinical observations that seem counterintuitive. Glasgov and his colleagues (12) were the first group to show from a pathologic study that the relationship between the progression of atherosclerosis and its effect on lumen compromise is more complex. In the early stages of atherosclerosis, there may actually be a compensatory enlargement, whereby the accumulation of additional atherosclerosis does not result in lumen compromise. Rather, the affected artery enlarges to accommodate the atherosclerotic burden without a reduction in lumen area. Based on serial angiography in same patient cohorts, others have also shown that the atherosclerotic lesions responsible for acute ischemic syndromes are those that were not flow-limiting on the initial angiogram (13,14). Furthermore, there may be a discrepancy between the measurable atherosclerosis "regression", such as seen on serial angiographic studies, and the clinical benefit from lipid reduction. Whereas the angiographic changes may take years to detect (15), the clinical benefit may occur much earlier (16). Thus, luminal narrowing is not the sole indicator of the overall atherosclerosis or clinical significance of the plaque volume.

Objective of the monograph:

The difficult question is how one should objectively document the progression or regression of atherosclerosis, either as a consequence of natural history of the disease or as a result of intervention, such as lipid reduction therapy. This monograph will examine two imaging modalities (angiography and intravascular ultrasound) and their merits in such important studies involving the coronary artery circulation.

SERIAL CORONARY ANGIOGRAPHY

The obvious choice and the gold standard thus far has been the serial coronary angiography. There have been many studies evaluating different treatment strategies to reduce serum cholesterol and their effects on serial angiography (17). Some of these studies (18-21) have shown that atherosclerosis can be stabilized, whereas other studies (22-26) showed that atherosclerosis is reversible. One study (22) showed that new lesion formation can be reduced. These studies have also demonstrated that changes in lesion morphology appear to be a continuum, with lesion progression, stability, and regression often occurring in different lesions within the same patient (27). The changes were only modest, with <0.3 mm change in absolute luminal dimension or 10% in diameter stenosis using both qualitative and quantitative measurements. Furthermore, there is no uniform methodology to accurately assess angiographic progression or regression of atherosclerosis. There are other limitations of serial coronary angiography in detecting atherosclerosis progression or regression (Table 1). These inherent limitations (28,29) include technical difficulties of reproducible data acquisition on serial studies, intra- and interobserver variability of interpreting the acquired data, and inability of angiograms to provide insight into the mechanism of atherosclerosis progression or regression. Coronary angiography does not measure atherosclerosis but rather the reduction in luminal caliber at the lesion site relative to adjacent "reference arterial segments" considered to be free of disease. Thus, there is a distinction between angiographic regression and true atherosclerotic regression resulting from a reduction in overall plaque mass.

Table 1. Limitations of Coronary Angiography on Detecting Atherosclerosis Progression or Regression.

I. Difficulties with Data Acquisition:
   Consistency on serial angiograms
II. Difficulties with Data Interpretation:
   Underestimates the extent of disease ;
   Intra- and inter-observer variability;
   Compensatory enlargement misinterpreted as regression
III. Mechanistic Aspects:
   Does not measure atherosclerosis;
   Cannot assess lesion composition;
IV. Other Limitations:
   Requires large sample size to demonstrate significant regression;
   Requires prolonged study duration.

Reprinted with permission from *Annals of Internal Medicine* (17). Please refer to reference 17 for further details.

INTRAVASCULAR ULTRASOUND

Rationale for the use of intravascular ultrasound:

Alternatively, intravascular ultrasound (30-32) is a recent development that permits detailed, high-quality, cross-sectional pictures of the coronary arteries *in vivo*, and is not subject to the same limitations as coronary arteriography. The normal coronary artery architecture (intima, media, and adventitia), the major components of the atherosclerotic plaque (lipid, fibrous connective tissue, and calcium), and the changes that occur in coronary arterial dimensions and anatomy with the atherosclerotic disease process can be studied *in vivo* in a manner previously not possible using any other imaging modality (Figure 1).

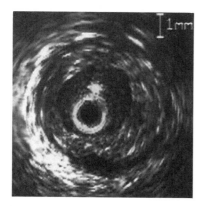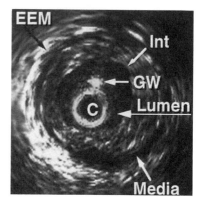

Figure 1. The left and right panels show identical intravascular ultrasound cross-sectional images to illustrate the typical appearance of an atherosclerotic coronary artery; the right panel is labeled. From inner to outer, there is the imaging catheter (Cath), guidewire (GW), lumen, intima (Int), media (M), and external elastic membrane (EEM), which represents the adventitia.

Intravascular ultrasound systems:

The miniaturization of ultrasound crystals and transducers has resulted in commercially available intravascular ultrasound imaging catheters. At present, the smallest catheters available are 2.9 Fr (0.96 mm outside diameter). Intravascular ultrasound catheters are side-looking and create a 360^0 tomographic image of the artery. One catheter system uses a modification of phased array technology (33), which contains 64 tiny transducer elements located circumferentially at the tip of the catheter and fired sequentially. The other catheter systems currently use a rotating transducer to generate the tomographic image. Intravascular ultrasound transducers used to image coronary arteries have a 20 to 30 MHz center carrying frequency. Lower frequencies have lower resolution and are more suited to imaging peripheral vessels, the aorta, and cardiac chambers. Although higher frequency transducers would improve resolution, current designs have limited penetration and produce images *in vivo* in which the artery is obscured by the spontaneous contrast effects of reflections from red blood cells. The accuracy of both phased array and mechanical systems has been validated *in vitro*. *In vivo* intravascular ultrasound studies of patients with coronary artery disease have reported findings that parallel many of the previous *in vitro* pathologic observations.

Quantification of atherosclerotic plaque by intravascular ultrasound:

Quantification of atherosclerosis requires accurate measurements of both cross-sectional and longitudinal dimensions. The ability of intravascular ultrasound to measure coronary arterial cross-sectional dimensions accurately has been validated *in vitro* (34-42). Routine planar measurements include total arterial cross-sectional area [defined as the arterial area contained within the boundary of the external elastic membrane (EEM)], lumen cross-sectional area, their difference (which is equal to the combined cross-sectional area of atherosclerotic plaque plus media), and percent cross-sectional narrowing (plaque + media cross sectional area/EEM cross sectional area, Figure 2). The correlation coefficients for these measurements range from 0.85 to 0.98 compared to histology. The ability of intravascular ultrasound to measure media thickness (and, therefore, quantify plaque cross-sectional area as opposed to plaque + media cross-sectional area) is variable. The media appears to thin or disappear completely behind some atheromas (41) either because of anatomic thinning of the media or because of attenuation of the ultrasonic beam by the atherosclerotic plaque. Alternatively, what is perceived to be media may instead be an acoustic effect of overlying plaque. Pathologically, media thickness does not change significantly in adolescents and young or mature adults (43). It is only with advanced atherosclerosis that media thins (44-46). As a result, the combined measurements of plaque + media is used as a measure of plaque cross-sectional area. Finally, intravascular ultrasound measured plaque + media cross-sectional area is not affected by coronary arterial vascular tone (47).

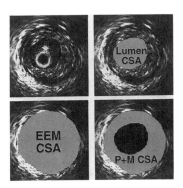

Figure 2. These four panels show identical cross-sectional images to illustrate the standard planar quantitative intravascular ultrasound image analysis. (Abbreviations: EEM CSA=external elastic membrane cross-sectional area; P + M=plaque + media; P + M CSA=EEM CSA - Lumen CSA).

244

Recently, a motorized transducer pullback device has been developed that permits accurate measurements of coronary arterial length (48). Using Simpson's rule and intravascular ultrasound measurements of equidistantly spaced arterial cross-sections (obtained at 1 mm intervals, for example), accurate quantification of plaque volume is a reality. Measurement of plaque volume has been validated *in vitro* using intravascular ultrasound imaging of phantoms constructed to resemble coronary arteries (49) and human coronary arteries obtained at necropsy (50), and analysis of serial cross sections at 1 mm intervals (intravascular ultrasound plaque volume = measured plaque volume + 0.53 ($r=0.97$, $p<0.001$). Alternatively, equidistantly spaced planar intravascular ultrasound cross-sections obtained using a constant transducer pullback rate can be digitized and used to reconstruct three-dimensional coronary artery architecture (51,52). Assuming cylindrical coronary artery geometry, interactive tracing of the EEM and intima could be used to calculate plaque volume. This approach would speed the analysis process considerably.

Determination of plaque composition by intravascular ultrasound:

Numerous investigators have validated the ability of intravascular ultrasound to determine plaque composition *in vitro* (30,34,36,39,53,54). By intravascular ultrasound gray scale analysis, plaque elements are categorized grossly as calcified, densely fibrotic, or soft (Figure 3). Calcium causes bright, highly reflective echoes (brighter than the reference adventitia) with acoustic shadowing of deeper arterial structures. Dense fibrous tissue causes bright, highly reflective echoes (as bright or brighter than the reference adventitia, but *without* acoustic shadowing). Soft plaque is less dense than the reference adventitia; soft plaque is lipid-rich, but may also contain loose connective tissue, intimal hyperplasia, and thrombus. In one study, intravascular ultrasound determined plaque composition *in vitro* with a diagnostic accuracy of 96% (36). The analysis of the raw radiofrequency signal holds promise as a more precise method of analyzing plaque components, such as the % lipid content in any diseased segment.

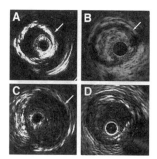

Figure 3. Panel A shows circumferential calcific atherosclerotic plaque (white arrow). Panel B shows fibrotic atherosclerotic plaque, which is as bright or brighter than the reference adventitia (white arrow) without acoustic shadowing of deeper arterial structures. Panel C shows soft atherosclerotic plaque, which is less dense compared to the reference adventitia (white arrow). Panel D shows a mixed lesion.

Detection of atherosclerosis in angiographically normal reference coronary arterial segments by intravascular ultrasound:

Many investigators have reported detecting significant atherosclerosis in angiographically normal reference segments either distal or proximal to a lesion targeted for transcatheter therapy (34,55-59). The incidence is as high as 93% (59) and the percent cross-sectional narrowing ranges from 35±23% (34) to 51±13% (59) (Figure 4). Atherosclerosis contained in angiographically normal proximal reference segments frequently is lipid-rich and eccentric (57,58), especially in patients who present with unstable coronary syndromes (60). In one study, the mean arc of fibrosis + calcification of the atherosclerosis within the angiographically normal segment was 45^0 as compared to target lesions that contained a mean arc of fibrosis + calcification that averaged 215^0 (61).

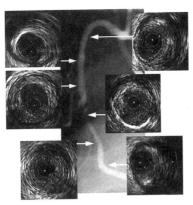

Figure 4. This is an intravascular ultrasound cross-sectional image of right coronary artery. There is extensive atherosclerotic plaque proximal and distal to the mid lesion.

Detection of atherosclerosis progression and regression by intravascular ultrasound:

The ability of intravascular ultrasound to detect early coronary atherosclerosis and its progression has been shown in animal models as early as 5 weeks after intimal injury. Angiography showed an initial decrease in lumen diameter after intimal injury, but no further evidence of plaque formation while intravascular ultrasound showed progressive plaque accumulation (62,63). Furthermore, intravascular ultrasound was able to detect regression of atherosclerosis in this model after 3, 6, and 9 months on a regression diet (64).

In humans, intravascular ultrasound can detect coronary artery intimal thickening in hearts soon after cardiac transplantation (65-68). Originally thought to be normal, a three-layered appearance of a coronary artery indicates abnormal intimal thickening that exceeds 178 um (69). The intravascular ultrasound measurements of intimal thickness correlate well with histologic measurements (r=0.91, p<0.001) (41). Intimal thickness has been shown to increase with patient age (70), to be a typical finding in otherwise normal coronary arterial segments in patients with hypercholesterolemia (71), and to be an early part of atherosclerotic disease process (72,73). Serial intravascular ultrasound observations have detected early progression of allograft atherosclerosis that correlated with the time elapsed post transplantation and that was not apparent angiographically (62,66,67). Table 2 summarizes the advantages of intravascular ultrasound in studying atherosclerosis progression or regression.

Table 2. Advantages of Intravascular Ultrasound in Detecting Atherosclerosis Progression or Regression.

I. Intravascular ultrasound (IVUS) can quantify the amount of atherosclerotic plaque (49).

II. IVUS can determine plaque composition (36).

III. IVUS routinely detects significant atherosclerosis in angiographically normal reference coronary arterial segments (34,55-59).

IV. IVUS can detect disease progression (62,63) and regression (64).

References are given in parenthesis.

Limitations of intravascular ultrasound for serial studies:

Despite the advantages listed above, there are several limitations of intravascular ultrasound for serial studies. One limitation is the requirement for intracoronary insertion of the catheter. Although this procedure is in general safe, there is a small percentage of patients (0.4%), who may experience complications related to the procedure (74). Furthermore, due to the catheter size (smallest catheter size of 0.96 mm), distal vessels or diseased arterial segments <1 mm cannot be accurately studied. Likewise, unlike coronary angiography, which can interrogate the entire epicardial segments of the major coronary arteries, it would be time-consuming and less than ideal to study all three major epicardial arteries at the same time, especially with the automatic pull-back system. Finally, there is additional cost of the intravascular ultrasound machines and the catheters.

CONCLUSIONS

In summary, intravascular ultrasound has the potential to answer many of the questions regarding atherosclerosis progression and regression, without the limitations inherent in coronary arteriography. Because intravascular ultrasound can measure the extent of disease, even in "angiographically normal" segments, it should be a more sensitive detector of atherosclerosis progression and regression than quantitative coronary arteriography. Likewise, changes in plaque volume may be detected earlier with intravascular ultrasound than changes in lumen dimensions can be detected with quantitative coronary arteriography (75). Furthermore, atherosclerotic plaque volume can be quantified, not just inferred. Assessment of lesion morphology in conjunction with changes in plaque burden may identify predictors of plaque regression and, therefore, aid in the selection of patients with target lesions amenable to pharmacologic and lifestyle interventions. Thus, although it is not without limitations, intravascular ultrasound should become the gold standard for the assessment of coronary atherosclerosis and the success of strategies designed to modify its progression and regression.

248

REFERENCES

,1. Goldman L, Cook EF. The decline in ischemic heart disease mortality rates: An analysis of the comparative effects of medical interventions and changes in lifestyle. Ann Intern Med. 1984;101:825-836.

2. Sytkowski PA, Kannel WB, D'Agostino RB. Changes in risk factors and the decline in mortality from cardiovascular disease: The Framingham Heart Study. N Engl J Med. 1990;322:1635-1641.

3. Kaplan GA, Cohen BA, Cohen RD, Guralnik J. The decline in ischemic heart disease mortality: Prospective evidence from the Alameda County Study. Am J Epidemiol. 1988;127:1131-1142.

4. Cohn BA, Kaplan GA, Cohen RD. Did early detection and treatment contribute to the decline in ischemic heart disease mortality? Prospective evidence from the Alameda County Study. Am J Epidemiol. 1988;127:1143-1144.

5. Sempos C, Cooper R, Kovar MG, McMillen M. Divergence of the recent trends in coronary mortality for the four major race-sex groups in the United States. Am J Public Health. 1988;78:1422-1427.

6. Weinstein MC, Coxson PG, Williams LW, Pass TM, Stason WB, Goldman L. Forecasting coronary heart disease incidence, mortality, and cost: The coronary heart disease policy model. Am J Public Health. 1987;77:1417-1426.

7. Deupree RH, Fields RI, McMahan CA, Strong JP. Atherosclerotic lesions and coronary heart disease: Key relationships in necropsied cases. Lab Invest 1973;28:252-262.

8. Daoud AS, Florentin RA, Goodale F. Diffuse coronary atherosclerosis versus isolated plaques in the etiology of myocardial infarction. Am J Cardiol 1964;13:69-74.

9. Wissler RW. Update on the pathogenesis of atherosclerosis. Am J Med 1991;91(Suppl 1B):3S-9S.

10. Stokes JI. Dyslipidemia as a risk factor for cardiovascular disease and untimely death: The Framingham Study. In: Stokes JI, Mancini M, ed. Atherosclerosis Reviews. New York: Raven Press Limited, 1988.

11. Simons LA. Interrelations of lipids and lipoproteins with coronary artery disease mortality in 19 counties. Am J Cardiol 1986;57:5G-10G.

12. Glagov S, Weisenberg E, Zarins CK, Stankunavicius R, Kolettis GJ. Compensatory enlargement of human atherosclerotic coronary arteries. N Engl J Med. 1987;316:1371-1375.

13. Ambrose JA, Tannenbaum MA, Alexopoulos D, Hjemdahl-Monsen CE, Leavy J, Weiss M, Borrico S, Gorlin R, Fuster V. Angiographic progression of coronary artery disease and the development of myocardial infarction. J Am Coll Cardiol 1988;12:56-62.

14. Little WC, Constantinescu M, Applegate RJ, Kutcher MA, Burrows MT, Kahl FR, Santamore WP. Can coronary angiography predict the site of subsequent myocardial infarction in patients with mild-to-moderate coronary artery disease? Circulation 1988;78:1157-1166.

15. Brown G, Albers J, Fisher LD, Schaefer SM, Lin JT, Kaplan C, et al. Regression of coronary artery disease as a result of intensive lipid-lowering therapy in men with high levels of apolipoprotein B. N Engl J Med. 1990;323:1289-1298.

16. The Pravastatin Multinational Study Group for Cardiac Risk Patients. Effects of pravastatin in patients with serum total cholesterol levels from .2 to 7.8 mmol/liter (200 to 300 mg/dl) plus two additional atherosclerotic risk factors. Am J Cardiol 1993;72:1031-1037.

17. Hong MK, Mintz GS, Popma JJ, Kent KM, Pichard AD, Satler LF, Leon MB. Limitations of angiography for analyzing coronary atherosclerosis progression or regression. Ann Intern Med 1994;121:348-354.

18. Buchwald H, Varco RL, Matts JP, Long JM, Fitch LL, Campbell GS, et al. Effect of partial ileal bypass surgery on mortality and morbidity from coronary heart disease in patients with hypercholesterolemia: Report of the program on the surgical control of the hyperlipidemias (POSCH). N Engl J Med. 1990;323:946-955.

19. Arntzenius A, Kromhout D, Barth JD, Reiber JHC, Bruschke AGV, Buios, B, et al. Diet, lipoproteins and progression of coronary atherosclerosis. N Engl J Med. 1985;312:805-811.

20. Brensike J, Levy R, Kelsey SF, Passamani, ER, Richardson, JM, Loh, IK, et al. Effects of therapy with cholestyramine on progression of coronary atherosclerosis. Results of the NHLBI Type II coronary intervention study. Circulation. 1984;69:313-324.

21. Schuler G, Hambrecht R, Schlierf G, Niebauer J, Hauser K, Neumann J, et al. Regular physical exercise and low-fat diet: Effects on progression of coronary artery disease. Circulation. 1992;86:1-11.

22. Ornish D, Brown SE, Scherwitz LW, Billings JH, Armstrong WT, Ports TA, et al. Can lifestyle changes reverse coronary heart disease? The Lifestyle Heart Trial. Lancet. 1990;136:129-133.

23. Blankenhorn D, Nessim SA, Johnson RL, San Marco ME, Azen AP, Cashin-Hemphill L. Beneficial effects of combined colestipol-niacin therapy on coronary atherosclerosis and coronary venous bypass grafts. JAMA. 1987;257:3233-3240.

24. Brown BG, Lin JT, Kelsey S, Passamani ER, Levy RI, Dodge HT, et al. Progression of coronary atherosclerosis in patients with probably familial hypercholesterolemia. Atherosclerosis. 1989;9(Suppl I):I-81-1-90.

25. Kane JP, Malloy MJ, Ports TA, Phillips NR, Diehl JC, Havel RJ. Regression of coronary atherosclerosis during treatment of familial hypercholesterolemia with combined drug regimens. JAMA. 1990;264:3007-3012.

26. Watts GF, Lewis B, Brunt JNH, Lewis ES, Coltart DJ, Smith LDR, et al. Effects on coronary artery disease of lipid-lowering diet, or diet plus cholestyramine, in the St Thomas Atherosclerosis Regression Study (STARS). Lancet. 1992;339:563-569.

27. Blankenhorn DH. Regression of atherosclerosis: What does it mean? Am J Med. 1991;90(Suppl 2A):42S-47S.

28. de Feyter PJ, Serruys PW, Davies MJ, Richardson P, Lubsen J, Oliver MF. Quantitative coronary angiography to measure progression and regression of coronary atherosclerosis: Value, limitations, and implications for clinical trials. Circulation. 1991;84:412-423.

29. Selzer RH, Hagerty C, Azen SP, Siebes M, Lee P, Shicore A, et al. Precision and reproducibility of quantitative coronary arteriography with application to controlled clinical trials. J Clin Invest. 1989;83:520-526.

30. Coy KM, Maurer G, Siegel RJ. Intravascular ultrasound imaging: A current perspective. J Am Coll Cardiol 1991;18:1811-1823.

31. Nissen SE, Gurley JC, Booth DC, DeMaria AN. Intravascular ultrasound of the coronary arteries: Current applications and future directions. Am J Cardiol 1992;69:18H-29H.

32. Liebson RP, Klein LW. Intravascular ultrasound in coronary atherosclerosis: A new approach to clinical assessment. Am Heart J 1992;123:1643-1660.

33. Bom N, ten Hoff H, Lancee CT, Gussenhoven WJ, Bosch JG. Early and recent intraluminal ultrasound devices. In J Cardiac Imaging 1989;4:79-88.

34. Tobis JM, Mallery J, Mahon D, Lehman K, Zalesky P, Griffith J, et al. Intravascular imaging of human coronary arteries in vivo: Analysis of tissue characteristics with comparison to histologic specimens. Circulation 1991;83:913-926.

35. Pandian N, Kreis A, Brockway B, Isner JM, Sacharaoff A, Boleza E, et al. Ultrasound angioscopy: Real-time, two-dimensional, intraluminal ultrasound imaging of blood vessels. Am J Cardiol 1988;62:493-494.

36. Potkin BN, Bartorelli AL, Gessert JM, Neville RF, Almagor Y, Roberts WC, et al. Coronary artery imaging with intravascular high-frequency ultrasound. Circulation 1990;81:1575-1585.

37. Nissen SE, Grines CL, Gurley JC, Sublett K, Haynie D, Diaz C, et al. Application of a new phased-array ultrasound imaging catheter in the assessment of vascular dimensions: In vivo comparison to cineangiography. Circulation 1990;81:660-666.

38. Tobis JM, Mallery JA, Gessert J, Griffith J, Mahon D, Bessen M, et al. Intravascular ultrasound cross-sectional arterial imaging before and after balloon angioplasty in vitro. Circulation 1989;80:873-882.

39. Nishimura RA, Edwards WE, Warnes CA, Reeder GS, Holmes DR, Jr, Tajik AJ, et al. Intravascular ultrasound imaging: In vitro validation and pathologic correlation. 1990;16:145-154.

40. Hodgson JM, Graham SP, Sarakus AD, Dame SG, Stephens DN, Dhillon PS, et al. Clinical percutaneous imaging of coronary anatomy using an over-the-wire ultrasound catheter system. In J Cardiac Imaging 1989;4:186-193.

41. Mallery JA, Tobis JM, Griffith J, Gessert J, McRae M, Moussabeck O, et al. Assessment of normal and atherosclerotic arterial wall thickness with an intravascular ultrasound imaging catheter. Am Heart J 1990;119:1392-1400.

42. Lonn E, Lockwood G, Gotlieb A, Foster S, Ryan L, Rakowski H, et al. Very high frequency intravascular ultrasound: In vitro identification and quantification of components of the human arterial wall. Circulation 1991;84:II-675.

43. Velican D, Velican C. Study of coronary intimal thickening. Atherosclerosis 1985;56:331-344.

44. Crawford T, Levene CI. Medial thinning in atheroma. J Path Bacterial 1953;66:19-23.

45. Isner JM, Donaldson RF, Fortin AH, Tischler A, Clarke RH. Attenuation of the media of coronary arteries in advanced atherosclerosis. Am J Cardiol 1986;58:937-939.

46. Gussenhoven E, Pijl A, Frietman P, Gerritsen P, Essed C, Roelandt J, et al. Thinning of the media in atherosclerosis: An in vitro/in vivo intravascular echographic study. Circulation 1990;82:III-458.

47. Yamagishi M, Nissen SE, Booth DC, Gurley JC, Fischer C, DeMaria AN. Impaired nitroglycerin induced vasodilation in coronary atherosclerosis: Evidence from intravascular ultrasound. J Am Coll Cardiol 1992;19:95A.

48. Mintz GS, Keller MB, Fay KG. Motorized IVUS transducer pullback permits accurate quantitative axial length measurements. Circulation 1992;86:I-323.

49. Galli FC, Sudhir K, Kao AK, Hargrave VK, Fitzgerald PF, Yock PG. Direct measurements of plaque volume by three-dimensional ultrasound: Potentials and pitfalls. J Am Coll Cardiol 1992;19:115A.

50. Matar FA, Mintz GS, Farb A, Douek P, Pichard AD, et al. The contribution of tissue removal to lumen improvement after directional coronary atherectomy. Am J Cardiol 1994;74:647-650.

51. Rosenfield K, Losordo DW, Ramaswamy K, Pastore JO, Langevin RE, Razvi S, et al. Three-dimensional reconstruction of human coronary arteries and peripheral arteries recorded during two-dimensional intravascular examination. Circulation 1991;84:1938-1956.

250

52. Coy KM, Park JC, Fishbein MC, Laas T, Diamond GA, Adler L, et al. In vitro validation of three-dimensional intravascular ultrasound for the evaluation of arterial injury after balloon angioplasty. J Am Coll Cardiol 1992;20:692-700.

53. Gussenhoven EJ, Essed CE, Lancee CT, Mastik F, Frietman P, van Egmond FC, et al. Arterial wall characteristics determined by intravascular ultrasound imaging: An in vitro study. J Am Coll Cardiol 1989;14:947-952.

54. Coy KM, Park JC, Siegel RJ. Intravascular ultrasound imaging: From experimental studies to clinical use. Cardiovasc Imaging 1991;3:7-11.

55. Nissen SE, Gurley JC, Grines CL, Booth DC, Fischer C, DeMaria AN. Coronary atherosclerosis is frequently present at angiographically normal sites: Evidence from intravascular ultrasound in man. Circulation 1990;82:III-459.

56. Keren G, Douek P, Hansch E, Milner MR, Pichard AD, Leon MB. Intravascular ultrasound characteristics of atheroma in angiographically "normal" segments. J Am Coll Cardiol 1991;17:217A.

57. Davidson CJ, Tenaglia AN, Buller CE, Kisslo K, Bauman R, Kisslo J. Coronary angiography underestimates post-interventional lesion stenosis and reference segment disease. Circulation 1991;84:II-437.

58. Nissen SE, Gurley JC, Booth DC, Yamagishi M, Berk MR, Fausch M, et al. Mechanisms of false negative coronary arteriography: Insights from intravascular ultrasound imaging. J Am Coll Cardiol 1992;19:140A.

59. Mintz GS, Painter JA, Pichard AD, Kent KM, Satler LF, Popma JJ, et al. Atherosclerosis in angiographically "normal" coronary artery reference segments: An intravascular ultrasound study with clinical correlations. J Am Coll Cardiol 1995;25:1479-1485.

60. Hodgson JM, Reddy KG, Suneja R, Sheehan HM, Lesnefsky EJ, Nair R. Intracoronary ultrasound plaque composition in non-lesional segments differs in unstable angina and stable angina patients: Evidence from intracoronary ultrasound. J Am Coll Cardiol 1992;19:79A.

61. Douek PC, Bonner RF, Mintz GS, Matar F, Keren G, Leon MB. Intravascular ultrasound observations in de novo and restenosis coronary lesions. Cath Cardiovasc Diag 1992;26:77.

62. Lassetter JE, Krall RC, Moddrelle DS, Jenkins RD. Intravascular ultrasound detects plaque progression earlier and more accurately than quantitative coronary arteriography. J Am Coll Cardiol 1991;17:156A.

63. Gupta M, Connolly AJ, Zhu BQ, Sievers RE, Sudhir K, Sun YP, et al. Quantitative analysis of progression of atherosclerosis by intravascular ultrasound: Validation in a rabbit model. Circulation 1992;86:I-518.

64. Lassetter JE, Krall RC, Moddrelle DS, Jenkins RD. Morphologic changes of the arterial wall during regression of experimental atherosclerosis. Circulation 1992;86:I-518.

65. St Goar FG, Pinto FJ, Alderman EL, Fitzgerald PJ, Stinson EB, Billingham ME, et al. Detection of coronary atherosclerosis in young adult hearts using intravascular ultrasound. Circulation 1992;86:756-763.

66. Ventura HO, Jain A, Mesa JE, Collins TJ, White CJ, Ramee SR, et al. Intravascular ultrasound: Progression of allograft coronary artery disease in cardiac transplantation recipients. J Am Coll Cardiol 1992;19:173A.

67. Pinto FJ, St Goar FG, Alderman EL, Valentine HA, Schroeder JS, Stinson EB, et al. Utility of a new classification of transplantation coronary artery disease using intravascular ultrasound. J Am Coll Cardiol 1992;19:173A.

68. St Goar FG, Pinto FJ, Alderman EL, Valentine HA, Schroeder JS, Gao SZ, et al. Intracoronary ultrasound in cardiac transplant recipients: In vivo evidence of "angiographically silent" intimal thickening. Circulation 1992;85:979-987.

69. Fitzgerald FJ, St Goar FG, Connolly AJ, Pinto FJ, Billingham ME, Popp RL, et al. Intravascular ultrasound imaging of coronary arteries. Is three layers the norm? Circulation 1992;86:154-158.

70. Nissen SE, Yamigishi M, Booth DC, Gurley JC, Berk MR, Bates M, et al. Coronary intimal thickness increases with age: Evidence from intravascular ultrasound in normal and CAD patients. J Am Coll Cardiol 1992;19:301A.

71. Zeiher AM, Grove A, Bleile T, Fritz R. Intravascular ultrasound characteristics of coronary arterial wall architecture of early lesions relate to risk factors for coronary artery disease. Circulation 1991;84:II-676.

72. Enos WF, Holmes RH, Beyer J. Coronary disease among United States soldiers killed in action in Korea. JAMA 1953;152:1090-1093.

73. McNamara JJ, Molot MA, Stremple JF, Cutting RT. Coronary artery disease in combat casualties in Vietnam. JAMA 1971;216:1185-1187.

74. Hausmann D, Erbel R, Alibelli-Chemarin MJ, Boksch W, Caracciolo E, Cohn JM, et al. The safety of intracoronary ultrasound: A multicenter survey of 2207 examinations. Circulation 1995;91:623-630.

75. Hong MK, Hoeg JM, Vossoughi J, Hoyt RF, Wong SC, Mintz GS, Zuckerman BD, Mehlman MD, Kent KM, Leon MB. Altered vascular biomechanical properties precede angiographically detectable disease in early atherosclerosis of LDL receptor deficiency. *J Am Coll Cardiol* 1995;Suppl A:290A.

11.

STENOSIS MORPHOLOGY AND RISK ASSESSMENT IN BALLOON ANGIOPLASTY

Koon-Hou Mak, M.B.B.S. and Stephen G. Ellis, M.D.
The Cleveland Clinic Foundation, Cleveland, Ohio

Dr. Mak is funded by an award from the Human Medical
Development Programme of the Ministry of Health, Singapore

Introduction

The risk of percutaneous transluminal balloon angioplasty (PTCA) includes acute vessel closure and perforation potentially leading to myocardial Infarction, need for emergency coronary artery bypass surgery and death. Factors such as the skill of the operators, availability of technology and patient selection are the major consideration in the risk assessment. From 1979-83, the operators from the National Heart, Lung and Blood Institute (NHLBI) PTCA Registry reported major adverse coronary events in 13.6% of their patients (1); with an emergent coronary artery bypass rate of 6.6% and non-fatal myocardial infarction rate of 5.5%. Subsequently, the 1985-86 NHBLI PTCA Registry documented that the emergency coronary artery by-pass and non-fatal myocardial infarction rates fell to 4.3 % and 4.3 % respectively (2). The higher incidence of the elderly, multivessel disease and poor left ventricular function in the latter group of patients may account for the lack of change in the mortality rate; which was about 1%. Hence, with more experienced operators and better technology, the risk for a patient was reduced. In 1988, lesion morphology described on coronary angiography became the basis of risk assessment in the guidelines set up by the American College of Cardiology and American Heart Association (3) (Table 1). This recommendation was first validated by Cragg et al (4) when it was used successfully to help select patients for early hospital discharge after PTCA. Ellis et al (5) further refined the system by sub-dividing the type B lesions into B1 and B2 - B1 lesions consist of only one B characteristic and B2 lesions consist of at least two B characteristics. They demonstrated a step-wise relationship between the lesion types (A, B1, B2 and C) with success and complication rates.

252

Table 1

American College of Cardiology/American Heart Association
Classification of Lesion Type

Type A Lesions (High Success, >85%; Low Risk)

- Discrete (<10 mm length)
- Concentric
- Readily accessible
- Nonangulated segment, <45°
- Smooth contour

- Little or no calcification
- Less than totally occlusive
- Nonostial in location
- No major branch involvement
- Absence of thrombus

Type B Lesions (Moderate Success, 60 to 85%; Moderate Risk)

- Tubular (10 to 20 mm length)
- Eccentric
- Moderate tortuosity of proximal segment
- Moderately angulated segment, >45°, <90°
- Irregular contour

- Moderate to heavy calcification
- Total occlusions <3 months old
- Ostial in location
- Bifurcation lesions requiring double guidewires
- Some thrombus present

Type C Lesions (Low Success, <60%; High Risk)

- Diffuse (>2 cm length)
- Excessive tortuosity of proximal segment
- Extremely angulated segments >90°

- Total occlusions >3 months old
- Inability to protect major side branches
- Degenerated vein grafts with friable lesions

From Ryan TJ, Bauman WB, Kennedy JD et al. Guidelines for percutaneous transluminal coronary angioplasty: A report of the American College of Cardiology/American Heart Association Task Force on Assessment of Diagnostic and Therapeutic Cardiovascular Procedures (Subcommittee on Percutaneous Transluminal Coronary Angioplasty). J Am Coll Cardiol 1993;22:2033-54.

Interventional cardiology has grown in complexity and maturity. The constant improvement of PTCA hardware and upgrading of operator skill have made this classification out-dated in some ways. In the experienced hands of Kahn and Hartzler (6), out of the 3398 lesions attempted, procedural failure rate was only 3.7%. Chronic total occlusion, "rigid" lesion and severe proximal tortuosity were the main reasons. Similarly, Myler et al (7) noted a 7.7% procedural failure rate with chronic total occlusion, unprotected bifurcation lesions, long lesions and thrombus as risk factors. Therefore, certain lesion characteristics are associated with higher risk and may be more important in predicting outcome (8). Furthermore, new and bail-out devices and pharmacologic interventions to make coronary intervention better and safer; which are now competing with and complimenting the humble balloon. In addition, there are now new windows of visualizing lesion morphology using intracoronary ultrasound and angioscopy. This chapter reviews the clinical importance and application of the information available on the angiographic appreciation of lesion morphology.

Total occlusion
The decision to treat a totally occluded vessel poses a management dilemma to the physician. Although lower success and higher complication rates deterred the early angioplasters from intervening these lesions, PTCA was in fact performed as early as in some of the initial patients of Andreas Gruentzig with a success rate was 62% (9). Subsequently, the NHLBI reported that about 10% of attempted PTCA were on totally occluded vessels (2). The early experience from the Thorax Center (10) and Mayo Clinic (11) demonstrated that the procedural success was higher in lesions which were totally occluded for less than 8 to 12 weeks. Kereiakes et al (12) estimated that the success rate for chronic occlusion less than 20 weeks to be 3 to 4 times higher than if it was more than 20 weeks. However, results from some investigators may not substantiate this relationship (13-15). This may be partly accounted by the difficulty in determining the exact duration of occlusion. It could also be likely that there was bias selection of patients with older lesions with more favorable anatomy for PTCA. In addition, success rates depend on the experience of the operators (16). From 1981 to 1989, the success rate for PTCA of totally occluded vessels was only 53% out of 73 lesions compared to 1992, it was 83% out of 180 lesions. Therefore, as a general guideline, the Task Force of the American College of Cardiology and American Heart Association (ACC/AHA) on PTCA suggested that total occlusion for a period of more than three months is probably technically difficult (3).

Although the site and location of the totally occluded vessel were not predictors for success of PTCA (13,15,17), there are several other factors that may influence the likelihood of success, including faint antegrade flow, presence of bridging collaterals, length of totally occluded segment and size of the vessel. Functional total occlusion consists faint contrast filling of a true central lumen associated with delayed distal coronary contrast enhancement and washout (Thrombolysis In Myocardial Infarction or TIMI flow grade I). In the earlier reports (10,17), the success rates for absolute total occlusion were 45 to 63% and functional total occlusion were 78 to 81%.

Although in some studies (13,14) did not show this association, most clinicians would still believe that this characteristic is an important determinant for success (18), especially when the vessel has a tapered morphology (19). The presence of tapering probably facilitates the passage of the guidewire into the true lumen.

Stone et al (13) found that the presence of bridging collaterals to be the most powerful predictor for procedural failure. The success rate was only 18% for those with and 85% without bridging collaterals. But in another large study of 353 patients (20), the success rate for lesions with bridging collaterals did not differ significantly from those without (71% versus 82%). The reason for this observation is uncertain. In general, these collaterals represent enlarged vaso vasorum are fragile and prone to perforation. In addition, it is difficult to manipulate the guidewire through the true lumen. For the same reason, success rate is also low for a totally occluded vessel which is very close to a branch. The guidewire would tend to enter the branch which is the path of least resistance.

Another feature that helps determine procedural success is the length of the occluded segment. The chance of crossing the lesion is greater if the segment is short. The non-visualized segment is estimated by measuring from the point of occlusion to the most proximal point of the distal vessel. This is visualized by collateral contrast filling in a view perpendicular to the direction of flow. Sometimes, a late freeze frame may be useful. Kereiakes et al (12) found that the mean length of non-visualized segments was 21 mm in patients who were successful in recanalization and 35 mm in patients who were unsuccessful. Comparing the length of the non-visualized segment, they found that the likelihood of success is about twice if it was less than 15 mm compared to when it was greater than 15 mm (78% versus 42%). In addition, PTCA was more likely to succeed in patients when the non-visualized segment is measurable (12,17) than when it is not. This observation was further substantiated by pathological examination of post-mortem specimens of chronic totally occluded vessels (21). Loose fibrous tissue penetrated the occluded segment in lesions less than 15 mm long such that a track could be easily formed. On the other hand, fibrous tissue was dispersed in the occluded segment when the lesions was longer than 15 mm.

One of the possible reasons that led the early operators to attempt to revascularize chronic occluded vessels was the belief that the complication rate was negligible. It was felt that it was difficult to make an occluded vessel worse, especially in the presence of adequate collateral flow (22). However, acute complications do occur. The risk is probably between that of diagnostic angiography and PTCA of a subtotally occluded vessel (table 2) and is higher in patients with acute coronary ischemia (12,28). Out of 500 consecutive patients who had PTCA for totally occluded vessels (28), 17 patients (3.4%) experienced major complications including Q wave myocardial infarction (1%), emergent coronary artery bypass surgery (1%) and death (2%). Most of the incidents are as a result of guide catheter, guidewire or balloon induced trauma, side branch closure, extensive dissection and distal embolization. Sometimes the ischemic events are due to treatment of other sites

Table 2

Balloon Angioplasty of Totally Occluded Vessels

Author	Year	No. of Pts.	Functional Occlusion (%)	Age of Occlusion (months)	Primary Success (%)	Collaterals (%)	Emergency CABG (%)	MI (%)	Intra-hospital death (%)	Mean follow-up period (mos.)	Recurrence (%)	Restenosis (%)	Reocclusion (%)	Angiography follow-up (%)	Long-term clinical improvement (%)
Dervan[23]	1983	13	69	1	54	100	0	0	0	6	43	39	4	100	86
Serruys[10]	1985	49	33	2	57	76	2	18	0	7	65	25	40	71	64
Kereiakes[12]	1985	76	10	7	53	NR	1	11	0	7	75	NR	NR	30	75
DiSciascio[14]	1986	46	50	2	63	100	4	0	0	8	48	NR	NR	100	52
Ellis[24]	1989	484	NR	3	NR	74	NR	NR	NR	8	77	56	21	53	NR
Warren[25]	1990	44	0	1	59	100	0	0	0	31	38	NR	NR	100	88
Stone[13]	1990	905	40	12	72	74	0.8	0.6	0.8	NR	38	NR	NR	NR	69
Stewart[26]	1991	95	NR	NR	47	NR	3	2	0	14	59	NR	NR	NR	83
Bell[15]	1992	354	0	2	66	40	3	2	3	32	59	45	14	NR	NR
Ivanhoe[17]	1992	480	45	NR	66	NR	10	2	1	48	54	38	16	53	67
Haine[27]	1993	500	NR	2	67	NR	1	1	2	NR	NR	NR	NR	NR	NR
Pooled		3046	32	6	67	69	3	1.8	1.3	26	54	46	18	53	70

CABG = coronary artery bypass graft
MI = myocardial infarction
NR = not reported
Pts = patients

during multi-vessel procedure (13,27) and the presence of intracoronary thrombus (12). To reduce the chance of guidewire trauma, most operators would use floppy guidewires first. When this fails in spite of adequate support from the guiding and balloon catheters, an intermediate or standard wire could be used.

Distal embolization occurred in as high as 10% of patients who were successfully recanalized in an early series of patients (12). Most of these are not associated with significant clinical sequelae. More recently, Haine et al (27) found that only 3 (0.6%) out of 500 patients had distal embolization following PTCA of totally occluded vessels. The reason for this low rate of embolization is not certain.

Therefore, PTCA of a totally occluded vessel is associated with reduced success and increased complication rates. Certain morphological characteristics are helpful in the assessment of risks and should be considered together with the potential benefits of revascularization before treating such a lesion.

Degree of Stenosis
The degree of stenosis in a lesion was associated with procedural success. High grade stenotic lesion probably has a greater plaque burden making dilatation more difficult and the chance for complications higher. Savage et al (29) demonstrated a step-wise association between primary success rate and severity of stenosis. The success rates for lesions with stenosis rate of 60% to 74%, 75% to 89%, 90% to 99% and 100% were 96%, 90%, 84% and 69% respectively. Recently, Tan et al (30) also found that the degree of stenosis correlated to the risk of acute vessel closure in a stepwise fashion. The relative risk for acute closure for a lesion of 80% to 99% was 10.7 (with a 95% confidence interval of 2.6 to 44.2) times that of a lesion with 51% to 79% narrowing.

Bifurcation Lesions
Stenotic lesions at bifurcations is another important risk factor during PTCA (5,7). The incidence of what ranged from 1.3 to 54.0% (5,31-35). Mathias et al (34) reported that the success rate when the ostium of a branch was involved was 74% in 119 of the lesions. But it was significantly higher, at 91%, when the ostium was not involved. In their patients, ostial involvement was defined as a stenosis within 3 mm of a major branch. Furthermore, they also found that the complication rate was about 2.5 times higher for patients with ostial involvement. In an early series, Meier et al (35), indicated that 54% of their 302 patients had side branches which may be in jeopardy for occlusion during PTCA. After PTCA, 20 of the 365 lesions (5.5%) were occluded. When the side branch originated from the lesion segment, the risk was 14% compared to only 1% when it originated from the vicinity of the stenosis.

Vetrovec et al (36) reported a much higher side branch occlusion rate, at 27%, when the ostium was involved. However, the side branches were smaller (not more than 1 mm) compared to the Meier's series of patients (1 to 2 mm). The commonest attributable mode of side branch occlusion is due to the "snow-plow" effect. This is when the inflated balloon "pushes" the atherosclerotic plaque from the target vessel to the side branch. Vessel spasm, dissection and embolism are the other possible causes. Fortunately, most patients with side branch closure were frequently associated with minimal chest pain and without significant electrocardiographic or enzyme changes (32,37). On the other hand, Arora et al (33) reported the incidence of myocardial infarction in patients after PTCA of the side branches to be 14%. However, closure of septal perforators in 26 occlusions in the three major epicardial arteries was not associated with myocardial infarction. Some of these occluded side branches recanalized on follow-up (37).

Introducing a guidewire into a significant branch vessel may offer some protection. However, more recently, in a study of PTCA of 1,157 lesions, the procedural success rates for 970 non-bifurcation, 135 "protected" bifurcation and 52 "unprotected" bifurcation lesions were 93%, 95% and 85% respectively ($p > 0.05$). In addition, the risks for abrupt vessel closure were similar (30). Weinstein et al (32) found that the salvage rate was 91% when the side branch closed compared to only 38% when this was not done.

Another problem with such lesions is the presence of significant residual stenosis after balloon dilatation in spite of adequate balloon sizing and prolonged inflation. This is probably due to elastic recoil created by the high and low wall shear stress at the apex of bifurcations (38). These forces lead to an increase in elastic tissue at the branches. Oversizing the balloon in the hope of overcoming this problem may result in an increase in complications. Newer technologies are now being tested.

Therefore, care must be exercised when treating these vessels especially noting the size of the branch and ostial involvement. The operator must determine amount of myocardium at risk if the side branch closes during the procedure and decide which technique he should employ.

Intracoronary thrombus
The presence of thrombus is another important morphological characteristic in risk assessment before PTCA because of its association with lower success and higher complication rates. It is identified by an intraluminal filling defect separate from the vessel wall or a radiolucency surrounded by contrast that is seen in multiple projections; usually in the absence of calcium within the defect (39). Sometimes, the presence is inferred from the persistence of contrast material within the defect, visible distal embolization of intraluminal material and convex contrast medium outline at a point of total occlusion with post-injection staining (39). In addition, haziness at the area of the lesion often implies the presence of a white thrombus with intimal disruption (40). The incidence of pre-procedural intracoronary thrombus is estimated to range from 4% to 11% (29,30,39) with a predisposition in patients with unstable angina or recent myocardial infarction. Success rates in these patients have been reported to be 74 to 92% (29,30,43). Hillegass et al (44) evaluated the effect of preprocedural intracoronary thrombus in 2,614 patients on the outcome after percutaneous coronary intervention. Procedural success rates for patients with stable

angina, unstable angina and unstable angina with intracoronary thrombus were 87%, 85% and 80% respectively. Using a multiple logistic regression model derived from various morphological characteristics in 1,156 lesions (30), the odds ratio for procedural success rate in lesions with intracoronary thrombus was 0.28 (95% confidence interval of 0.13 to 0.58) that of those without.

One of the major concerns regarding risk with thrombus arose from a high closure rate of 73% from the very early Mayo Clinic experience (39). Unlike lesions with total occlusion, acute closure usually occurred in the catheterization laboratory rather than outside (39,43). This could be due to dislodgement of atheromatous or thrombotic material or propagation of the thrombus (39). Coronary artery spasm and dissection were less commonly identified. Later studies (41,47) reported a closure rate of 6 to 31%. Non-surgical recanalization could still be achieved in half of these patients. The incidences of acute closure rate for patients with stable angina, unstable angina and unstable angina with thrombus were 4%, 6% and 11% respectively (44).

Distal embolization is another concern associated with intracoronary thrombus. Although the rate for distal embolization was 24% in an early report (41), subsequently it was reduced to 1% (43). However, this rate was still higher than the overall 0.1% chance of embolization in the group of patients reported by the National Heart, Lung and Blood Institute PTCA Registry (46). Fortunately, most of these patients did not require emergent coronary artery bypass surgery.

The risk for emergent coronary artery by-pass surgery for PTCA in lesion with intracoronary thrombus was high initially at 9% (41). Subsequently, the risk was reduced to 3.5% (43) and Arora et al (42) did not even find that the risk for emergent coronary artery by-pass was higher for patients with intracoronary thrombus compared to those without.

The characteristics of the intracoronary thrombus, such as angiographic appearance and size of thrombus, may also have an impact on outcome. Data from 2,686 patients who underwent PTCA at the Cleveland Clinic (unpublished) from December 1992 to June 1994, showed that the complication rates were 2.5% in lesions which did not appear hazy angiographically and 5.0% in lesions which were angiographically hazy. When there was a definite intraluminal filling defect, the complication was increased to 11.6%. Ellis et al (45) examined 140 procedures complicated by acute closure. The presence of 2 mm or larger filling defect observed before PTCA was associated with a 3.9 times higher risk of acute closure compared to its absence.

To overcome these problems, Mooney et al (43) suggested using intracoronary heparin and prolonged balloon inflation with relatively oversized balloons (balloon to vessel ratio of 1.2:1). Although pre-treatment with intravenous heparin has been shown to be useful, the results from the Thrombolysis and Angioplasty in Unstable Angina (TAUSA) Trial (47) did not support this strategy. Similarly, intracoronary thrombolytic agents (48) improved results in some patients, but the results from the TAUSA Trial (49) showed that the complication rates were higher. This trial consisted of 469 patients with unstable angina pectoris who were randomized to receive intracoronary urokinase or placebo at the time of PTCA. Out of the 240 patients who had urokinase administered and with complex angiographic lesions, the risk for post-PTCA acute closure was 10.6% and ischemia was 9.8% compared to 2.7% for each of the complications in patients who received placebo. Newer pharmacological agents have also been used as adjunctive therapy in the treatment of lesions with high possibility of thrombus. By administering a monoclonal antibody directed against Fab fragment (c7E3) directed against the platelet glycoprotein IIb/IIIa integrelin during PTCA and atherectomy in 2099 patients, the EPIC (Evaluation of c7E3 in the Prevention of Ischemic Complications) investigators (50) demonstrated a reduction of about 30% reduction of ischemic complications.

One of the major difficulties with analysis of the results of PTCA in lesions with intracoronary thrombus is the subjectivity in its identification. Den Heijer et al (51) showed that angiography could only detect 22% of protruding thrombus which was visualized by angioscopy. On the other hand, dissection, tissue frons or bulky plaque may be misidentified as thrombus (52).

Although lesions with intracoronary thrombus are unlikely to reduce procedural success rates, they would still constitute an increase risk of complications at PTCA (7), especially if the filling defect is greater than 2 mm. In situations whereby percutaneous revascularization is mandatory, pretreatment with intravenous heparin or use of the monoclonal antibody c7E3 may reduce complication rates.

Proximal tortuosity and angulated stenosis

The problem with proximal vessel tortuosity is the difficulty in accessing the stenosis to be dilated. By one definition, if there are two bends greater than 60 degrees proximal to the lesion, then the amount of tortuosity was considered to be moderate. When there are three or more bends greater than 60 degrees then tortuosity is excessive. In the MAPS Study Group (5), dilatation failure was more than 1.5 times when tortuosity was severe. From December 1992 to June 1994, out of 3,262 PTCAs performed at the Cleveland Clinic, the proximal vessels were severely tortuous in 114 (3.5%) lesions. The procedural success rate for these lesions was 72% compared to 88% for the remaining lesions. The odds ratio for a successful outcome at PTCA in patients with severe proximal tortuosity was only 0.35 (with a 95% confidence interval of 0.23 to 0.54) compared to those without.

In addition, when the guidewire transverses across tortuous vessels, its characteristics change. This reduces its maneuverability and increases the chance of injury to the vessel wall, thereby increasing the complication rate (5). At the Cleveland Clinic, the rate for major complications in lesions with severe proximal tortuosity was 6.1% compared to 3.1% for those without. However, this difference was not significant statistically.

Therefore, only severe proximal vessel tortuosity is associated with a reduction in procedural success rate and may increase complication rates. Large diameter flexible tip guidewires may assist in crossing the lesions and facilitate balloon advancement. In addition, the choice of guide catheters is also important in providing support. Low profile balloons may be useful to negotiate through the proximal tortuosity. Newer interventional devices are generally less flexible, steerable and trackable and therefore unlikely to be suitable for these lesions.

Angulated lesions have also been associated with a higher complication incidence (45). A bend point is considered to be present in any angiographic projection it appears when the balloon, in the position to dilate, is located in a portion of the vessel that has a 45 degree or greater angulation at end-diastole (45). Care has to be taken that the view of the vessel is not fore-shortened. The MAPS Study Group (5) found this type of lesion in 21.6% of their patients and about a quarter of these (4.8%) had angulation greater than 60 degrees. Ellis et al (53) subsequently reported the success rate for patients with angulated lesions to be 70% compared to 89% for those without. As expected, the complication rate was 13% and 3.5% for patients with and without angulated stenoses respectively. Lesions with angulation greater than 60 degrees has a even lower success rate of 53% (5). More recently, Savas et al (54) used long balloons for PTCA in 69 lesions with angulation greater than 45 degrees. The success rate was 88%.

The overall complication rate was 13% compared to only 3.5% for patients without angulated lesions (5). This was due to a higher chance of dissection on a fixed atherosclerotic plaque from non-coaxial stress as the balloon straightened and stretched the lesion (45). Tan et al (30) found that the rate for abrupt vessel closure was 13% for lesion greater than 90 degrees, 8.8% for lesions between 45 and 90 degrees and 2.2% for lesions less than 45 degrees. In addition, the presence of an associated thrombus, lesion length of greater than 10 mm or age at least 65 years led to an even greater risk of major complications (45). Using long balloons for lesions with bends greater than 45 degrees, the rates for dissection, abrupt closure and ischemic complications were 20%, 7% and 1% respectively. Therefore, PTCA of such lesions should only be undertaken after careful consideration and selection of patients.

Calcified lesions
Calcified lesions occurred only in about 4% to 14% of patients in which PTCA was attempted (29,55), probably due to the insensitive detection by angiography. Using intravascular ultrasound, the incidence has been noted to be as high as 83% (56). Due to the difficulty in expanding calcified lesions, the success rate for calcified lesions was lower at 74% to 92% compared to 90 to 95% for non-calcified lesions (29,30). Using a multiple logistic regression model, the odds ratio for procedural success for calcified lesions was 0.27 (95% confidence interval of 0.15 to 0.48) that of non-calcified lesions (30).

Calcification changes the elastic properties of the arteriosclerotic plaque or vessel wall such that dissections tended to occur at the region of transition between non-calcified and calcified areas due to non-uniform stress distribution (56). Recently, intravascular ultrasonography during PTCA (55) validated this hypothesis. In addition, in animal studies, vessels exposed to higher inflation pressure had a significantly higher incidence of mural thrombus, dissection and medial necrosis (57). These factors account for the 1.5 times higher complication rate which was shown in clinical studies (5,7). In a more recent study, Tan et al (30) showed that the risk for abrupt vessel closure for calcified lesions was 14% compared to 2.5% for non-calcified lesions.

The severity of calcification may also influence the success of PTCA. From December 1992 to June 1994, PTCA was performed in 2,675 lesions, of which 454 were calcified. The amount of calcification in these lesions were further categorize semiquantitatively into absent, mild, moderate or severe. There were 23 patients with severe, 135 patients with moderate, 296 patients with mild and 2221 patients with no calcification at the treated lesions. The acute complication rates were 0%, 4.4%, 3.4% and 2.9% respectively. The differences were not statistically significant. This observation may be due to the small number of patients with calcified lesions who underwent PTCA because other newer devices are utilized for most patients with moderate or severe calcification. In addition, the amount of calcium deposits is difficult to quantify angiographically. Intravascular ultrasound may help to define the amount of calcification better by delineating the site, arc, length and distribution patterns. This may influence the choice of device (58).

Lesions with mild to moderate calcification require higher inflation pressure to "crack" them (30). Although non-compliant balloons using polyethylene terephthalate (PET) are often necessary, the chance of balloon rupture with the accompanying risk of vessel trauma, balloon entrapment and distal embolization remain. Furthermore, calcium can occur as a discrete deposit resulting in an increase stress on a small area of the balloon surface. This increases the stress on the balloon and may increase the likelihood for rupture. It was suggested that the distal third of the balloon be positioned in the lesion. If the balloon ruptures, less material would be trapped within the lesion and therefore facilitating withdrawal. In severely calcified lesions, newer interventional devices such as high-speed rotational atherectomy (59) or excimer laser (60) have been used with improved results.

Lesion eccentricity
At angiography, an asymmetrically positioned stenosis is deemed eccentric. In the various studies (5,7,61), the amount of lesion occupying the lumen used to define eccentricity ranged from a quarter to three-quarters. Early experience of PTCA showed that eccentric lesions were associated with lower success rates (80% versus 89%) compared to concentric lesions (61). The early investigators also showed that the risk for acute complications such as dissection and coronary occlusion were increased (62). However, more recent studies (5,7,30) did not find that eccentric lesions were associated with lower success or higher complication rates unless it

occurred in the presence of a "complex" lesion (eccentric lesion or with irregular borders), whereby the acute closure rate was 2.9 times higher (63).

Another possible reason for the differences in results is that angiography does not identify eccentric lesions well. Intravascular ultrasonic images have demonstrated angiographically concentric lesions having significant eccentric plaques. Only severely eccentric lesions visualized by intravascular ultrasound are identified as eccentric angiographically. When intravascular ultrasound was used to define eccentricity, success (64) and complication (65) rates were similar.

In general, mild to moderate eccentric lesions could be treated with good results and low complication rates with PTCA. When eccentricity is marked or the lesion calcified and long, newer devices like directional atherectomy would be helpful (66).

Lesion length
Long lesions are commonly associated with a lower success rate and a higher complication rate (61). The reason for these associations may be that the area to be treated is larger for longer lesions and therefore the chance for intimal disruption is higher. By convention, the length of a lesion is measured by caliper as the distance from the proximal to distal "shoulder" in the projection that best elongated the stenosis (5). Stenosis of 10 to 20 mm in length were defined as tubular and those greater than 20 mm in length were defined as diffuse. These definitions corresponded to the ACC/AHA score of "B" and "C" respectively. Various early reports (7,30) demonstrated a step-wise success rate for this semi-quantitation of lesion length; 95% for discrete, 85% to 91% for lesions tubular and 78% to 89% for diffuse lesions. With increasing experience and improved technology, success rate exceeded 90% for lesions more than 10 mm long (67). Goudreau et al (68) showed that even in diffusely diseased coronary artery segments, clinical success was achieved in 91 out of 98 patients (93%).

The NHLBI PTCA Registry (69) reported that a diffuse lesion was 2.6 times more likely for occlusion during PTCA than a single discrete lesion (8.5% versus 3.3%). However, results from several investigators (7,30,68) did not show a consistent relationship between lesion length and complications rates. Measurement errors could be magnified as lesion length can be as much as 7 to 10 catheter diameters. Instead of using absolute units of measurement, Ellis et al (45) demonstrated that when the lesion length was greater than two luminal diameters, the chance of acute closure was about two times higher.

By convention, the "shoulder to shoulder" definition is most commonly used. The shoulder is sometimes difficult to determine and other authors have used a pre-determined amount of narrowing as the margins for measurement (45,67). Ellis et al (45) used 30%, 50% and 70% narrowings as the margins for measurement and found that the length of stenosis greater than 50% was a significant predictor for acute vessel closure.

In addition, long balloons were used in the later studies. Longer balloons were believed to improve results and reduce complication rates by distributing pressure more evenly along the entire length of the diseased segment (54,56,67). Cannon et al (70) evaluated the use of long balloons. Using 30 mm and 40 mm balloons, they achieved angiographic success in 77 (90%) out of 86 patients. In addition, the high pressure and prolonged inflation produced smoother and larger arterial wall lumens. Even though the risk of intimal tear was high at 35%, this was also not associated with major complications. However, mortality rate was 2.4% and 7% of the patients had myocardial infarction. Emergent coronary artery bypass surgery was needed in one patient (1.2%). The authors did not find that lesion length was correlated with complication rate. More recently, Cates et al (71) used 80 mm balloons to dilate lesions longer than 40mm. They achieved a success rate of 91% with a 4% rate of coronary artery bypass surgery.

With improved balloon technology, the success rate for long lesions is approaching that of discrete lesions. On the other hand, the complication rates are probably still higher. Fortunately, most of these complications are non flow limiting dissections.

Aorto-ostial lesions
Aorto-ostial lesions are uncommon manifestation of symptomatic coronary artery disease. They are more likely to be calcified and have greater elastic tissue compared to non-ostial lesions. When it occurs, it poses a challenge to the interventionalist. Choice and control of guide catheters are important to minimize the problems of catheter impaction and trauma. Furthermore, extra care must to put in during balloon positioning and inflation to avoid the "water melon-seed effect". With these additional technical difficulties, it was not surprising that the success rate for PTCA in an early series at the ostium of the right coronary artery to be 79% with a 9.4% risk for emergent coronary artery bypass surgery and 5.7% risk of myocardial infarction (72). Subsequently, with better equipment, Bedotto et al (73) reported the angiographic success rate for patients with lesions at the ostium of the right coronary artery and saphenous venous grafts to be 85%. They did not encounter any major complications.

More recently, Tan et al (30) showed that the success rate for PTCA in 77 lesions with ostial disease was 94% compared to 93% in 1,080 lesions without ostial disease. In addition, none of the lesions with ostial disease had abrupt vessel closure compared to 3.5% in lesions without ostial disease. The improvement of results is probably brought about by improved balloon technology, greater operator experience and use of newer technological devices such as rotational atherectomy.

Coronary artery bypass grafts
Although coronary artery bypass surgery is effective in relieving ischemic symptoms and improving survival in certain subgroups (74), disease in native vessels progresses and grafts, too, can suffer from atherosclerosis. Re-operation is associated with increased morbidity and mortality and less relief of ischemic symptoms (75). With limited supply of conduits, the percutaneous approach to revascularization is

attractive and viable.

Unlike native vessel PTCA, grafts often have unusual origins and courses. These may lead to difficulties in obtaining adequate guide support. The overall success for PTCA of venous grafts ranged from 76% to 97% (76-88). Overall major complication rate ranged from 2.2% to 4.5% (76-78,80,89) with an emergent bypass rate of 0% to 2.5%, myocardial infarction rate of 1.6% to 4.5% and mortality rate of less than 1% (76-78,80). More recently, the second trial of Coronary Angioplasty versus Excisional Atherectomy Trial (CAVEAT-II) (90) randomized 305 patients with de novo vein graft lesions to atherectomy or angioplasty. Of the 151 patients who underwent PTCA, the success rate was 79%. On the other hand, the results of PTCA at arterial grafts were more encouraging and success rates were reported to be 82% to 100% (89,91,92).

As with native vessel PTCA, lesion morphological characteristics, such as degree of stenosis, presence of thrombus, total occlusion, severe vessel tortuosity and angulation especially at anastomotic sites, remain as an important determinant for procedural success (84,89,92-94). The site of the lesion was another factor that was associated with procedural success. Out of a total of 216 lesions at proximal anastomotic sites, the success rate was 86% compared to 91% of 388 lesions at non-proximal sites (76,79,81-83,86-88). Greater elastic recoil at the proximal site may be the reason for the lower success rate. The number of graft lesions treated (81), time period from bypass surgery to PTCA (85) and the number of previous bypass surgeries (88) were not found to be associated with procedural success.

An important consideration for risk assessment in vein graft PTCA is the age of the graft. Generally, vein grafts older than three years old, especially when they were degenerated, were more likely to be associated with complications. A total of 541 vein graft lesions were studied with regards to graft age and complication rates (83,85). There was no major complications associated with PTCA of 142 vein graft lesions which were less than three years old. On the other hand, PTCA of 399 vein graft lesions which were more than three years old carried on overall major complication rate of 6.5%. More recently, when older vein grafts were treated, as in the CAVEAT-II study (90), the overall complication rate was 12.2% in the patients who underwent PTCA. The risks for emergent bypass, myocardial infarction and mortality were 0.6%, 11.5% and 1.9% respectively.

One of the major complications associated with PTCA of vein grafts was distal embolization, especially when the grafts were more than three years old (76,79,85). The difference in plaque composition may account for the higher risk of distal embolization in vein grafts compared to native vessels. Atherosclerotic plaques in vein grafts were usually larger and commonly associated with thrombus (95,96). They consisted of foam cells with focal erosions into the intima by plaque lesions leaving behind thin areas of fibrous cap (95,97). With less collagenous fibers and calcification, the plaques were softer, more fragile and friable and therefore more likely to dislodge and embolize. The incidence of distal embolization in 2% to 6%

of patients with vein graft angioplasty (80,88). In totally occluded grafts (94), Kahn et al reported the incidence of embolization to be 11%. More recently, in the CAVEAT-II study (98), old vein grafts with a mean age of 10 years were treated. The rate of distal embolization was 5.1% in the 156 patients randomized to PTCA compared to 13.4% for those randomized to directional atherectomy. Patients who had evidence for distal embolization were about nine times more likely to suffer from an in-hospital complication, which included death, myocardial infarction, repeat intervention or bypass surgery. In addition, clinical event rates were also marginally higher at 12 months. Distal embolization occurred more commonly in lesions with thrombus (80,96,98) or when the lesion was irregular or ulcerated (99). Diffusely diseased grafts with a large plaque volume were also independent predictors for distal embolization.

The decision to treat lesions at vein grafts must be carefully considered. Diffuse disease, chronically occluded or aged grafts and the presence of thrombus are the major morphological characteristics associated with low success and high complication rates.

Inter-observer Variability in Lesion Morphology Assessment
One of the limitations of using a morphological classification is observer variability. Interobserver variability is well-documented in the visual assessment of the degree of stenosis (100) and TIMI flow grade 101). The MAPS Study Group (5) found that the agreement between observers to describe lesion morphology using the modified ACC/AHA classification for 57 lesions was 58%. Disagreement by one score was 35%, two scores was 7% and three scores was 0%. As 93% of the scores did not differ more than one score, the authors concluded that interobserver variability was unlikely to make an impact on prognosis. More recently, Kleiman et al (102) demonstrated that in 150 consecutive angiograms that the interobserver agreement was 61% but the reproducibility was only fair (kappa=0.24). Though the agreement between A and non-A and C and non-C lesions were even higher at 79% and 81% respectively, the reproducibility were moderate (kappa=0.45) and poor (kappa=0.18).

The data from many of the studies in the literature were not from a quality-controlled core laboratory. In addition, the definitions of morphological characteristics and experience of the observers making such determinations were uncertain. These factors would further increase observer variability and affect the application of their results to daily practice.

Instead of using broad categories of classification, specific lesion morphology may improve agreement between observers. In addition, specific lesion morphology may be more important in risk stratification in the light of improved balloon technology. Ellis et al (45) reported the discordance rate for lesion length, bifurcation, angulation and eccentricity to be 22%, 20%, 12% and 24% respectively. Popma et al (103) proceeded further to demonstrate that the reproducibility for total occlusion was perfect and for other morphologies such as eccentricity, angulation, presence of thrombus, tortuosity and calcification was substantial.

Relevance of ACC/AHA Classification

The modified ACC/AHA classification for lesion morphology is widely used for risk stratification for patients before PTCA. With numerous changes in technology and experience since the first publication of these guidelines in 1988 (104), procedural results have improved tremendously . Nonetheless, recent studies still demonstrated the stepwise reduction of success rates (χ^2 trend, p<0.0001) and increment of complication rates (χ^2 trend, p<0.0013) with increasing lesion score (tables 3,4). However, the differences between each score diminished.

There was no significant difference in procedural success and complication rates between type A and B1 lesions. The success rate for B2 lesions remained lower than B1 lesions with a relative risk for success of 0.69 (95% confidence interval, 0.52 to 0.91) but the complication rates were similar. Similarly, the success rate for C lesions remained lower than B lesions with a relative risk for success of 0.50 (0.42 to 0.61) but the complication rates were not significantly different. However, the risk for complication was 3.11 times (1.30-7.42) higher for C2 lesions compared to C1 lesions.

Therefore, the modified ACC/AHA classification is able to only provide with a crude estimate of procedural success. It is also an insensitive predictor for complications. The improvement of balloon technology has enabled certain lesion morphological characteristics such as long lesions to be effectively treated. The advent of lesion-specific new devices may have also brought about better results. For example, a heavily calcified lesion is more readily treated with high speed rotational atherectomy than PTCA. In addition, suboptimal results, threatened or acute closure can be effectively treated with coronary stents in selected patients. Hence, specific lesion morphology rather than a broad lesion classification may be more useful and precise in the risk assessment for patients undergoing PTCA. However, there are lesions with multiple characteristics and these lesion morphologies may need to be arranged in a hierarchical fashion in order to interpret the risk more meaningfully.

Conclusion

Lesion morphology is indeed useful in the assessment of procedural success and complication rates. However, there are still several limitations. Variation between observers and differences in definitions have resulted in difficulties in interpreting and extrapolating results to patients. Tenaglia et al (105) attempted to generate a formula based on empirically weights for each characteristic in order to quantify the risk of abrupt closure for an individual patient succeeded partially. This is due to the complexity of lesion morphologies and therefore a very large number of patients was needed. Furthermore, this approach has to be validated by a large prospective trial. Other authors (5,107) used a scoring system for risk assessment. These are based on the number of diseased vessels (69) and the amount of myocardium at risk.

Table 3

Procedural Success Rates Based on the Modified American College
of Cardiology/American Heart Association Classification for Lesion Morphology

	Ellis[5]	Myler[7]	Favereau[8]	Tan[30]	Total
A	172/189 (91.0)	81/82 (98.8)	152/162 (93.8)	185/193 (95.9)	590/626 (94.2)
B	327/393 (83.2)	436/474 (92.0)	525/553 (94.9)	737/794 (92.8)	2024/2214 (91.5)
B1	198/230 (86.1)	204/215 (94.9)	310/329 (94.2)	351/369 (95.1)	1063/1143 (93.0)
B2	129/163 (79.1)	232/259 (89.6)	215/224 (95.9)	386/425 (90.8)	962/1071 (89.8)
C	54/80 (67.5)	401/444 (90.3)	209/269 (77.7)	210/261 (80.5)	874/1054 (82.9)
C1	-	340/373 (91.2)	-	196/240 (81.7)	536/613 (87.4)
C2	-	61/71 (85.9)	-	14/21 (66.7)	75/92 (81.5)
Total	553/662 (83.5)	918/1000 (91.8)	886/984 (90.0)	1132/1248 (90.7)	3489/3894 (89.6)

observed/total (percentage)

268

Table 4

Major Complication Rates Based on the Modified American College
of Cardiology/American Heart Association Classification of Lesion Morphology

Lesion Score	Ellis[5]	Myler[7]	Favereau[8]	Tan[30]	Total
A	4/189 (2.1)	1/82 (1.2)	0/162 (0)	4/193 (2.1)	9/626 (1.4)
B	34/393 (8.7)	9/474 (1.9)	8/553 (1.4)	21/794 (2.6)	72/2214 (3.3)
B1	18/230 (7/8)	3/215 (1.4)	6/329 (1.8)	4/369 (1.1)	31/1143 (2.7)
B2	16/163 (9.8)	6/259 (2.3)	2/224 (0.9)	17/425 (4.0)	41/1071 (3.8)
C	14/80 (17.5)	9/444 (2.0)	5/269 (1.9)	13/261 (5.0)	41/1054 (3.9)
C1	-	5/373 (1.3)	-	10/240 (4.2)	15/613 (2.4)
C2	-	4/71 (5.6)	-	3/21 (14.0)	7/92 (7.6)
Total	52/662 (7.9)	19/1000 (1.9)	13/984 (1.3)	38/1248 (3.0)	142/3894 (3.6)

observed/total (percentage)

In addition to lesion morphology, the clinical status and scenario of each patient have to be taken into account before providing the final risk assessment. In a multicenter prospective trial (105), Wolfe et al found that the age of patient, presence of multi-vessel disease and whether if the patient was in acute ischemia were the major determinants for outcome. Similarly, it was clinical parameters (108) that were the main predictors for long term outcome in patients who had PTCA.

Another factor that may affect the success and complication rates is the variability of operator experience. Using various mathematical models, Ellis et al (109) found that the volume of workload was useful in identifying operators with poor outcome.

Based on the 1993 Cleveland Clinic Interventional Database, only 7% of the variance in PTCA complications were accounted by angiographic factors using the modified ACC/AHA classification and left ventricular ejection fraction. An additional of 2% is contributed by lesion morphology characteristics; for example vessel size, thrombus or degenerated vein graft, which were under-represented in the modified ACC/AHA classification. Clinical factors, such as acute myocardial infarction, age, gender and prior restenosis accounted for another 3%. Therefore, 88% of the variance in PTCA complications remained unaccounted for. This fact may partly explained the unpredictability of PTCA outcome.

Lesion morphology forms only a small part of the risk assessment for a patient for PTCA. However, with the information available at present, it is probably the best determinant. The interventionalist can wisely use these parameters as a guide in the practice of the art of angioplasty.

Acknowledgements
The authors wish to thank Patti Durnwald for her expert secretarial assistance.

270

References

1.   Cowley MJ, Dorros G, Kelsey SF, van Raden M, Detre KM. Acute coronary events associated with percutaneous transluminal coronary angioplasty. Am J Cardiol 1984; 53:12C-16C.

2.   Detre K, Holubkor R, Kelsey S, et al. Percutaneous transluminal coronary angioplasty in 1985-1986 and 1977 to 1981: the National Heart, Lung, and Blood Institue. N Engl J Med 1988; 318:265-70.

3.   Ryan TJ, Bauman WB, Kennedy JW, et al. Guidelines for percutaneous transluminal coronary angioplasty: A report of the American College of Cardiology/ American Heart Association Task Force on Assessment of Diagnostic and Therapeutic Cardiovascular Procedures (Committee on Percutaneous Transluminal Coronary Angioplasty). J Am Coll Cardiol 1993; 22:2033-54.

4.   Cragg DR, Friedman HZ, Almony SC, et al. Early hospital discharge after percutaneous transluminal coronary angioplasty. Am J Cardiol 1989; 64:1270-4.

5.   Ellis SG, Vandormael MG, Cowley MJ, et al. Coronary morphologic and clinical determinants of procedural outcome with angioplasty for multivessel coronary disease. Implication for patient selection. Circulation 1990; 82:1193-202.

6.   Kahn JK, Hartzler GO. Frequency and causes of failure with contemporary balloon coronary angioplasty and implications for new technologies. Am J Cardiol 1990; 66:858-60.

7.   Myler RK, Shaw RE, Stertzer SH, et al. Lesion morphology and coronary angioplasty: current experience and analysis. J Am Coll Cardiol 1992; 19:1641-52.

8.   Favereau X, Corcos T, Zimarino M, et al. Is ABC classification for PTCA obsolete? Circulation 1993; 84:I-217.

9.   Meier B. Chronic total coronary occlusion angioplasty. Cathet Cardiovasc Diagn 1989; 17:212-7.

10.   Serruys PW, Umans V, Heyndrickx GR, et al. Elective PTCA of totally occluded coronary arteries not associated with acute myocardial infarction; short-term and long-term results. Eur Heart J 1985; 6:2-12.

11.   Holmes DR Jr, Vlietstra RE, Reeder GS, et al. Angioplasty in total coronary occlusion. J Am Coll Cardiol 1984: 3:845-9.

12. Kereiakes DJ, Selmon MR, McAuley BJ, McAuley DB, Sheehan DJ, Simpson JB. Angioplasty in total coronary artery occlusion: Experience in 76 consecutive patients. J Am Coll Cardiol 1985; 6:526-33.

13. Stone GW, Rutherford BD, McConahay DR, et al. Procedural outcome of angioplasty for total coronary artery occlusion: an analysis of 971 lesions in 905 patients. J Am Coll Cardiol 1990; 15:849-56.

14. DiSciascio G, Vetrovec GW, Cowley MJ, Wolfgang TC. Early and late outcome of percutaneous transluminal coronary angioplasty for subacute and chronic total coronary occlusion. Am Heart J 1986; 111:833-9.

15. Bell MR, Berger PB, Bresnahan JF, Reeder GS, Bailey KR, Holmes Jr DR. Initial and long-term outcome of 354 patients after coronary balloon angioplasty of total coronary artery occlusions. Circulation 1992; 85:1003-11.

16. Shimizu M, Kato O, Otsuji S, et al. Progress in initial outcome of PTCA for complete occlusion. Circulation 1993; 88:I-504.

17. Ivanhoe RJ, Weintraub WS, Douglas JS Jr, et al. Percutaneous transluminal coronary angioplasty of chronic total occlusions: Primay success, restenosis, and long-term clinical follow-up. Circulation 1992; 85:106-15.

18. Safian RD, McCabe CH, Sipperly ME, McKay RG, Baim DS. Initial success and long-term follow-up of percutaneous transluminal coronary angioplasty in chronic total occlusions versus conventional stenoses. Am J Cardiol 1989;61:23G-28G.

19. Tan KH, Sulke AN, Taub NA, Watts E, Sowton E. Coronary angioplasty of chronic total occlusion: determinants of procedural success. J Am Coll Cardiol 1993; 21:76A.

20. Kinoshita I, Kato O, Kamide K, et al. Coronary angioplasty (PTCA) of chronic total occlusion with bridging collaterals. Circulation 1993; 88:I-505.

21. Katsuragawa M, Fujiwara H, Miyamae M, Sasayama S. Pathological background of percutaneous transluminal coronary angioplasty for chronic total occlusion. J Am Coll Cardiol 1993; 21:76A.

22. Meier B. "Occlusion angioplasty": light at the end of the tunnel or dead end? Circulation 1992;85:1214-1216.

23. Dervan JP, Baim DS, Cherniles J, Grossman W. Transluminal angioplasty of occluded arteries: use of a movable guide wire system. Circulation 1983; 68:776-84.

272

24.   Ellis SG, Shaw RE, Gershony G, et al. Risk factors, time course and treatment effect for restenosis after successful percutaneous transluminal coronary angioplasty of chronic total occlusion. Am J Cardiol 1989; 63:897-901.

25.   Warren RJ, Black AJ, Valentine PA, Manolas EG, Hunt D. Coronary angioplasty for chronic total occlusion reduces the need for subsequent coronary bypass surgery. Am Heart J 1990; 120:270-4.

26.   Stewart JT, Williams MG, Mulcahy DA,et al. Angioplasty in chronic occlusions: risks and benefits. Circulation 1991; 84:II-332.

27.   Haine E, Urban P, Dorsaz P-A, Meier B. Outcome and complications of 500 consecutive chronic total occlusion coronary angioplasties. J Am Coll Cardiol 1993; 21:138A.

28.   Piante S, Laarman G, de Feyer PJ, et al. Acute complications of percutaneous transluminal coronary angioplasty for total occlusion. Am Heart J 1991: 121:417-26.

29.   Savage MP, Goldberg S, Hirshfeld JW, et al. Clinical and angiographic determinants of primary coronary angioplasty success. J Am Coll Cardiol 1991; 17:22-8.

30.   Tan K, Sulke N, Taub N, Sowton E. Clinical and lesion morphology determinants of coronary angioplasty success and complication: current experience. J Am Coll Cardiol 1995; 25:855-65.

31.   Pinkerton CA, Slack JD, van Tassel JW, Orr CM. Angioplasty for dilation of bifurcation stenoses. Am J Cardiol 1985;55:1626-8.

32.   Weinstein JS, Baim DS, Slipperly ME, McCabe CH, Lorell BH. Salvage of branch vessels during bifurcation lesion angioplasty: acute and long-term follow-up. Cathet Cardiovasc Diagn 1991; 22:1-6.

33.   Arora RR, Raymond RE, Dimas AP, Bhadwar K, Simpfendorfer C. Side branch occlusion during coronary angioplasty: incidence, angiographic characteristics, and outcome. Cathet Cardiovasc Diagn 1989; 18:210-2.

34.   Mathias DW, Mooney JF, Lange HW, Goldenberg IF, Gobel FL, Mooney MR. Frequency of success and complications of coronary angioplasty of a stenosis at the ostium of a branch vessel. Am J Cardiol 1991; 67:491-5.

35.   Meier B, Gruentzig AR, King SB III, et al. Risk of side branch occlusion during coronary angioplasty. Am J Cardiol 1984; 53:10-4.

36.   Vetrotec GW, Cowley MJ, Wolfgang TC, Ducey KC. Effects of percutaenous transluminal coronary angioplasty on lesion-associated branches. Am Heart J 1985; 109:921-5.

37.   Shiu MF, Singh A. Spontaneous recanalisation of side branches occluded during percutaenous transluminal angioplasty. Br Heart J 1985; 54:215-7.

38.   Saltissi S, Webb-Peploe MM, Coltart DJ. Effect of variation in coronary artery anatomy on distribution of stenotic lesions. Br Heart J 1979; 42:186-91.

39.   Mabin TA, Holmes DR Jr, Smith HC, et al. Intracoronary thrombus: role in coronary occlusion complicating percutaneous transluminal coronary angioplasty. J Am Coll Cardiol 1985; 5:198-202.

40.   Manzo K, Nesto R, Sassower M, et al. Coronary lesion morphology by angioscopy vs angiography: the ability of angiography to detect thrombi. J Am Coll Cardiol 1994; 23:406A.

41.   Deligonul U, Gabliani GI, Caralis DG, Kern MJ, Vandormael MG. Percutaneous transluminal coronary angioplasty in patients with intracoronary thrombus. Am J Cardiol 1988; 62:474-6.

42.   Arora RR, Platko WP, Badwar K, Simpfendorfer C. Role of intracoronary thrombus in acute complications during percutaneous transluminal coronary angioplasty. Cathet Cardiovasc Diagn 1989; 16:226-9.

43.   Mooney MR, Mooney JF, Goldenberg IF, Almquist AK, Van Tassel RA. Percutaneous transluminal coronary angioplasty in the setting of large intracoronary thrombi. Am J Cardiol 1990; 65:427-31.

44.   Hillegass WB, Ohman EM, O'Hanesian MA, et al. The effect of preprocedural intracoronary thrombus on patient outcome after percutaneous coronary intervention. J Am Coll Cardiol 1995; 25:94A.

45.   Ellis SG, Roubin GS, King III SB, et al. Angiographic and clinical predictors of acute closure after native vessel coronary angioplasty. Circulation 1988; 77:372-9.

46.   Kent KM, Bentivoglio LG, Block PC, et al. Percutaneous transluminal coronary angioplasty: report from the Registry of the National Heart, Lung, and Blood Institute. Am J Cardiol 1982; 49:2011-9.

47.   Ambrose JA, Almeida OD, Ratner D, et al. Heparin adminstered prior to angioplasty does not decrease angioplasty complications - TAUSA trial results. Circulation 1994; 90:I-374.

48.   Schieman G, Cohen BM, Kozina J, et al. Intracoronary urokinase for intracoronary thrombus accumulation complicating percutaneous transluminal coronary angioplasty in acute ischemic syndromes. Circulation 1990; 82:2052-60.

49.   Torre SR, Ambrose JA, Sharma SK, et al. Adjuvant intracoronary urokinase worsens the procedural outcome for PTCA of complex lesions in unstable angina: results of the Throbolysis and Angioplasty in Unsatble Angina Trial (TAUSA). J Am Coll Cardiol 1994; 23:105A.

50.   The EPIC Investigators. Use of a monoclonal antibody directed against the platelet glycoprotein IIb/IIIa receptor in high-risk coronary angioplasty. N Engl J Med 1994; 330:956-61.

51.   Den Heijer P, Foley DP, Escaned J, et al. Angioscopic versus angiographic detection of intimal dissection and intracoronary thrombus. J Am Coll Cardiol 1994; 24:649-54.

52.   Teirstein PS, Schatz RA, Johnson AD, et al. Angioscopic versus angiographic detection of thrombus and dissection during coronary intervention. J Am Coll Cardiol 1993; 21:79A.

53.   Ellis SG, Topol EJ. Results of percutaneous transluminal coronary angioplasty of high-risk angulated stenoses. Am J Cardiol 1990; 66:932-7.

54.   Savas V, Puchrowicz S, Williams L, Grines CL, O'Neill WW. Angioplasty outcome using long balloons in high risk lesions. J Am Coll Cardiol 1992; 19:34A.

55.   Honye J, Mahon DJ, Jain A, et al. Morphological effects of coronary balloon angioplasty in vivo assessed by intravascular ultrasound imaging. Circulation 1992; 85:1012-25.

56.   Richardson PD, Davies MJ, Born GVR. Influence of plaque configuration and stress distribution on fissuring of atherosclerotic plaque. Lancet 1989; 2:941-4.

57.   Sarembock IJ, LaVeqau PJ, Sigal SL, et al. Influence of inflation pressure and balloon size on the development of intimal hyperplasia after balloon angioplsty: a study in the atherosclerotic rabbit. Circulation 1989; 80:1029-40.

58.   Mintz GS, Popma JJ, Pichard AD, et al. Patterns of target lesion calcification in coronary artery disease. A statistical analysis of intravascular ultrasound and coronary angiography in 1155 lesions. Circulation 1995; 91:1959-65.

59.   MacIsaac AI, Bass TA, Buchbinder M, et al. High speed rotational atherectomy: outcome of calcified and non-calcified cornary artery lesions. J Am Coll Cardiol (accepted).

60.   Levine S, Mehta S, Krauthamer D, Margolis JR. Excimer laser coronary angioplasty of calcified lesions. J Am Coll Cardiol 1991; 17:206A.

61.   Meier B, Gruentzig AR, Hollman J, Ischinger T, Bradford JM. Does length or eccentricity of coronary stenoses influence the outcome of transluminal diatation? Circulation 1983; 67:497-9.

62.   Fitzgerald PJ, Ports PA, Yock PG. Contribution of localized calcium deposits to dissection after angioplasty. An observational study using intravascular ultrasound. Circulation 1992; 86:64-70.

63.   de Feyter PJ, van den Brand M, Jaarman G, et al. Acute artery occlusion during and after percutaneous transluminal coronary angioplasty. Frequency, prediction, clinical course, management, and follow-up. Circulation 1991; 83:927-36.

64.   The SHK, Gussenhoven EJ, van Strijen M, et al. Can intravascular ultrasound predict clinical outcome following percutaneous transluminal angioplasty. J Am Coll Cardiol 1994; 23:242A.

65.   Tenaglia AN, Buller CE, Kisslo KB, Stack RS, Davidson CJ. Mechanisms of balloon angioplasty and directional atherectomy as assessed by intracoronary ultrasound. J Am Coll Cardiol 1992;20:685-691.

66.   Hinohara T, Rowe MH, Robertson GC, et al. Effect of lesion characteristics on outcome of directional coronary atherectomy. J Am Coll Cardiol 1991; 17:1112-20.

67.   Tenaglia AN, Zidar JP, Jackman JD Jr, et al. Treatment of long coronary artery narrowings with long angioplasty balloon catheters. Am J Cardiol 1993; 71:1274-7.

68.   Goudreau E, DiSciascio G, Kelly K, et al. Coronary angioplasty of diffuse coronary artery disease. Am Heart J 1991; 121:12-9.

69.   Detre KM, Holmes DR Jr, Holubkov R, et al. Incidence and consequences of periprocedural occlusion. The 1985-1986 National Heart, Lung, and Blood Institute Percutaneous Transluminal Coronary Angioplasty Registry. Circulation 1990; 82:739-50.

70.   Cannon AD, Roubin GS, Hearn JA, et al. Acute angiographic and clinical results of long balloon percutaneous transluminal coronary angioplasty and adjuvant stenting for long narrowings. Am J Cardiol 1994; 73:635-41.

71.   Cates CU, Knopf WD, Lembo NJ, et al. The 80 mm ballon: the first 95 vessel cumulative experience. J Am Coll Cardiol 1994; 23:58A.

72.   Topol EJ, Ellis SG, Fishman J, et al. Multicenter study of percutaneous transluminal angioplasty for right coronary artery ostial stenosis. J Am Coll Cardiol 1987; 9:1214-8.

73.   Bedotto JB, McConahay DR, Rutherford BD, et al. Balloon angioplasty of aorta coronary ostial stenosis revisited. Circulation 1991; 84:II-251.

74.   CASS Principal Investigators and their Associates. Coronary artery surgery study (CASS): a randomized trial of coronary bypass surgery: survival data. Circulation 1983; 68:939-50.

75.   Loop FD, Lytle BW, Cosgrove DM, et al. Reoperation for cornary atherosclerosis. Changing practice in 2509 consecutive patients. Ann Surg 1990; 212:378-84.

76.   Douglas JS Jr, Gruentzig AR, King SB III, et al. Percutaneous transluminal coronary angioplasty in patients with prior coronary bypass surgery. J Am Coll Cardiol 1983; 2:745-54.

77.   Block PC, Cowley MJ, Kaltenbach M, Kent KM, Simpson J. Percutaneous angioplasty of stenoses of bypass grafts or of bypass graft anastomotic sites. Am J Cardiol 1984; 53:666-8.

78.   El Gamal M, Bonnier H, Michels R, Heijman J, Stassen E. Percutaneous transluminal angioplasty of stenosed aortocoronary bypass grafts. Br Heart J 1984; 52:617-20.

79.   Corbelli J, Franco I, Hollman J, Simpfendorfer C, Galan K. Percutaneous transluminal coronary angioplasty after previous coronary artery bypass surgery. Am J Cardiol 1985; 56:398-403.

80.   Cote G, Myler RK, Stertzer SH, et al. Percutaneous transluminal angioplasty of stenotic coronary artery bypass grafts: 5 years' experience. J Am Coll Cardiol 1987; 9:8-17.

81.   Pinkerton CA, Slack JD, Orr CM, Vantassel JW, Smith ML. Percutaneous transluminal angioplasty in patients with prior myocardial revascularization surgery. Am J Cardiol 1988; 61:15G-22G.

82. Cooper I, Ineson N, Demirtas E, et al. Role of angioplasty in patients with previous coronary artery bypass surgery. Cathet Cardiovasc Diagn 1989; 16:81-6.

83. Platko WP, Hollman J, Whitlow PL, Franco I. Percutaneous transluminal angioplasty of saphenous vein graft stenosis: long-term follow-up. J Am Coll Cardiol 1989; 14:1645-50.

84. Douglas JS Jr, Weintraub WS, Liberman HA, et al. Update of saphenous vein graft (SVG) angioplasty: restenosis and long term outcome. Circulation 1991; 84:II-249.

85. Miranda CP, Rutherford BD, McConahay DR, et al. Angioplasty of older saphenous vein grafts continues to be a sound therapeutic option. J Am Coll Cardiol 1992; 19:350A.

86. Webb JG, Myler RK, Shaw RE, et al. Coronary angioplasty after coronary bypass surgery: initial results and late outcome in 422 patients. J Am Coll Cardiol 1990; 16:812-20.

87. Meester BH, Samson M, Suryapranata H, et al. Long-term follow-up after attempted angioplasty of saphenous vein grafts: the Thoraxcenter experience 1981-1988. Eur Heart J 1991; 12:648-53.

88. Dorros G, Lewin RF, Mathiak LM, et al. Percutaneous transluminal coronary angioplasty in patients with two or more previous coronary artery bypass grafting operations. Am J Cardiol 1988; 61:1243-7.

89. Dimas AP, Arora RR, Whitlow PL, et al. Percutaneous transluminal angioplasty involving internal mammary artery grafts. Am Heart J 1991; 122:423-9.

90. Holmes DR Jr, Topol EJ, Califf RM, et al. A multicenter, randomized trial of coronary angioplasty versus direnctional atherectomy for patients with saphenous vein bypass graft lesions. Circulation 1995; 91:1966-74.

91. Pinkerton CA, Slack JD, Orr CM, VanTassel JW. Percutaneous transluminal angioplasty involving internal mammary artery bypass grafts: a femoral approach. Cathet Cardiovasc Diagn 1987; 13:414-8.

92. Hill DM, McAuley BJ, Sheehan DJ, et al. Percutaneous transluminal angioplasty of internal mammary artery bypass grafts. J Am Coll Cardiol 1989; 13:221A.

278

93. de Feyter PJ, Serruys P, van den Brand M, et al. Percutaneous transluminal angioplasty of a totally occluded venous bypass graft: a challenge that should be resisted. Am J Cardiol 1989; 64:88-90.

94. Kahn JK, Rutherford BD, McConahay DR, et al. Initial and long-term outcome of 83 patients after balloon angioplasty of totally occluded bypass grafts. J Am Coll Cardiol 1994; 23:1038-42.

95. Smith SH, Geer JC. Morphology of saphenous vein-coronary artery bypass grafts. Seven to 116 months after surgery. Arch Pathol Lab Med 1983; 107:13-8.

96. Neitzel GF, Barboriak JJ, Pintar K, Qureshi I. Atherosclerosis in aortocoronary bypass grafts. Morphologic study and risk factor analysis 6 to 12 years after surgery. Arteriosclerosis 1986; 6:594-600.

97. Waller BF, Rothbaum DA. Gorfinkel HJ, et al. Morphologic observations after percutaneous transluminal balloon angioplasty of early and late aortocornary saphenous vein bypass grafts. J Am Coll Cardiol 1984; 4:784-92.

98. Lefkovits J, Holmes DR Jr, Califf RM, et al. Predictors and sequelae of distal embolization during saphenous vein graft intervention from the CAVEAT-II Trial. Circulation 1995 (accepted).

99 Liu MW, Douglas JS Jr, Lembo NJ, King SB III. Angiographic predictors of a rise in serum creatine kinase (distal embolization) after balloon angioplasty of saphenous vein coronary artery bypass grafts. Am J Cardiol 1993; 72:514-7.

100. Zir LM, Miller SW, Dinsmore RE, Gilbert JP, Harthorne JW. Interobserver variability in coronary angiography. Circulation 1976; 53:627-32.

101. Hackworthy RA, Sorensen SG, Fitzpatrick PG, et al. Dependence of assessment of coronary artery reperfusion during acute myocardial infarction on angiographic criteria and interobserver variability. Am J Cardiol 1988; 62:538-42.

102. Kleiman WS, Rodriguez AR, Raizner AE. Interobserver variability in grading of coronary arterial narrowings using the American College of Cardiology/ American Heart Association grading criteria. Am J Cardiol 1992; 69:413-5.

103. Popma JJ, Kennard E, Yeh W, et al. Reproducibility of qualitative and quantitative angiographic findings in the New Approaches to Coronary Intervention (NACI) Registry. J Am Coll Cardiol 1995; 25:153A.

104. Ryan TJ, Faxon DP, Gunnar RM, et al. ACC/AHA guidelines for percutaneous transluminal coronary angioplasty: a report of the American College of Cardiology/ American Heart Association Task Force on assessment of diagnostic and therapeutic cardiovascular procedures. J Am Coll Cardiol 1988; 12:529-45.

105. Tenaglia AN, Fortin DF, Califf RM, et al. Predicting the risk of abrupt vessel closure after angioplasty in an individual patient. J Am Coll Cardiol 1994; 24:1004-11.

106. Bergelson BA, Jacobs AK, Cupples LA, et al. Prediction of risk for hemodynamic compromise during percutaneous transluminal coronary angioplasty. Am J Cardiol 1992; 70:1540-5

107. Wolfe MW, Leya F, Bonan R, et al. Predictors of outcome after balloon angioplasty: a prospective multicenter study. Circulation 1993; 88:I-300.

108. Mick MJ, Piedmonte MR, Arnold AM, Simpendorfer C. Risk stratification for long term outcome after elective coronary angioplasty: a multivariate analysis of 5000 patients. J Am Coll Cardiol 1994; 24:74-80.

109. Ellis SG, Omoigui N Bittl JA, et al. Analysis of operator specific outcomes in interventional cardiology from a multicenter database of 4860 quality-controlled procedures. Circulation 1995 (accepted).

12.

INTRAVASCULAR ULTRASOUND-GUIDED SELECTION OF NEW CORONARY DEVICES IN CORONARY INTERVENTION

Stuart T. Higano, M.D. and David R. Holmes, Jr., M.D.
Mayo Clinic, Rochester, MN

INTRODUCTION

The beginning of coronary angiography in 1960 ushered in a new era in the diagnosis and management of coronary artery disease. Without coronary angiography, current treatment strategies for coronary artery disease, including coronary artery bypass surgery and catheter-based interventions, would most likely not have been developed. However, there are several inherent limitations of angiography for diagnosing and quantitating coronary atherosclerosis. In essence, angiography produces an x-ray silhouette of the coronary lumen, sometimes referred to as a "luminogram".(1) Atherosclerosis is detected when the column of x-ray contrast in the vessel lumen is indented by plaque. The severity of coronary atherosclerosis is estimated by comparing the lumen diameter at the stenosis to the diameter of the normal reference segment. The "luminogram" yields almost no qualitative information about plaque constituents. It is inaccurate for quantitating the severity of atherosclerosis for several reasons, including diffuse disease, geometric remodeling, and complex lesion morphologies. A normal reference segment is not present when there is diffuse disease resulting in an underestimation of stenosis severity. Geometric remodeling, or compensatory enlargement, occurs early in the development of atherosclerosis allowing for the development and growth of plaque with minimal luminal narrowing (see Figure 1).(2, 3) Significant atherosclerotic plaque can be present which is not appreciated by angiography. Complex lesion morphologies such as those seen after angioplasty, with splits, micro-tears, and dissections, make the angiographic "luminogram" even more difficult to assess.

Intravascular ultrasound (IVUS) is a relatively new technology for obtaining cross-sectional images of coronary arteries with catheters equipped with miniaturized ultrasound transducers. Images are obtained that are similar to pathologic sections; Lumen area and wall thickness can be accurately measured.(4) The typical coronary artery has a three layered appearance by IVUS (see Figure 2), including a thin echo-dense intima, a sonolucent media (outside the internal elastic lamina, which is not visible), and a more echo-dense adventitia (outside the external elastic lamina, which is also not visible). If the intimal thickness is less than 175 microns, it may not be visible by IVUS. As the intimal thickness increases with age and is usually greater than 175 microns in most adult patients, the intima is usually visible by IVUS.(5)

282

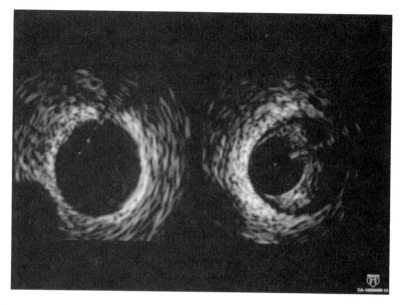

Figure 1. Serial IVUS images approximately 2 mm apart obtained during catheter pullback demonstrating compensatory enlargement at an atherosclerotic plaque. There is minimal luminal narrowing (approximately 35% diameter stenosis) despite a large plaque.

Arterial plaque is readily identified and quantified by IVUS. Plaque area is measured by subtracting the lumen area from the total vessel area, i.e. the area inside the echodense adventitia. This area includes the media and is termed "plaque plus media". The underlying media is often not be distinguishable from plaque and cannot be separately measured in most lesions. Calcium in the plaque is easily recognized as it is highly echo-dense creating a shadowing effect in the far field (see Figure 3).

There are basically two types of IVUS transducer designs currently available: mechanical and solid-state.(6) The mechanical transducers have a single ultrasound crystal which is rotated by a drive shaft connected to motor drive, usually outside the body. Imperfections in the rotation along the drive shaft can lead to significant, sometimes undetectable, artifacts in the image.(7) Recently, micro-motors have been adopted from watch technology and incorporated into the catheter tip thereby minimizing drive shaft length and artifacts. The solid-state system uses a 32 or 64 ultrasound crystal array arranged around the catheter tip circumference. Each crystal is controlled by a series of miniaturized integrated circuits arranged just proximal to the crystal array. Each crystal is sequentially activated to electronically sweep the ultrasound around the catheter tip. The returning ultrasound signal is processed by the system computer creating a synthetic or dynamic aperture array. Both mechanical and solid-state systems have inherent limitations. The rotating shaft of the mechanical catheter can produce artifacts when ideal 1:1 rotation along the length of the shaft does not occur.(7) These rotational artifacts, termed non-uniform rotational defects or NURD, can produce significant errors in image reconstruction dissections, left main coronary artery disease, ostial disease. Three-dimensional reconstruction will also be useful for assessing longitudinal stent-vessel wall

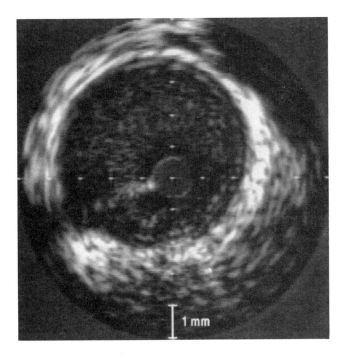

Figure 2. IVUS of a normal left anterior descending coronary artery demonstrating the three layered appearance.

relationships. Further development of catheters will inevitably take place with the and quantitation. Rotational artifacts have been minimized by reducing rotational friction. Solid-state catheters have had significant problems with "ring-down" artifact which have been minimized with electronic subtraction techniques.

The development of IVUS catheters has been a remarkable feat requiring tremendous component miniaturization.(8) After the initial catheter development, further advances occurred primarily in image quality with current generation catheters having very high resolution images. Future developments will focus on new display methods and unique catheter designs. New display methods will include color B-mode displays, color flow imaging and three-dimensional reconstruction. Color B-mode displays use various color scales instead of gray scales to display the 256 levels of signal intensity and are widely used in echocardiography to enhance image recognition.(9) The human eye is much more sensitive to changes in colors than gray scales. Color flow imaging is a novel non-Doppler imaging method where flowing blood can be displayed as a distinct color. The lumen is made more obvious with this method. Three dimensional reconstruction can now be performed immediately in the catheterization lab with only a simple "pull-back" of the catheter

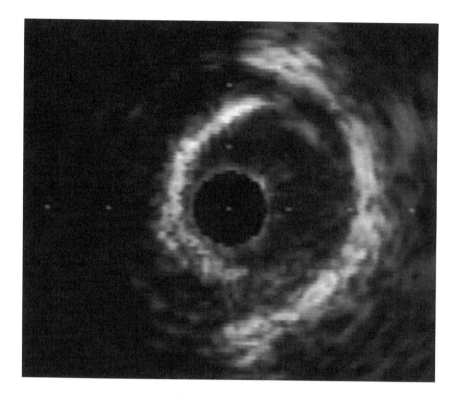

Figure 3. IVUS image of a heavily calcified plaque.

and a specialized computer system.(10, 11) Three-dimensional reconstruction will likely improve the assessment of complex longitudinal type disease, such as development of imaging cores and guidewires. Cost considerations will also promote the development of reusable, recyclable, or "resposable" catheters, which will have a disposable outer sheath with a reusable core.

PTCA

Morphologic Features – Intravascular ultrasound has confirmed the previously described pathologic findings following angioplasty. Successful PTCA often induces atherosclerotic plaque disruption, described as plaque "fracturing", "tearing", "splitting", and "cleaving" (12-20) which makes the silhouette technique of coronary angiography particularly inaccurate. There is a poor correlation between angiographic and histologic measurements of lumen diameter after both in-vitro and in-vivo balloon angioplasty.(21) Unfortunately, the angiographic silhouette does not fully display the cracks and fissures induced by balloon angioplasty. Intravascular ultrasound provides a tomographic image analogous to the pathologic section; Not surprisingly, there is a good correlation between ultrasound and histologic measurements of lumen diameter after balloon angioplasty (22-24) and a poor correlation between ultrasound and angiographic measurements of lumen diameter after PTCA.(22, 23, 25-28) There is a good correlation between ultrasound and angiographic measurements of lumen diameter before PTCA, however. In addition, angiography is insensitive to lesion eccentricity and calcification. Compared to angiography, IVUS detects more eccentric lesions (77 vs. 33%) and calcification (62 vs. 35%) .(29)

Angiography underestimates the severity of plaque burden following angioplasty. When the angiogram shows a residual 20 to 30 percent diameter stenosis, the IVUS frequently shows a 50 to 60 percent area stenosis.(23) It must be remembered that percent diameter stenosis and percent area stenosis are not equivalent measurements of stenosis severity. They are related to each other given that area is proportional to the diameter squared (See Figure 4):

$$\text{Area stenosis} = 1 - \left(1 - \frac{\text{Diameter stenosis}}{100}\right)^2 \times 100$$

In addition, percent diameter stenosis uses an adjacent "normal" site for reference *lumen* diameter whereas percent area stenosis usually uses the lesion site for reference *vessel* area. Alternatively, the *lumen* area at a proximal or distal reference site can be

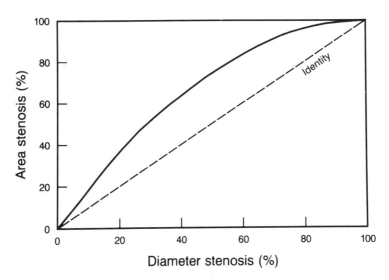

Figure 4. Relationship of percent area and diameter stenosis. Percent diameter stenosis and the percent area stenosis are not equivalent, but rather are related to each other because the area is a squared function of the diameter. They are equivalent at 0 and 100 percent stenoses only. At all other values, the percent area stenosis is greater than the percent diameter stenosis. At 30 percent diameter stenosis, the percent area stenosis equals 51 percent. At 50 percent diameter stenosis, the difference between percent diameter stenosis and percent area stenosis is maximal with the percent area stenosis equaling 75 percent. Between 28 and 72 percent diameter stenosis, the percent area stenosis is at least 20 percentage points higher than the percent diameter stenosis.

used for calculating percent area stenosis. The presence of diffuse disease and geometric remodeling makes the plaque burden further underestimated by angiography. When diffuse disease is present, a normal reference segment does not exist. When there is disease in the "normal" reference segment, the reference lumen diameter will be small relative to the true vessel size resulting in an underestimated angiographic percent diameter stenosis.(30) When there is geometric remodeling, the vessel area at the lesion is larger than vessel area at an adjacent site.(2, 3, 31-33) The growing atherosclerotic plaque primarily expands outward without significant luminal narrowing. Angiography reveals information about the lumen but gives little information about the vessel wall architecture (see Figure 5).

Before intravascular ultrasound, the mechanism of PTCA in humans could only be studied by angiography and by examining pathologic material, usually obtained at autopsy. Initially, lumen enlargement after PTCA was thought to be due to compression of soft components of atherosclerotic plaque.(34) Subsequent pathologic studies have demonstrated that plaque disruption accompanies most successful PTCA procedures.(16, 19, 35) In addition, vessel stretching has also been considered a possible mechanism of PTCA. The relative contribution of plaque disruption and vessel wall stretch could not be determined by angiography alone.

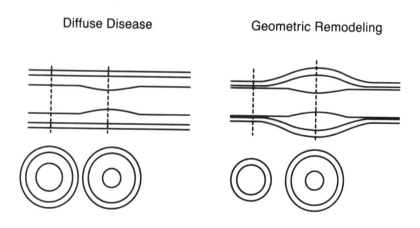

Figure 5. Illustrations of geometric remodeling and diffuse disease.

Autopsy studies were also not very helpful as pre-PTCA vessel dimensions were needed to assess changes in vessel wall morphology induced by PTCA. Intravascular ultrasound has been quite useful for assessing changes in vessel wall morphology induced by PTCA in-vivo. The high incidence of plaque disruption seen at autopsy has been confirmed with IVUS.(29, 36-39)

Serial IVUS studies before and after successful PTCA have shown that lumen area enlarges both from vessel enlargement (or stretch) and plaque reduction (See Table 1). Plaque fracture may accompany both processes. Interestingly, there is conflicting data as to whether the dominant mechanism of lumen enlargement is vessel stretch or plaque reduction. However, the mechanism of lumen enlargement is undoubtedly related to the underlying atherosclerotic plaque which in turn may be related to the presenting symptoms. When compared with patients with stable angina, patients with unstable angina more often have "soft" lesions (74 vs. 41%) and fewer intra-lesional calcium deposits (16 vs. 45%, both p<0.01).(40) Patients with unstable angina and "soft" plaques appear to have a reduction in plaque area as the main contributor to lumen enlargement. A reduction in plaque area, also called plaque "compression", may occur either by longitudinal displacement of plaque or by expression of liquid material from plaque; Actual compression of plaque is unlikely to occur given its low compressibility index. It has previously been shown that lipid containing plaque, or "soft" plaque, is reduced in weight after application of pressure, presumably a result of fluid expression.(41) Conversely, patients with stable angina or "hard", calcific plaques appear to have an improvement in lumen area predominantly by vessel stretching. It has been hypothesized that atherosclerotic plaque produces a cicatrizing effect on the vessel wall which is released by PTCA-induced plaque disruption. Balloon dilatation has been shown to increase the distensibility of the stenotic segment.(42) In summary, the mechanism of luminal enlargement appears to be plaque compression in patients with soft plaques with unstable syndromes and vessel stretch in patients with hard plaques with stable angina.

Table 1. Serial IVUS studies pre and post-PTCA

Authors, Source	Lesions	Δ Lumen Area	Contribution to Δ Lumen Area, %	
			Δ Vessel Area	Δ Plaque area
Suneja, *AHJ 1993*	84% UAP 76% soft	2.4 to 5.5 mm^2 (229%)	6%	94%
Braden, *JACC 1994*	17% UAP 40% Ca^{++}	2.6 to 5.4 mm^2 (212%)	81%	19%
DiMario, *AJC 1995*	50% UAP 56% soft	1.7 to 6.4 mm^2 (376%)	48%	52%

UAP, unstable angina pectoris; Ca^{++}, calcified lesion; soft, soft lesion.
References (38, 39, 43)

In the majority of cases, successful PTCA depends on a controlled disruption or tear of the atherosclerotic plaque (see Figure 6). If too little or no tear occurs then there may be inadequate dilatation with an increased tendency for elastic recoil and restenosis.(44-47) Conversely, extensive tearing or dissection with medial extension often portends a poor outcome, with a 6.5 fold increase in risk of major complication.(48) Angiography is inaccurate at assessing the extent of dissection and can be improved upon with IVUS.(21, 49) After PTCA, approximately 50% of patients will have dissections by IVUS with only 22% by angiography. The presence of dissection appears to improve the efficiency of PTCA as expressed as the neolumen: balloon ratio (NLBR). The single most important predictor of a high NLBR after PTCA was the presence of dissection.(29) Lesions with dissection had NLBR of 0.90 vs. 0.74 without dissection (p<0.001). Calcium, which can readily be detected by IVUS, plays an important role in the genesis of plaque tearing and dissection. Almost 90% of dissections detected by IVUS after PTCA are adjacent to calcification.(50) There is an abrupt change in biomechanical properties at the plaque-calcium interface which increases local wall stress and risk of dissection during PTCA.(51-55) Intravascular ultrasound studies have shown that calcified plaques have larger dissections after PTCA.(50)

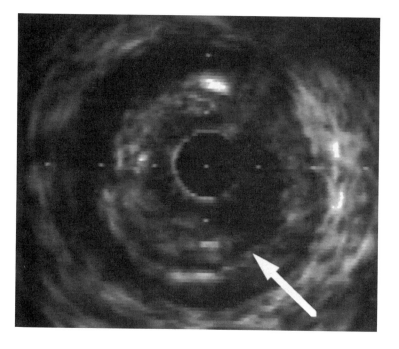

Figure 6. IVUS example of dissection post-PTCA. Arrow marks site of intimal tear. The dissection runs along a calcified segment at the base of the plaque, the most common site of dissections

Trial Data – Several classification schemes have been developed for describing the angioplasty result by IVUS.(37, 56) Honye et al classified the angioplasty result by the degree of plaque disruption (see Table 2).(37) Tears or splits are disruptions of the plaque only without dissection, defined as separation of plaque from underlying media. Dissections are further sub-classified based on the degree circumferential separation. In a small series of patients, those without plaque fracture detected by IVUS had a higher rate of restenosis (approximately 50%) compared to those with fracture (12%) supporting the concept that some tearing is necessary for adequate dilation.(37) However, other investigators have found that an IVUS-detected dissection carries an increased risk for adverse cardiac events (death, CABG, MI, restenosis).(36) Waller et al has suggested that dissections that are >180° (type D dissections) or are >1 cm in length are inherently unstable.(57) Other classification schemes have also been developed for assessing the IVUS result post-PTCA.(58) Although these classification schemes provide a nice conceptual framework for understanding extent of arterial injury post-PTCA, they have yet to find clinical usefulness.

An important question to ask is whether IVUS can improve the outcome of patients undergoing PTCA. However, IVUS is a diagnostic tool and can not improve patient outcome unless it is followed by additional catheter-based therapy, such as stenting. The ability of IVUS to improve patient outcome therefore is related not only to its ability to predict adverse outcomes but also on the success of additional catheter-based therapy. It is tempting to design studies combining IVUS with additional catheter-based therapies to test the hypothesis that IVUS can improve patient outcome. However, what IVUS derived morphology should be used to prompt additional catheter-based therapy? Inadequate lumen area, residual percent area stenosis, absence of plaque rupture, or some other criteria? The natural history of IVUS morphologies post-PTCA is unknown at this time. It would therefore be premature to design a therapeutic study based on IVUS morphologies. Phase II of the Guidance by Ultrasound Imaging for Decision Endpoints Trial (GUIDE Trial Phase II) will examine the natural history of IVUS findings post-PTCA. In this study, IVUS was performed after angiographically successful PTCA or stent placement. The operators were blinded to the results of the IVUS so that subsequent treatment would not be altered in any way based on the IVUS findings. Patients were then followed for adverse clinical endpoints (recurrent angina, target vessel revascularization, MI, or death) with a subpopulation having angiography at 6 months for restenosis.

Preliminary results from the GUIDE II Trial have shown that the degree of residual stenosis is predictive of outcome. Approximately halfway through the trial, multivariate analysis revealed that IVUS percent plaque area following

Table 2. Morphologic patterns of PTCA by IVUS

Type	Pattern
A	Linear, partial tear of plaque
B	Split in plaque, extends to media
C	Dissection behind plaque, < 180°
D	Extensive dissection, > 180°
E	No evidence of fracture

E1, concentric; E2, concentric
Reference(37)

angiographically successful PTCA was associated with angiographic restenosis. In the same analysis, IVUS MLD was associated with the primary clinical endpoints, including death, Q-wave myocardial infarction, or target vessel revascularization (see Figure 7). While these data are compelling and may allow for the subsequent rational design of a therapeutic trial, they must be critically examined. For example, although lumen area post-PTCA is significantly lower in those with adverse clinical outcomes, there is likely to be a large overlap between those without adverse clinical outcomes. As such, it will be difficult to select any one optimal "cut-off" value above which would indicate a low risk and below which would indicate a high risk. Any "cut-off" value would likely have a low predictive accuracy and therefore a low relative risk of adverse clinical event. If this "cut-off" value were used to determine who required additional catheter-based therapy, such as coronary stenting, then many truly low risk patients may receive stents while some truly high risk patients may not receive additional therapy. The same would be true for any of the post-PTCA IVUS morphologies reported thus far.

Several other trials are in progress which will help define the morphologic predictors of outcome, including: Post IntraCoronary Treatment Ultrasound Result (PICTURE), Serial Ultrasound REstenosis (SURE), and INtravascular ultraSound PredIctors REstenosis (INSPIRE). These trials are not yet published and only preliminary data is available in abstract form. While some studies are in accord with the GUIDE II trial, others show no relationship of IVUS morphologies with patient outcome. In the PICTURE trial, a multicenter trial from the Netherlands, there have been no IVUS morphologies predictive of restenosis to date.(59)

Future Implications - IVUS has been useful as research tool to study for the first time in-vivo the mechanisms of lumen enlargement post-PTCA and restenosis, and the morphologies predictive of adverse clinical outcome. Widespread clinical use will only occur if the additional information obtained by IVUS can translate into improved patient outcome. When the morphologic predictors of outcome are further defined in the studies listed above, then further studies can be performed with randomization of the "high risk" groups to additional therapy, such as coronary stenting. Only then will the effect of IVUS on patient outcome become apparent. Although it may be obvious, any improvement in patient outcome is in large part related to the efficacy of the added therapy. New interventional technologies will add to the armamentarium to be used for these "high risk" morphologies. In addition, new interventional technologies may also change the natural history of IVUS morphologies post-PTCA. For example, local gene therapy post-PTCA will undoubtedly change the response of the vessel to balloon-induced injury.

Intravascular ultrasound may also been useful for determining balloon size. Angiographic and IVUS measurements of lumen diameter correlate well at the reference segment when the lumens are round, so the benefit of IVUS for balloon sizing is not immediately apparent. However, the angiogram gives little information about the presence of diffuse disease which may be present in the reference segment. If diffuse disease is present, then our angiographically-sized balloon will be appropriate for the reference *lumen* but will be undersized relative to the reference *vessel*. In this case, we may be able to improve our angioplasty result by using balloons that are somewhat larger than angiography would indicate. Previous

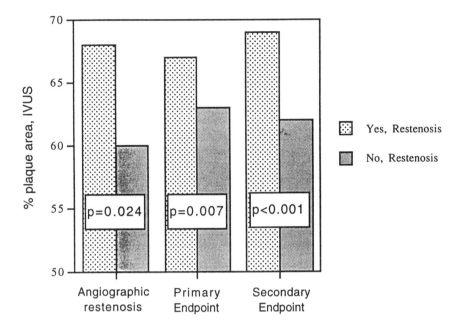

Figure 7. Preliminary data from the GUIDE II trial demonstrating increased percent plaque areas in patients with angiographic restenosis, primary and secondary clinical endpoints.

angiographic studies have clearly shown that oversized balloons increase the risk of dissection. However, in the presence of diffuse disease, the vessel size is larger which may allow the safe use of larger balloons and improve the PTCA result. In the CLOUT pilot trial, IVUS-guided balloon sizing resulted in upsizing in 85% of patients compared to angiographic sizing (balloon: artery ratio 1.04 to 1.18, p<0.001). Balloon upsizing resulted in an improvement in angiographic (MLD 1.7 to 2.0 mm, % diameter stenosis 33 to 20%, p<0.001 for both) and IVUS result (lumen area 3.4 to 4.5 mm2, p<0.001) without an increase in adverse outcomes. It has yet to be determined if this will translate into an improvement in patient outcome.(60)

DIRECTIONAL CORONARY ATHERECTOMY

Morphologic Features - Directional coronary atherectomy (DCA) has a unique advantage over PTCA in that it removes atheromatous tissue. The device is placed into the vessel and atheroma is pushed through the cutter window during balloon inflation. The cutter is passed along the length of the window amputating plaque which protrudes through the window. By IVUS, DCA treated plaque frequently has a "scalloped" appearance in places where the cutter has removed plaque.

The mechanism of lumen enlargement has not been defined with angiographic studies. Theoretically, an improvement in lumen area and angiographic dimension is due to the removal of atheroma. However, there may also be a significant "Dottering" or dilating effect induced by DCA catheter passage and balloon inflation. Although atheromatous tissue is usually removed with DCA, this finding does not preclude the dilating effect as the major mechanism of lumen enlargement. Angiography is unable to fully define the mechanism of DCA as it provides no information about the quantity of plaque or degree of wall stretch. IVUS has been used to define the mechanism of lumen enlargement with DCA and the mechanism has been contrasted with the mechanism of PTCA.(38, 39, 61) The mechanism of luminal enlargement with DCA has consistently been due to reductions in plaque area and presumably plaque removal, with a very small component coming from increases in vessel area or vessel stretch (see Table 3). In contrast, the mechanism of lumen enlargement with PTCA varies considerably with IVUS plaque morphology (see Table 1). The degree of plaque removal can be expressed quantitatively as the atherectomy index:

$$\text{Atherectomy index} = \frac{\text{Pre}_{P+M} - \text{Post}_{P+M}}{\text{Post}_{\text{Lumen}} - \text{Pre}_{\text{Lumen}}},$$

where Pre_{P+M} and Post_{P+M} are the plaque plus media areas before and after DCA, and $\text{Pre}_{\text{Lumen}}$ and $\text{Post}_{\text{Lumen}}$ are the lumen areas before and after DCA. In essence, the atherectomy index tells what part of the improvement in lumen area is accounted for by a reduction in plaque plus media area, and is shown in the Plaque Area Change column in Table 3.

Other IVUS derived morphologic data has shown that when the treated site is compared to the reference site, there is very little change in the vessel dimension after DCA. After PTCA, however, there is a significant increase in the vessel dimension at the treated site compared to the reference site. Additionally, dissection occurs only rarely following DCA yet it commonly occurs after PTCA (7% vs 50%, p<0.01). Both of these findings indicate that the dominant mechanism of DCA is plaque removal which occurs with minimal dilation of the vessel. Even gentle predilation (with 2 mm balloon) does not appear to result in significant vessel expansion.(63)

IVUS guidance of DCA procedures - Intravascular ultrasound has been used during DCA procedures to localize plaque and direct the DCA cutter towards eccentric plaque. Unfortunately, angiography does not accurately define the true eccentricity of plaque relative to the vessel wall.(29) Angiography can show the degree of eccentricity of the plaque relative to the surrounding lumen, but in most cases the plaque anatomy is not accurately displayed.

When IVUS identifies an eccentric plaque, the operator must then attempt to use the IVUS data to correctly position the DCA cutter flouroscopically into the eccentric plaque. Several skills are required to do this step properly. First, the IVUS image orientation must be understood. By convention, all IVUS images are displayed as though looking down the catheter from proximal to distal. Therefore, if an anterior septal branch is seen at six o'clock, the diagonal branches should be seen between nine o'clock and 12 o'clock. Second, the location of the plaque relative to these

Table 3. Serial IVUS studies pre and post-DCA

Authors, Study size, *Source*	Residual Stenosis (% Diameter or % Area)*	Contribution to Δ Lumen Area		
		Lumen Area Change (Pre to post, mm²; Δ Lumen Area, mm²)	Vessel Area Change (Pre to post, mm²; Δ Area, mm²; % Δ lumen area)	Plaque area Change (Pre to post, mm² Δ Area, mm² % Δ lumen area)
Suneja, et al n=40 *AHJ 1993*	Angio: 18% IVUS: 54%	2.2 to 7.7 +5.5	16.0 to 16.9 +0.9 16%	13.8 to 9.2 -4.6 84%
Braden, et al n=25 *JACC 1994*	Angio: N.R. IVUS: 40%	2.4 to 7.0 +4.7	16.7 to 17.5 +0.8 17%%	14.3 to 10.5 -3.8 83%
Matar, et al n=47 *JACC 1995*	Angio: 21% IVUS: 68%	1.7 to 6.6 +4.9	20.0 to 20.6 + 0.6 12%	18.3 to 14.0 -4.3 88%
Nakamura, et al n=28 *AHJ 1995*	Angio: 19% IVUS: 61%	2.9 to 7.0 +4.1	17.1 to 18.7 +1.6 39%	14.2 to 11.7 -2.5 61%

*Residual stenosis: angio = % diameter, IVUS = % area, N.R.= not recorded.
References (38, 39, 61, 62)

structures must be ascertained. Slight advancement or withdrawal of the catheter may be required to identify the location of a known landmark relative to the angiographic stenosis. With this knowledge, the operator knows immediately, for example, whether an eccentric lesion in the LAD is on the left or right side of the vessel. Third, the DCA catheter must be placed flouroscopically into the eccentric plaque. If one has a stable landmark (good examples are the circumflex branch for the proximal LAD, diagonal branches for the mid-LAD, obtuse marginal branches for the left circumflex, and acute marginal branches for the right coronary artery), then the DCA catheter window can be placed adjacent to the landmark. The DCA catheter may then need to be rotated if the plaque was not exactly in line with the landmark. For example, if the lesion was 90° *clockwise* to the landmark on the IVUS image, then 90° of *clockwise* torque on the DCA catheter will re-align the window onto the plaque. With these maneuvers, additional plaque can be removed over flouroscopic guidance alone.(64)

Other investigators have also proposed the "single pass" technique where a single pass is performed with the catheter in a known flouroscopic location. IVUS is the performed to examine the location of the plaque relative this first pass, if it can be identified. Subsequent passes can then be made with either additional clockwise or counter-clockwise torque on the DCA catheter.

Trial Data - Despite the consistency of the findings in the four IVUS studies reported in Table 2, the response to DCA is clearly dependent on plaque morphology. Plaques can be broadly separated into echogenic and echolucent plaques with echogenic plaques having higher collagen and calcium content and echolucent plaques having higher levels of fibrin, nuclei, and lipids.(65) Echogenic plaques have a smaller degree of plaque reduction with DCA than echolucent plaques (60±18% vs

76±21%, p<0.05) and are likely somewhat more difficult to cut. Interestingly, the degree of plaque reduction correlated well with the weight of resected material (r=0.62, p<0.01). Despite the improvement in plaque reduction in the echolucent plaque patients, the incidence of restenosis was 100% (vs 33% for echogenic plaques. The number of patients in this study was small (n=22), so no firm conclusions can be made until additional data is available. The inability to remove tissue in echogenic plaques was most likely related to the calcium content.

Plaques that are heavily calcified are not cut well by the device, particularly when the calcium is superficial, or adjacent to the luminal surface. Calcified lesions (with ≥90° of calcium) have larger residual plaque areas and smaller residual lumen areas after DCA compared to lesions with minimal or no calcium (plaque area; 16.9±5.5 vs 11.9±4.6 mm2, p<0.007, and lumen area; 7.5±2.5 vs 10.3±4.5. p=0.08).(66) In this study, calcium was often not present angiographically and therefore could not have been identified without IVUS. Conversely, deep calcium seen along the media-adventitia border, may actually prevent sub-intimal resection and protect against deep adventitial injury. The amount of tissue removed is equivalent for lesions with deep calcification and for non-calcified lesions (19.7±6.9 vs 22.5±7.2 mg, respectively). However, lesions with superficial calcium had approximately half as much tissue removed (10.3±6.8 mg, p<0.001).(29)

In a multivariate analysis of 170 patients undergoing DCA, clinical, procedural, angiographic, and IVUS variables were studied to identify predictors of success.(62) The endpoint used was lumen cross-sectional area and residual cross-sectional narrowing determined by the final IVUS image. Of the multiple variables examined, the pre-intervention lesion arc of calcium was the most consistent predictor of the success of DCA. Even after correction for reference vessel size, both arc of calcium and pre-atherectomy plaque plus media cross-sectional area were associated with larger lumen cross-sectional areas (p=0.02 and p=0.0003, respectively). Arc of calcium (p=0.0002), pre-atherectomy plaque plus media cross-sectional area (p=0.0001), lesion length (p=0.01) were all associated with a larger post-atherectomy residual cross-sectional narrowing. Interestingly, the presence of superficial calcium did not predict outcome in this multivariate analysis. However, the overall message is that the more highly calcified the lesion, the less suited the lesion is for DCA.

In the Optimal Atherectomy Restenosis Study (OARS), a strategy of "optimal" atherectomy with IVUS was examined.(67) Repetitive IVUS was used to facilitate the atherectomy technique with a goal of achieving a residual angiographic stenosis less than 15%. The average angiographic stenosis achieved was 7% with 81% of patients achieving the goal of <15% stenosis. By IVUS, the percent area stenosis was reduced from 81% to 14% when the lesion lumen area was compared to the reference segment lumen area. However, when the cross-sectional area stenosis was measured at the lesion site, there was still a residual 56% area stenosis. This discrepancy is likely due to a combination of diffuse disease and compensatory enlargement. The aggressive IVUS guided atherectomy strategy did not increase the complication rate and resulted in a reasonably low restenosis rate of 30%. These results were significantly improved from the CAVEAT and CCAT results which used a more timid atherectomy protocol. The large residual plaque burden by IVUS raises the question if better results could be obtained with even more complete atherectomy. IVUS guidance would be required to avoid deep injury.

Combined DCA/IVUS Device - A more direct approach for guiding DCA with IVUS is to mount the IVUS imaging system onto the DCA catheter tip. The plaque can be directed into the DCA cutting window with cuts taken under direct ultrasonic observation. In addition, the operator would be able to treat and image with the same catheter thereby avoiding catheter exchanges. Several strategies for combining DCA and IVUS have been developed. The first catheter to be used in animal models and humans for guided DCA (GDCA) has incorporated the ultrasound transducer onto the rotating cutter (see Figure 8). An image is produced in only one quadrant of the image screen where the ultrasound "looks out" the cutter window. The metal housing prevents imaging of the other quadrants. Imaging only occurs when the cutter is activated and rotating. An image of the lesion is created as the cutter is withdrawn. The cutter housing can be rotated towards plaque if the window is up against normal vessel wall. In addition, higher balloon inflation pressures could be used to push plaque further into the window while insuring that the depth of the cut is not sub-intimal. In the first five patients treated with the GDCA catheter, all procedures were angiographically successful with only one patient having media in the resected tissue.(68) With conventional DCA, approximately 50% of samples have media and 10% of samples have adventitia. It would appear that GDCA can remove plaque while minimizing deep wall injury.

Future Implications - Improvements in the DCA technique has the potential to significantly improve the clinical outcome. As outlined above, initial DCA technique was quite timid and more aggressive strategies have indeed improved the outcome. These results are consistent with current thinking regarding restenosis as outlined by Kuntz and Baim.(69) The paradigm proposes that a certain degree of late lumen loss will occur following all coronary interventional procedures, presumably due to a combination of recoil and intimal hyperplasia. The amount of late lumen loss approximates half of the acute gain. Kuntz and Baim state that "bigger *is* better" implying that larger acute gains, although associated with larger late lumen loss, end up with a final lumen that does not compromise coronary flow reserve.

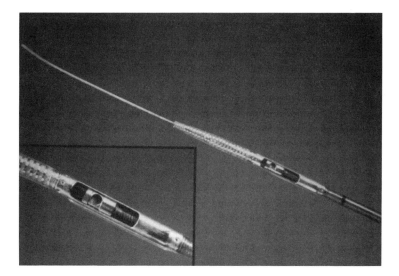

Figure 8. Guided-directional coronary atherectomy catheter (GDCA) catheter.

As shown in the OARS study above, more aggressive DCA strategies can clearly improve the initial result which is translated into a reduced restenosis rate compared to CAVEAT and CCAT data. Unfortunately, increasingly aggressive DCA strategies that are not IVUS-guided may result in an increase in deep arterial injury. While this may increase acute lumen gain, it may also add to the risk of the procedure. Deep arterial injury can increase the degree of intimal proliferation (70) and indeed conventional DCA has been associated with more late lumen loss compared to PTCA. Deep arterial injury may also predispose the artery to focal constriction, or negative remodeling. However, the added risk of deep arterial injury remains controversial. Fishman et al found an improvement in restenosis if the final minimal lumen diameter was greater than 3.0 mm (risk ratio 0.63, p=0.047).(71) Surprisingly, there was a trend towards lower restenosis if adventitia was retrieved (risk ratio 0.63, p=0.176).

IVUS guided DCA should allow for plaque removal with a minimum of deep arterial injury. With the GDCA catheter, it in fact may be possible to produce residual stenoses below zero without deep injury which, in theory, should significantly reduce the restenosis rate.

STENTS

Morphologic Features - One of the most important applications of IVUS may be for guiding stent implantation. Angiography has specific weaknesses when used for assessing the adequacy of stent deployment. First, most stent are radiolucent and are not visible even with high resolution flouroscopy. The presence of the stent is usually inferred by the angiographic appearance. The proximal and distal ends of the stent are often not well appreciated by angiography. Second, when there is a minimal residual stenosis (<20%), a small change in angiographic diameter (which are not usually detectable) can result in large changes in lumen area (see Table 4).

Table 4. Theoretical changes in area vs. diameter during stent optimization

	Reference segment	Stent Initial	Stent Final	% change
Diameter, mm	3.8	3.5	3.7	6%
Area, mm^2	11.34	9.62	10.75	12%
% Diameter Stenosis	–	8%	3%	
% Area Stenosis	–	15%	5%	

Assuming reference lumen dimensions of 3.8 mm and an initial stent dimension of 3.5 mm which is further improved 3.7 mm with additional inflation. The percent change in area (IVUS) is larger than the percent change in diameter (angiography). These numbers would likely be further exaggerated with non circular stent lumens whose dimensions may be overestimated by angiography

Therefore, small residual stenoses that require additional treatment may not be apparent angiographically. Third, the relationship of the stent to the vessel wall can not be determined by angiography. For example, individual stent tines or wires may not be in contact with the vessel wall which is termed incomplete apposition. Additionally, the Palmaz-Schatz stents often expand asymmetrically with most of the tines on one side of the lumen. Angiography can not resolve these details. Fourth, small "filling defects" within the stent are difficult to discern angiographically. Tissue prolapse through the articulation site of Palmaz-Schatz stents can be obstructive and are the main site of stent restenosis.(72) Due to their focal nature, only a truly orthogonal angiographic image will accurately display the prolapse. Fifth, margin tears or dissections are more difficult to visualize angiographically because one end is tacked down by the stent. However, the dissections may be obstructive and require additional treatment. Without question, IVUS shows more details regarding stent location, deployment, and vessel wall interactions than angiography, which although not proven , likely improves the clinical outcome.

Metallic stents can be easily imaged with IVUS due to their echogenicity. The individual wires or tines appear echodense on the image. The tines can be confused with either the coronary guidewire or superficial "specks" of calcium. The guidewire can usually be traced proximal and distal to the stent to identify its location within the stent. In addition, many IVUS imaging systems now require guidewire removal prior to imaging eliminating any confusion. Although occasionally calcium can appear as a stent tine, the typical ultrasound signature of the stent is usually recognizable.(73) Slotted tube stents (Palmaz-Schatz) have pairs of tines which appear to spread apart and then come together again during pullback through the stent. Coronary Palmaz-Schatz stents have six pairs of tines while biliary Palmaz-Schatz stents have seven pairs of tines. At the articulation site in the middle of the stent, all tines except one disappear. Newer Palmaz-Schatz stent designs will not have this finding. Wire stents (e.g. Gianturco-Rubin, Wiktor) have a much different signature due to the serpiginous course of the stent wire. The typical image shows the refractile wire along a portion of the intimal surface which undulates back and forth during pullback (see Figure 9).

The IVUS assessment includes measurements of the proximal and distal reference segments with measurements made of the lumen and vessel area and maximum and minimum diameter. Vessel area measurements are made along the outer edge of the sonolucent media at the presumed external elastic lamina. Vessel and lumen areas may be quite different in patients with diffuse disease in the reference segments. Some investigators average the proximal and distal measurements to derive the reference segment values. Similar measurements are made within the stent at the point of smallest area. The stent is interrogated for any regions of incomplete apposition. Most IVUS catheters have some signal blooming along stent tine edges due to lateral resolution abnormalities which can sometimes mimic incomplete apposition. A careful search for filling defects within the stent is made paying particular attention to the articulation site. Importantly, the inflow and outflow portions of the stent must be carefully screened for any obstruction, including proximal or distal extension of dissection. Multiple criteria for successful stent implantation have been used in the past.

Trial Data - Initially, stents were used as bail-out devices for treating abrupt closure or threatened abrupt closure, where they were found to be very effective at

298

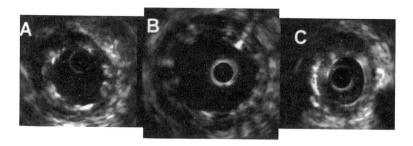

Figure 9. Stent examples; A, Johnson and Johnson coronary stent; B, Johnson and Johnson biliary stent; C, Gianturco -Rubin stent.

reducing the need for emergency CABG. More recently, stents have been shown to be effective at reducing the restenosis rate, raising the question of whether stent use should be widespread. Unfortunately, major complications of stenting were reported with stent thromboses occurring in 3-4 % of elective cases and 8-16% of emergency or bail-out cases. Aggressive anticoagulation strategies to prevent stent thrombosis led to a vascular complication rate of 4-10 % and with an increased need for blood transfusion thereby limiting the widespread application of stents.

Perhaps the greatest contribution of IVUS to invasive cardiology has been to improve stent deployment techniques which have significantly reduced the overall complication rate. Seminal IVUS observations were made by Dr. Antonio Colombo and colleagues in 1993 which clearly demonstrated that angiography was inadequate for assessing stent deployment.(74-76) Despite having an excellent angiographic result (< 10% diameter stenosis), only 13 % of patients had an adequate IVUS result.(75) However, with additional balloon inflations with either larger balloons or higher pressures, both the angiographic and IVUS dimensions could be improved (angiographic % diameter stenosis from 9% to -4% and IVUS stent lumen area from 6.6 mm^2 to 8.8 mm^2, p<0.0001 for both).(74, 76) Other investigators have found similar results.(77) In the Optimal Stent Implantation (OSTI) study, there was an improvement in lumen diameter by IVUS with increasing inflation pressure from 12, 15, to 18 ATM, without any change in angiographic dimension.(see Figure 10)(78)

Dr. Colombo proposed that anticoagulation would no longer be required if the stent dimensions were optimized with IVUS confirmation. Perhaps the prior problems with stent thrombosis were related to inadequate stent deployment rather than inherent thrombogenicity of metallic stents. With IVUS optimization, the rate of stent thrombosis was only 0.9% (0.6% acute and 0.3% sub acute) despite the fact that no anticoagulation was used post-procedure. Antiplatelet therapy was used following the procedure (indefinite aspirin and ticlopidine for 1-2 months). The lack of anticoagulant could theoretically have increased mural thrombus formation post-procedure and contributed to an increased restenosis rate. However, the long term results were also excellent with only 13% of patients having a repeat PTCA. The angiographic restenosis rate is not available in this cohort of patients. A comparison of the patients with IVUS-guided stent implantation with the non-IVUS guided stent implantation is shown in Table 5. Although not necessarily a fair comparison because of baseline and procedural differences that may have been present between studies, IVUS guided stent deployment without anticoagulation resulted in a significant reduction in bleeding and/or vascular complications while not compromising the acute or long term stent results. Other differences between the studies may have included larger reference vessels, balloon/artery ratios, and higher balloon inflation pressures. However, the Colombo data does include all elective stent cases and not just those eligible for study randomization.

The criteria for optimal stent expansion used by Dr. Colombo's group evolved significantly over time and with additional clinical experience. Initially, the goal was to achieve a minimal stent area of 60% of the average of the proximal and distal *vessel* cross-sectional areas. This goal was set in an effort "to accommodate the compensatory dilation that occurs with early atheroma deposition". Unfortunately, this strategy resulted in an oversizing of balloons and an increased complication rate.

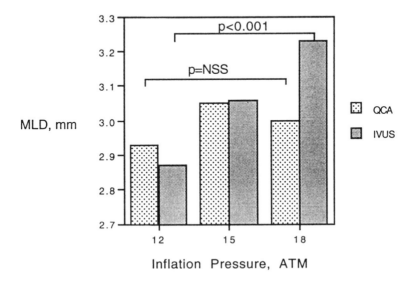

Figure 10. Stent minimal lumen diameter (MLD) measurements by IVUS and QCA with sequential increments in balloon inflation pressure from the OSTI study.(78)

Table 5. Comparison of Colombo, STRESS, and Benestent results

	Standard stent deployment	IVUS-guided stent deployment	
	STRESS n=205 pts	Benestent n=259 pts	Colombo n=359 pts
All Deaths, 6-8 mos	1.5%	0.8%	1.9%
MI			
In-Hospital	N.A.	3.5%	3.9%
Late, 7 mos.	N.A.	4.2%	1.7%
All	6.3%	.7.7%	5.7%
CABG	4.9%	8.1%	6.4%
Bleeding and/or vascular complication.	7.3%	13.5%	0.6%
Subacute thrombosis	3.4%	3.5%	1.4%
Ref. vessel size, mm	3.0	3.0	3.3
%DS, post-procedure	19%	33%	-7%
MLD, post-procedure	2.5	2.5	3.4
Balloon pressure, ATM	N.A.	10	14.9
Balloon/artery ratio	N.A.	1.12	1.17
Restenosis	32%	22%	N.A.

N.A.=Not available

Later, the goal was reset to achieve at least 100% of the distal *lumen* area. The same excellent results were obtained with a lower acute complication rate using appropriately sized balloons with very high inflation pressures. The results are summarized in Table 6.

The criteria for optimal stent implantation are still in evolution and have been developed primarily from clinical experience rather than randomized controlled studies. However, the following four criteria are suggested for optimal stent implantation by IVUS (see Table 7). First, there must be good stent apposition with all components of the stent in contact with the vessel wall. This is a qualitative observation which requires careful stent interrogation during IVUS catheter pullback. Second, optimal stent expansion should occur with the stent achieving at least 90% of the distal reference lumen cross-sectional area. Larger vessels may not require such a large stent area given the large lumen cross-sectional area even with residual 20% stenoses. Tobis has suggested that a sliding scale method be used with the acceptable final stent cross-sectional area being a function of the reference lumen size (see figure 11). Third, tissue prolapse through the articulation site must be treated if significant obstruction is present. The articulation site is usually the smallest site following stent deployment due to tissue prolapse and most restenosis occurs focally at this site. The obligatory neointimal proliferation is less well tolerated if the articulation site is already narrowed. Typical treatment requires placing a second stent or half a stent within the first stent covering the articulation site. Fourth, the inflow and outflow portions of the stent should be free of obstructing plaque or dissection. If the lumen area is compromised by 60% or greater compared to the adjacent reference

Table 6. Comparison of two strategies of optimal stent expansion

	Oversize Final Balloon 339 lesions, 263 patients	Appropriate -Size Final Balloon 113 lesions, 96 patients	P
Proximal reference, mm	3.30±0.57	3.30±0.47	0.97
Final stent MLD, mm	3.44±0.54	3.21±0.49	.0001
Final % stenosis	-9±15	1±10	.0001
Balloon diameter, mm	3.91±0.52	3.42±0.47	.0001
Ratio Balloon/Reference	1.20±0.19	1.05±0.14	.0001
Maximal inflation pressure, atm	14.7±2.9	15.7±3.1	.009
Intraprocedural event, n (%)	15 (5.7%)	1 (1.0%)	.042
Coronary rupture, n (%)	4 (1.2%)	0 (0%)	.28
Stent thrombosis, n (%)	2 (0.8%)	1 (1.0%)	.82

From (76)

segment, then additional stents should be placed. The same is true for margin tears, also termed "pocket tears", although short, non-obstructing tears can be left alone.

Other criterion have been used and generally found to be ineffective, such as the symmetry index defined as the minor diameter divided by the major diameter. Despite inflation with oversized and high pressure balloons, the symmetry index could not be significantly improved.(74, 79) Another criterion was to reduce the percent area stenosis at the stent site by compressing the plaque with the stent. This strategy did not take into account either the non-compressibility of the plaque or compensatory enlargement. Another criterion was to achieve 70% of the nominal PTCA balloon area. Even with high pressure balloon inflations, this criterion is frequently not met.

Future Implications - IVUS has the potential to improve the acute results, by reducing the subacute thrombosis rate and the need for anticoagulation, as well as the long term results, by reducing the restenosis rate. IVUS has clearly proven that our initial stent deployment strategies, which were based on angiographic findings, were often inadequate. High pressure balloon inflations resulted in significant improvements in our acute stent results, with anticoagulation now no longer routinely required. Many questions regarding the clinical utility of IVUS in stent deployment remain. Has IVUS just been an instrument to improve our stent deployment techniques or is it still required in every stent patient to tailor therapy, particularly if high pressure balloon inflation has already been performed? Should all patients have high pressure balloon inflations and are there any adverse effects? High pressure balloon inflations are generally well tolerated but acute complications such as rupture or dissection extension can occur. If high pressure balloon inflation has already been performed and the angiographic result is satisfactory, what else can IVUS find that would require additional treatment? All of the findings in Table 7, including incomplete stent apposition or expansion, tissue prolapse, or inflow and outflow problems may exist despite a satisfactory angiographic result and can be treated with additional inflations with higher pressure or balloon size or additional stents. Are these IVUS findings clinically relevant and do they all need additional

302

Table 7. IVUS criteria for successful stent implantation

1	Stent apposition	Complete apposition
2	Stent expansion	Small vessels; 90% distal lumen area Large vessels; 80% distal lumen area (using sliding scale method)
3	Tissue prolapse	None allowed
4	Inflow and outflow portions	Margin tears or plaque must be less than 60% of adjacent reference lumen area

treatment? The natural history of these IVUS findings is unknown but will be examined in the STRUT registry. In this registry, IVUS abnormalities following stent deployment were not acted upon and the patients were followed for clinical events at six months. There was a high incidence of IVUS abnormalities in this cohort of stent patients approximately 50% of patients having incomplete expansion, 10% incomplete apposition, and 20% margin tears. Other trials are in progress to further assess the utility of IVUS in stent deployment. Further advancements in stent technology, such as heparin coating, local gene delivery, or irradiation may further change the risk profile of coronary stents altering the potential benefits of IVUS.

ROTATIONAL ATHERECTOMY

Morphologic Features - Percutaneous transluminal coronary rotational atherectomy (PTCRA) is a unique method of coronary revascularization in which plaque is removed with an abrasive mechanism. In vitro studies have shown that the mechanism of lumen enlargement with PTCRA is due to selective removal of non-compliant material, especially calcium. As such, the morphology of lesions after PTCRA is expected to be quite different than after PTCA. IVUS studies after PTCRA have demonstrated that the lumens created are circular with a symmetry index approaching unity (1.1 ± 0.1).(80) Deviations from circular lumens only occurred in regions of soft plaque or where significant tissue disruption of calcified plaque occurred. The lumen-plaque interfaces were described as unusually sharp, clear, and distinct. Although the mechanism for this finding is not defined, it is likely due to the abrasive action on the calcified plaque. With the endothelium denuded, the calcium may be in direct contact with the lumen. Alternatively, there may be changes in the vessel wall acoustical properties following PTCRA which result in these findings. The micro-cavitations created in the lumen by the rotating burr might conceivably effect the ultrasonic characteristics of the lumen-plaque interface. The lumens created were larger than the largest burr size both for stand alone and adjunctive balloon procedures (1.19 ± 0.19 and 1.30 ± 0.15, respectively). Additional lumen may have been created by radial movement, or shimmy, of the burr or due to vessel spasm during passage. Vessel spasm is a common feature during PTCRA procedures. The removal of calcium may release the vessel from a cicatrizing effect of the plaque allowing additional dilation following the procedure.

Serial IVUS studies during PTCRA procedures in patients with mostly heavily calcified arteries have shown that the mechanism of lumen enlargement is entirely plaque removal with no evidence of barotrauma (see Table 8).(81) In contrast to

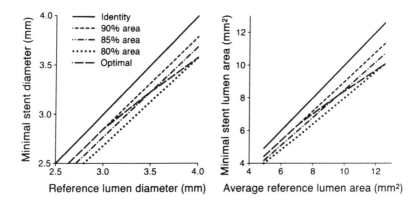

Figure 11. Sliding scale for stent optimization.

PTCA, vessel area decreased following PTCRA, perhaps due to vasospasm. After adjunctive PTCA, there is further improvement in lumen area due primarily to vessel stretch, with no significant reduction in plaque area. Despite achieving an excellent angiographic result of 20% stenosis, the lumen cross-sectional area stenosis by IVUS was 71%. The underestimation of disease by angiography is undoubtedly due to a combination of compensatory enlargement and diffuse disease. Decalcification did occur with the procedure with the arc of calcium being reduced from 227±107° to 209±107° (p=0.048). Quantitation of vessel calcification with IVUS is difficult due to acoustical shadowing which makes measuring the thickness of the calcium deposit problematic. Therefore, IVUS is not sensitive to changes in calcium deposit thickness which may have occurred following PTCRA.

After PTCRA alone, dissections occurred in 26% of lesions by IVUS and in 6% by angiography. By contrast, PTCA in heavily calcified arteries results in dissections in the majority of lesions (73 to 100%).(82, 83) After PTCRA alone, dissections occurred predominantly within the calcium deposit, a distinctly different pattern than that seen after PTCA where dissections occur primarily adjacent to the calcium deposit.(50) With adjunctive PTCA, the incidence of dissection increased to 77% by IVUS and 18% by angiography. The additional dissections seen were now more like primary PTCA dissections with the greatest number occurring adjacent to the calcium deposit.

Future Implications - PTCRA is ideally suited for treating heavily calcified arteries which may not be successfully treated with PTCA alone. IVUS is more sensitive at detecting coronary calcification than angiography. Even in a patient population with mostly heavily calcified arteries, flouroscopic calcification was detected in only 69% while IVUS detected calcium in 92%. In theory, IVUS could

Table 8. Serial IVUS studies pre and post-PTCRA and post-adjunctive PTCA

| | Residual Stenosis (% Diameter or % Area)* | Contribution to Δ Lumen Area | | |
		Lumen Area Change (Pre to post, Δ Lumen Area)	Vessel Area Change (Pre to post, Δ Area, % Δ lumen area)	Plaque area Change (Pre to post, Δ Area, % Δ lumen area)
Post-PTCRA	Angio: 37% IVUS: 74%	1.8 to 3.9 mm^2 +2.1 mm^2	17.4 to 16.7 mm^2 -0.6 mm^2 -29%	15.7 to 13.0 mm^2 -2.7 mm^2 129%
Post-adjunctive PTCA	Angio: 20% IVUS: 71%	3.9 to 5.0 mm^2 +1.3 mm^2	16.7 to 18.8 mm^2 +2.1 mm^2 162%	13.0 to 13.7 mm^2 +0.7 mm^2 -54%

*Residual stenosis: angio = % diameter, IVUS = % area.
Reference (81)

be used to identify patients with calcified arteries who might benefit the most from PTCRA. Unfortunately, no prospective, randomized trial testing this strategy has been performed.

IVUS AND DEVICE SELECTION

Catheter-based intervention now includes a vast array of tools for recanalizing stenotic and occluded arteries. Different tools or devices have fundamentally different mechanisms for enlarging the vessel lumen. The interventionalist must decide which mechanism or device will be most successful for a given lesion. Until recently, this decision was based primarily on the angiographic anatomy, as well as the patients clinical situation. It is unlikely that any new imaging modality will replace angiography for making this decision. In addition providing to details about the lesion, angiography yields information about the entire coronary tree, such as proximal disease, vessel tortuosity, branch vessels, and distal run-off. However, the interventionalist relying solely on the angiogram may have many misconceptions about the anatomy which can be further clarified with IVUS. For example, one of the most important predictors of the response to catheter intervention is vessel calcification. Angiography underestimates the degree of calcification and can not identify. Adapted from reference (85) the location of calcium within the vessel, i.e. superficial or deep. Angiography correlates poorly with IVUS when assessing lesion eccentricity. This finding indicates that the plaque may be eccentric relative to the reference lumen but may be concentric at the level of the plaque. The converse may also occur. If DCA is used to treat such a lesion based on the angiogram, the interventionalist will not know where to direct the cutter to maximize safe plaque removal. By further defining the plaque morphology, IVUS may be useful as an adjunctive imaging modality to guide device selection.(84)

Pre-intervention IVUS imaging frequently result in a change in intended therapy. In 313 lesions in 301 patients imaged prior to intervention, there was a change in therapy in 40%.(85) The IVUS imaging resulted in device selection or a change in device selection in 26% of lesions. In 7% of lesions, revascularization was canceled as no significant plaque was found. Devices were selected on the basis of lesion calcification, eccentricity, and the presence of thrombus. Lesions with significant superficial calcium were treated with rotational atherectomy, excimer laser angioplasty or surgery. Eccentric lesions without significant superficial calcium were treated with DCA. Dissections and true aneurysms were treated with stent placement even if calcified. Thrombus-containing lesions in vein grafts were treated with thrombolytic therapy or extraction atherectomy, or both. Fibrotic vein graft lesions were treated with balloon angioplasty or stent placement. Potential strategies for device selection after IVUS imaging are shown in Table 9.

While this data is intriguing, it represents a series of patients without controls to know if the best treatment was indeed performed. To date, no randomized trials have been performed to demonstrate an improvement in patient outcome with pre-intervention IVUS imaging. The smallest catheter size is approximately 1 mm, a size larger than most minimal lumen diameters. IVUS imaging alone does result in some dilatation, or "Dottering", of the lesion which could theoretically destabilize the plaque and change its subsequent response to catheter intervention.(86) While widely considered a safe procedure overall, the complication rate is clearly increased in interventional cases.(87, 88) These factors need to be taken into account when considering the overall benefit of IVUS imaging in device selection.

SUMMARY

Interventional Cardiology is a dynamic rapidly changing field. The changes have been made possible by advancements in technology and improved understanding of the potential responses of the vascular tree to the arterial trauma, as well as the development of new drugs. In the early days of interventional cardiology, the knowledge base was small and the procedure was notable for many successes, but relatively frequent major complications requiring urgent CABG. Major complications also had an increased rate of acute myocardial infarction and mortality. Since the early experiences, there have been significant changes. There is increased emphasis on a more rational approach to therapy with consideration of matching strategies and lesions. IVUS has been a fundamentally important addition to the armamentarium. It has served several functions. It has been invaluable in furthering

Table 9. IVUS imaging preintervention for device selection

IVUS finding	Proposed device
Calcium (superficial)	Rotational atherectomy Excimer laser CABG
Eccentric lesion	Directional atherectomy
Plaque disruption or dissection	Stent
Thrombus, especially in vein grafts	Thrombolytic Transluminal extraction atherectomy Both
Fibrotic lesions, including vein grafts	PTCA Stent Both
Severe left main disease	CABG or deferred procedure

our understanding of vascular anatomy including calcification, response to arterial injury, and long-term effects of therapy. Without IVUS, the clinical relevance of recoil and remodeling would have remained unexplained. In addition, the role of calcium in predicting outcome of different interventions, e.g., PTCA or Rotablator, would have been poorly understood. Monitoring the acute outcome of therapy would have also been problematic; IVUS has served as the impetus to change the way stenting is performed. Without IVUS, stenting would still be characterized by its need for intense anticoagulants with increased bleeding. The "added value" of IVUS is somewhat difficult to measure. Laboratories without access to the technology can continue to provide superb patient care, and patients in whom IVUS is not used can still be treated optimally. In both of these situations, however, the operators and patients have benefited from lessons learned from IVUS.

References

1. Topol EJ, Nissen SE. Our preoccupation with coronary luminology. The dissociation between clinical and angiographic findings in ischemic heart disease. [Review]. Circulation 1995;92(8):2333-42.

2. Glagov S, Weisenberg E, Zarins CK, Stankunavicius R, Kolettis GJ. Compensatory enlargement of human atherosclerotic coronary arteries. New England Journal of Medicine 1987;316(22):1371-5.

3. Stiel GM, Stiel LS, Schofer J, Donath K, Mathey DG. Impact of compensatory enlargement of atherosclerotic coronary arteries on angiographic assessment of coronary artery disease. Circulation 1989;80(6):1603-9.

4. Nishimura RA, Edwards WD, Warnes CA, et al. Intravascular ultrasound imaging: in vitro validation and pathologic correlation. Journal of the American College of Cardiology 1990;16(1):145-54.

5. Velican C, Velican D. Study of coronary intimal thickening. Atherosclerosis 1985;56(3):331-44.

6. Higano ST, Nishimura RA. Intravascular ultrasonography. [Review]. Current Problems in Cardiology 1994;19(1):1-55.

7. ten Hoff H, Korbijn A, Smith TH, Klinkhamer JF, Bom N. Imaging artifacts in mechanically driven ultrasound catheters. International Journal of Cardiac Imaging 1989;4(2-4):195-9.

8. Bom N, ten Hoff H, Lancee CT, Gussenhoven WJ, Bosch JG. Early and recent intraluminal ultrasound devices. [Review]. International Journal of Cardiac Imaging 1989;4(2-4):79-88.

9. Comess KA, Beach KW, Hatsukami T, Strandness D Jr., Daniel W. Pseudocolor displays in B-mode imaging applied to echocardiography and vascular imaging: an update. Journal of the American Society of Echocardiography 1992;5(1):13-32.

10. Matar FA, Mintz GS, Douek P, et al. Coronary artery lumen volume measurement using three-dimensional intravascular ultrasound: validation of a new technique [see comments]. Catheterization & Cardiovascular Diagnosis 1994;33(3):214-20.

11. Mintz GS, Pichard AD, Satler LF, Popma JJ, Kent KM, Leon MB. Three-dimensional intravascular ultrasonography: reconstruction of endovascular stents in vitro and in vivo. Journal of Clinical Ultrasound 1993;21(9):609-15.

12. Mizuno K, Kurita A, Imazeki N. Pathological findings after percutaneous transluminal coronary angioplasty. British Heart Journal 1984;52(5):588-90.

13. Chin AK, Kinney TB, Rurik GW, Shoor PM, Fogarty TJ. A physical measurement of the mechanisms of transluminal angioplasty. Surgery 1984;95(2):196-201.

14. Castaneda-Zuniga WR, Formanek A, Tadavarthy M, et al. The mechanism of balloon angioplasty. Radiology 1980;135(3):565-71.

15. Block PC, Myler RK, Stertzer S, Fallon JT. Morphology after transluminal angioplasty in human beings. New England Journal of Medicine 1981;305(7):382-5.

16. Waller BF. Early and late morphologic changes in human coronary arteries after percutaneous transluminal coronary angioplasty. Clin Cardiol 1983;6:363-72.

17. Soward AL, Essed CE, Serruys PW. Coronary arterial findings after accidental death immediately after successful percutaneous transluminal coronary angioplasty. American Journal of Cardiology 1985;56(12):794-5.

18. Waller BF, McManus BM, Gorfinkel HJ, et al. Status of the major epicardial coronary arteries 80 to 150 days after percutaneous transluminal coronary angioplasty. Analysis of 3 necropsy patients. American Journal of Cardiology 1983;51(1):81-4.

19. Farb A, Virmani R, Atkinson JB, Kolodgie FD. Plaque morphology and pathologic changes in arteries from patients dying after coronary balloon angioplasty. J Am Coll Cardiol 1990;16:421-9.

20. La Delia V, Rossi PA, Somers S, al e. Coronary histology after percutaneous transluminal coronary angioplaasty. Texas Heart Institute Journal 1988;15:113-6.

21. Waller BF. Morphologic correlates of coronary angiographic patterns at the site of percutaneous transluminal coronary angioplasty. Clinical Cardiology 1988;11(12):817-22.

22. Tobis JM, Mallery JA, Gessert J, et al. Intravascular ultrasound cross-sectional arterial imaging before and after balloon angioplasty in vitro. Circulation 1989;80(4):873-82.

23. Tobis JM, Mallery J, Mahon D, et al. Intravascular ultrasound imaging of human coronary arteries in vivo. Analysis of tissue characterizations with comparison to in vitro histological specimens. Circulation 1991;83(3):913-26.

24. Gussenhoven EJ, The SH, Gerritsen P, et al. Real-time intravascular ultrasonic imaging before and after balloon angioplasty. Journal of Clinical Ultrasound 1991;19(5):294-7.

25. Nissen SE, Grines CL, Gurley JC, et al. Application of a new phased-array ultrasound imaging catheter in the assessment of vascular dimensions. In vivo comparison to cineangiography. Circulation 1990;81(2):660-6.

26. Siegel RJ, Chae JS, Forrester JS, Ruiz CE. Angiography, angioscopy, and ultrasound imaging before and after percutaneous balloon angioplasty. American Heart Journal 1990;120(5):1086-90.

27. Werner GS, Sold G, Buchwald A, Kreuzer H, Wiegand V. Intravascular ultrasound imaging of human coronary arteries after percutaneous transluminal angioplasty: morphologic and quantitative assessment. American Heart Journal 1991;122(1 Pt 1):212-20.

28. Davidson CJ, Sheikh KH, Kisslo KB, et al. Intracoronary ultrasound evaluation of interventional technologies. American Journal of Cardiology 1991;68(13):1305-9.

29. Fitzgerald PJ, Yock PG. Mechanisms and outcomes of angioplasty and atherectomy assessed by intravascular ultrasound imaging. [Review]. Journal of Clinical Ultrasound 1993;21(9):579-88.

30. Dietz WA, Tobis JM, Isner JM. Failure of angiography to accurately depict the extent of coronary artery narrowing in three fatal cases of percutaneous transluminal coronary angioplasty. Journal of the American College of Cardiology 1992;19(6):1261-70.

31. Ge J, Erbel R, Zamorano J, et al. Coronary artery remodeling in atherosclerotic disease: an intravascular ultrasonic study in vivo. Coronary Artery Disease 1993;4(11):981-6.

32. Hermiller JB, Tenaglia AN, Kisslo KB, et al. In vivo validation of compensatory enlargement of atherosclerotic coronary arteries. American Journal of Cardiology 1993;71(8):665-8.

33. McPherson DD, Sirna SJ, Hiratzka LF, et al. Coronary arterial remodeling studied by high-frequency epicardial echocardiography: an early compensatory mechanism in patients with obstructive coronary atherosclerosis. Journal of the American College of Cardiology 1991;17(1):79-86.

34. Dotter CT, Judkins MP. Transluminal treatment of arteriosclerotic obstruction: description of a new technique and a preliminary report of its application. Circulation 1964;30:654-70.

35. Virmani R, Farb A, Burke AP. Coronary angioplasty from the perspective of atherosclerotic plaque: morphologic predictors of immediate success and restenosis. Am Heart J 1994;127:163-79.

308

36. Tenaglia AN, Buller CE, Kisslo KB, Phillips HR, Stack RS, Davidson CJ. Intracoronary ultrasound predictors of adverse outcomes after coronary artery interventions. Journal of the American College of Cardiology 1992;20(6):1385-90.

37. Honye J, Mahon DJ, Jain A, et al. Morphological effects of coronary balloon angioplasty in vivo assessed by intravascular ultrasound imaging. Circulation 1992;85(3):1012-25.

38. Suneja R, Nair RN, Reddy KG, Rasheed Q, Sheehan HM, Hodgson JM. Mechanisms of angiographically successful directional coronary atherectomy: evaluation by intracoronary ultrasound and comparison with transluminal coronary angioplasty. American Heart Journal 1993;126(3 Pt 1):507-14.

39. Braden GA, Herrington DM, Downes TR, Kutcher MA, Little WC. Qualitative and quantitative contrasts in the mechanisms of lumen enlargement by coronary balloon angioplasty and directional coronary atherectomy. Journal of the American College of Cardiology 1994;23(1):40-8.

40. Hodgson JM, Reddy KG, Suneja R, Nair RN, Lesnefsky EJ, Sheehan HM. Intracoronary ultrasound imaging: correlation of plaque morphology with angiography, clinical syndrome and procedural results in patients undergoing coronary angioplasty. Journal of the American College of Cardiology 1993;21(1):35-44.

41. Kaltenbach M, Beyer J, Walter S, Klepzig H, Schmidts L. Prolonged application of pressure in transluminal coronary angioplasty. Catheterization & Cardiovascular Diagnosis 1984;10(3):213-9.

42. Botas J, Clark DA, Pinto F, Chenzbraun A, Fischell TA. Balloon angioplasty results in increased segmental coronary distensibility: a likely mechanism of percutaneous transluminal coronary angioplasty. Journal of the American College of Cardiology 1994;23(5):1043-52.

43. Di Mario C, Gil R, Camenzind E, et al. Quantitative assessment with intracoronary ultrasound of the mechanisms of restenosis after percutaneous transluminal coronary angioplasty and directional coronary atherectomy. American Journal of Cardiology 1995;75(12):772-7.

44. Waller BF. PTCA: mechanisms of dilatation and causes of acute and late closures. Cardiovasc Rev Rep 1989;10:35-44.

45. Waller BF. Pathology of transluminal balloon angioplasty used in the treatment of coronary heart disease. [Review]. Cardiology Clinics 1989;7(4):749-70.

46. Matthews BJ, Ewels CJ, Kent KM. Coronary dissection: a predictor of restenosis? American Heart Journal 1988;115(3):547-54.

47. Leimgruber PP, Roubin GS, Anderson HV, et al. Influence of intimal dissection on restenosis after successful coronary angioplasty. Circulation 1985;72(3):530-5.

48. Bredlau CE, Roubin GS, Leimgruber PP, Douglas J Jr., King S3, Gruentzig AR. In-hospital morbidity and mortality in patients undergoing elective coronary angioplasty. Circulation 1985;72(5):1044-52.

49. Holmes D Jr., Vlietstra RE, Mock MB, et al. Angiographic changes produced by percutaneous transluminal coronary angioplasty. American Journal of Cardiology 1983;51(5):676-83.

50. Fitzgerald PJ, Ports TA, Yock PG. Contribution of localized calcium deposits to dissection after angioplasty. An observational study using intravascular ultrasound [see comments]. Circulation 1992;86(1):64-70.

51. Cheng GC, Loree HM, Kamm RD, Fishbein MC, Lee RT. Distribution of circumferential stress in ruptured and stable atherosclerotic lesions. A structural analysis with histopathological correlation. Circulation 1993;87(4):1179-87.

52. Lee RT, Richardson SG, Loree HM, et al. Prediction of mechanical properties of human atherosclerotic tissue by high-frequency intravascular ultrasound imaging. An in vitro study. Arteriosclerosis & Thrombosis 1992;12(1):1-5.

53. Lee RT, Loree HM, Cheng GC, Lieberman EH, Jaramillo N, Schoen FJ. Computational structural analysis based on intravascular ultrasound imaging before in vitro angioplasty: prediction of plaque fracture locations. Journal of the American College of Cardiology 1993;21(3):777-82.

54. Lee RT, Loree HM, Fishbein MC. High stress regions in saphenous vein bypass graft atherosclerotic lesions. Journal of the American College of Cardiology 1994;24(7):1639-44.

55. Loree HM, Tobias BJ, Gibson LJ, Kamm RD, Small DM, Lee RT. Mechanical properties of model atherosclerotic lesion lipid pools. Arteriosclerosis & Thrombosis 1994;14(2):230-4.

56. Tobis JM. Clinical utility of intravascular ultrasound imaging [editorial; comment]. Catheterization & Cardiovascular Diagnosis 1994;33(3):221-3.

57. Waller BF, Orr CM, Pinkerton CA, Van Tassel J, Peters T, Slack JD. Coronary balloon angioplasty dissections: "the good, the bad and the ugly" [editorial; comment]. Journal of the American College of Cardiology 1992;20(3):701-6.

58. Gerber TC, Erbel R, Gorge G, Ge J, Rupprecht HJ, Meyer J. Classification of morphologic effects of percutaneous transluminal coronary angioplasty assessed by intravascular ultrasound. American Journal of Cardiology 1992;70(20):1546-54.

59. Picture trial. Journal of the American College of Cardiology 1995;35A.

60. Hodgson JM, Stone GW, Linnemeier TJ, Sheehan HM, St. Goar FG, Berry JL. Intravascular ultrasound guided "oversized" balloon angioplasty: initial results from the CLOUT pilot trial. J Invas Cardiol 1995;7(Suppl C):31C.

61. Nakamura S, Mahon DJ, Leung CY, et al. Intracoronary ultrasound imaging before and after directional coronary atherectomy: in vitro and clinical observations. American Heart Journal 1995;129(5):841-51.

62. Matar FA, Mintz GS, Pinnow E, et al. Multivariate predictors of intravascular ultrasound end points after directional coronary atherectomy. Journal of the American College of Cardiology 1995;25(2):318-24.

63. Tenaglia AN, Buller CE, Kisslo KB, Stack RS, Davidson CJ. Mechanisms of balloon angioplasty and directional coronary atherectomy as assessed by intracoronary ultrasound. Journal of the American College of Cardiology 1992;20(3):685-91.

64. Kimura BJ, Fitzgerald PJ, Sudhir K, Amidon TM, Strunk BL, Yock PG. Guidance of directed coronary atherectomy by intracoronary ultrasound imaging. American Heart Journal 1992;124(5):1365-9.

65. Suarez de Lezo J, Romero M, Medina A, et al. Intracoronary ultrasound assessment of directional coronary atherectomy: immediate and follow-up findings. Journal of the American College of Cardiology 1993;21(2):298-307.

66. Popma JJ, Mintz GS, Satler LF, et al. Clinical and angiographic outcome after directional coronary atherectomy. A qualitative and quantitative analysis using coronary arteriography and intravascular ultrasound. American Journal of Cardiology 1993;72(13):55E-64E.

67. Simonton CA. Acute and late clinical and angiographic results of directional atherectomy in the Optimal Atherectomy Restenosis Study (OARS). Circ 1995;92:I-545 (abstract).

68. MacIsaac AI, Yock PG, Fitzgerald PJ, et al. Initial in vivo and in vitro testing of an ultrasound-guided directional coronary atherectomy catheter. Journal of the American College of Cardiology 1995;:(abstract).

69. Kuntz RE, Baim DS. Defining coronary restenosis. Newer clinical and angiographic paradigms. Circulation 1993;88((3)):1310-23.

70. Schwartz RS, Huber KC, Murphy JG, et al. Restenosis and the proportional neointimal response to coronary artery injury: results in a porcine model. Journal of the American College of Cardiology 1992;19((2)):267-74.

71. Fishman RF, Kuntz RE, Carrozza J Jr., et al. Long-term results of directional coronary atherectomy: predictors of restenosis. Journal of the American College of Cardiology 1992;20(5):1101-10.

72. Dussaillant GR, Mintz GS, Pichard AD, et al. Small stent size and intimal hyperplasia contribute to restenosis: a volumetric intravascular ultrasound analysis. Journal of the American College of Cardiology 1995;26(3):720-4.

73. Slepian MJ. Application of intraluminal ultrasound imaging to vascular stenting. International Journal of Cardiac Imaging 1991;6((3-4)):285-311.

74. Nakamura S, Colombo A, Gaglione A, et al. Intracoronary ultrasound observations during stent implantation. Circulation 1994;89(5):2026-34.

310

75. Goldberg SL, Colombo A, Nakamura S, Almagor Y, Maiello L, Tobis JM. Benefit of intracoronary ultrasound in the deployment of Palmaz-Schatz stents. Journal of the American College of Cardiology 1994;24(4):996-1003.

76. Colombo A, Hall P, Nakamura S, et al. Intracoronary stenting without anticoagulation accomplished with intravascular ultrasound guidance [see comments]. Circulation 1995;91(6):1676-88.

77. Gorge G, Haude M, Ge J, et al. Intravascular ultrasound after low and high inflation pressure coronary artery stent implantation. Journal of the American College of Cardiology 1995;26(3):725-30.

78. Stone G. IVUS and stent implantation. IVUS Stanford meeting 1996;.

79. Hall P, Colombo A, Almagor Y, et al. Preliminary experience with intravascular ultrasound guide Palmaz-Schatz coronary stenting: the acute and long term results on a consecutive eries of patients. J Intervent Cardiol 1994;7:141-159.

80. Mintz GS, Potkin BN, Keren G, et al. Intravascular ultrasound evaluation of the effect of rotational atherectomy in obstructive atherosclerotic coronary artery disease. Circulation 1992;86(5):1383-93.

81. Kovach JA, Mintz GS, Pichard AD, et al. Sequential intravascular ultrasound characterization of the mechanisms of rotational atherectomy and adjunct balloon angioplasty. Journal of the American College of Cardiology 1993;22(4):1024-32.

82. Potkin BM, Mintz GS, Keren G, Douek PC, Matar FA, Satler LF. Ultrasound assessment of lesion composition predicts mechanism of PTCA. Circulation 1991;84:II-722.

83. Potkin BN, Keren G, Mintz GS, et al. Arterial responses to balloon coronary angioplasty: an intravascular ultrasound study. Journal of the American College of Cardiology 1992;20(4):942-51.

84. Baptista J, Di Mario C, Escaned J, et al. Intracoronary two-dimensional ultrasound imaging in the assessment of plaque morphologic features and the planning of coronary interventions. American Heart Journal 1995;129((1)):177-187.

85. Mintz GS, Pichard AD, Kovach JA, et al. Impact of preintervention intravascular ultrasound imaging on transcatheter treatment strategies in coronary artery disease. American Journal of Cardiology 1994;73(7):423-30.

86. Alfonso F, Macaya C, Goicolea J, et al. Angiographic changes (Dotter effect) produced by intravascular ultrasound imaging before coronary angioplasty. American Heart Journal 1994;128:244-51.

87. Alfonso F, Macaya C, Goicolea J, al. e. Acute coronary closure complicating intravascular ultrasound examination. European Heart Journal 1994;15((5)):710-2.

88. Hausmann D, Erbel R, Alibelli-Chemarin MJ, et al. The safety of intracoronary ultrasound. A multicenter survey of 2207 examinations. Circulation 1995;91((3)):623-30.

13.

LESION MORPHOLOGY AND COMPOSITION: RISK OF RESTENOSIS FOLLOWING CORONARY INTERVENTIONS

Bradley H. Strauss MD, FRCP(C), PhD and Madhu K. Natarajan MD, FRCP(C)

University of Toronto, Division of Cardiology, Terrence Donnelly Heart Center, St. Michael's Hospital, 30 Bond Street, Toronto, Ontario, Canada

1. Introduction

In the past 10 years, there has been significant progress in our understanding of the clinical problem of restenosis following balloon angioplasty. This is due to a combined approach to determine the pathophysiology and complex biologic mechanisms that contribute to restenosis and the introduction and use of measurement systems in documenting and assessing the process. It should be recalled that in the early angioplasty years (1980-1985), angiographic assessment of restenosis was entirely on a categorical basis, the value of angiographic follow-up questionnable and clinical cardiologists were largely unaware of the use of quantitative angiography. Although quantitative coronary angiography (QCA) has been predominantly a research tool in interventional cardiology, it has raised the standards of interventional practice from purely "an art" to a more scientific level that can be evaluated by evidence-based medicine. QCA has altered our perceptions of restenosis and has served as the gold standard for comparing restenosis therapies (drugs and devices).

Investigators have used quantitative angiographic analysis to assess the contribution of lesion morphology to PTCA outcome. The importance of lesion morphology to the immediate outcome of balloon angioplasty has been recognized for many years. In 1988, a combined American College of Cardiology/ American Heart Association Task Force published a classification of specific lesion types (types B and C) that were associated with both decreased immediate success and increased rates of procedural complications (Table 1)[1]. A subclassification of B lesions into B1 and B2 by Stephen Ellis has attempted to more precisely quantify risk [2].

Many of the morphologic features associated with adverse immediate procedural outcomes have also been implicated as risk factors for restenosis. Until recently, quantitative coronary angiography (QCA) has been the only reliable means to assess the short and long term effects of coronary interventions. Sequential QCA studies have been critical to our knowledge of restenosis, as a tool to not only objectively establish criteria for restenosis, but also as a means to accurately measure the contribution of various lesion morphologies to restenosis. Although still in quite nascent stages of development, new imaging modalities, such as intravascular ultrasound (IVUS) and angioscopy, have begun to be utilized in coronary interventional studies. These newer technologies have provided unique observations from a perspective quite different than quantitative angiography.

The objectives of this chapter are two-fold. First, the relationship between lesion morphology and composition (based predominantly on QCA but supplemented by IVUS and angioscopy studies where available) and restenosis following balloon angioplasty will be reviewed. Second, the role of alternative interventional coronary devices on altering the risk of restenosis in these particular morphologies will be discussed.

2. What is restenosis and how should restenosis be evaluated?

The use of the term "restenosis" in this chapter refers specifically to the measurement of loss of luminal diameter in the vessel wall after an initially successful (ie. <50% residual diameter stenosis) interventional procedure. This is certainly a complex process that involves multiple mechanisms that are beyond the scope of this chapter. The problem of restenosis with its requirement for reintervention was recognized in the early days of angioplasty [3]. However, the early descriptions of this phenomenon were based on visual analysis (and occasionally caliper based measurements) of coronary angiograms, which were unreliable due to significant interobserver and intraobserver variability [4-6]. Since the mid 1980's, more sophisticated computerized analysis systems have been developed to more accurately measure coronary arteriograms. Several systems are currently available and appear to provide essentially comparable data [7]. Nevertheless, quantitative coronary angiography remains predominantly a research tool since the vast majority of cases are not evaluated beyond a simple visual assessment. Outside of multicenter restenosis trials, routine angiographic follow-up is rarely practised. Therefore, our knowledge of the relationship between morphologic features and restenosis is quite limited to a relatively small number of cases that have been evaluated in a handful of centers active in this area of research. Furthermore, newer imaging techniques such as intravascular ultrasound and angioscopy have been studied in even much fewer patients than QCA, and only limited data related to restenosis are available.

A variety of angiographic definitions of restenosis have been devised (Table 2.). The vast majority of these have never been popular or enjoyed widespread use. The clinician, whose predominant interest is in decision making, has typically regarded restenosis more as a binary event (restenosis yes/no) and this is reflected in the popularity of restenosis definition #5 (diameter stenosis >50% at follow-up) [8,9]. This definition is based on the experimental observation that this particular stenosis will blunt reactive hyperemia and thus limit coronary flow reserve in canine coronary arteries [10,11]. Its relevance to the physiologic significance in human coronary arterial lesions has never been adequately demonstrated, particularly when one considers the complexities of human coronary lesions that contribute to flow characteristics of a stenosis (eg. lesion length, diffuseness of disease, assumption that the reference diameter can be accurately measured by coronary angiography). Despite these limitations, clinicians and investigators have been unable to agree on a more suitable definition and thus, this particular criterion continues in popular use.

Is late renarrowing a binary event or a process that occurs to a variable extent in all lesions, with "restenosis" arbitrarily defined by the subgroup with the most extensive renarrowing? Using data collected from 1427 patients in 2 large restenosis trials, Rensing et al have shown that the follow-up minimal luminal diameter after balloon angioplasty follows a near Gaussian distribution with "restenotic" lesions located at the tail end [12]. From this perspective, restenosis is not a separate disease entity (occurring in some lesions but not in others) but rather part of a continuum. This continuous approach to restenosis has been further supported by the work of Richard Kuntz and Donald Baim in their comparisons of device-specific effects [13]. Recently, the Thoraxcenter group has challenged their previously held notion that restenosis (ie. luminal renarrowing) follows a normal distribution [14]. By increasing their cohort to 3093 patients (from 4 large restenosis trials), several measurements of late renarrowing (ie. late loss, loss index, diameter stenosis at follow-up) superficially resemble but do not actually statistically conform to a normal distribution, due to an excess frequency of lesions that fall into two groups: lesions that experience little change (late loss of 0.0 mm±0.3 mm, ie." nonrestenosers") and lesions with a more marked change (late loss 1.0-2.0 mm, ie."restenosers") [14]. They offer an alternative model of restenosis in which there are two subpopulations of lesions. This model is consistent with the bimodal distribution previously suggested by Spencer King's group [15]. Due to the measurement errors inherent in quantitative coronary angiography, these two types of lesions ("restenosers" and "nonrestenosers") will show variability in the determination of late loss that could mask the bimodal distribution. In fact, this bimodal model provided a better representation of the observed data than the "Gaussian distribution" model.

What conclusions about the restenosis process can be made based on these quite contradictory results? Despite careful attention to the acquisition and analysis of coronary angiograms, quite different observations were found when the original patient cohort was increased from 1427 patients to 3093 patients. Cynics may suggest that a different conclusion will emerge when the cohort is further extended! However, these studies appear to highlight the shortcomings and limitations of quantitative coronary angiography to adequately describe the biological processes that result in late renarrowing. The acceptance of either of two quite conflicting descriptions of biological behavior is really dependent on our confidence in the variability and error of this measurement technique. Furthermore, there is evidence that the error of this technique is not consistent at various lesion diameters. Keane et al have shown with all QCA systems, (including the CAAS system used in these large restenosis trials), that the baseline minimal luminal diameter may be overestimated and the acute gain in minimal luminal diameter actually underestimated after coronary intervention [7]. Thus, all currently available QCA systems, while clearly superior to visual or caliper-based measurements, have technical limitations that must be considered in evaluating the biological concepts of restenosis advanced by various investigators.

3. A Current View on QCA-Derived Restenosis Definitions: suboptimal dilatation versus aggressive renarrowing

Two important and related observations in the last 5 years have altered our view on how to evaluate restenosis.

a. Acute Gain:

In 1992, Beatt and Serruys introduced the concept that procedural luminal gain is the greatest single determinant of subsequent luminal narrowing or loss [16]. A similar relationship was reported concurrently by Kuntz and Baim [17]. This observation was subsequently repeated in studies of coronary stents and directional atherectomy in which much larger luminal gains and losses were seen compared to previously published reports of balloon angioplasty [18-20]. The randomized trials of directional atherectomy and stents versus balloon angioplasty confirmed this relationship between acute luminal gain at the time of the procedure and the subsequent development of late luminal loss at 6 month follow-up [21-24]. Thus, the more you gain initially (in minimal luminal diameter), the greater the loss will be over the ensuing months. This is a particularly important concept if one is comparing devices that differentially dilate coronary arteries. For example, over a 6 month follow-up period, stents have been shown to result in approximately 2x more luminal loss than balloon angioplasty (0.65 mm versus 0.32 mm) [21]. However, the residual diameter stenosis at 6 months is significantly greater in stented vs PTCA treated lesions since the acute gain is so much greater with stenting [21,22]. Despite a more aggressive renarrowing process in lesions treated with coronary stents, these devices improve "restenosis rates" since the initial effect of the stent (ie.larger minimal luminal diameter) is maintained.

b. Residual Stenosis/Minimal Luminal Diameter:

Kuntz et al have also demonstrated a related observation that a large post-procedure lumen (with minimal residual diameter stenosis) is the principal determinant of an optimal angiographic and clinical outcome at 6 months [17], leading to the 1990's interventional dictum "bigger is better". This group showed that three new devices (Palmaz-Schatz stenting, directional atherectomy and laser balloon) were able to provide a larger acute gain and a lower residual diameter stenosis than conventional balloon angioplasty [13]. The strongest predictor of restenosis (minimal luminal diameter or diameter stenosis at follow-up) was the postprocedural lumal dimension [25]. They found a consistent relationship between the acute gain and late loss, irrespective of the device studied (balloon angioplasty, stent implantation, directional atherectomy or excimer laser angioplasty) [17,25,26]. Essentially, for every 1 mm of luminal gain, a corresponding 0.5 mm of late loss in luminal diameter was observed [27]. In comparing the various devices, it is not really clear whether the relationship between acute gain and late loss is consistent for all devices at all levels of gain. Foley and colleagues have also suggested that there may be a device- specific effect of excimer laser angioplasty on restenosis with relatively more late narrowing for a given acute gain [28,29].

Thus, "restenosis" or significant luminal narrowing at 6 months post procedure can be due to a suboptimal angioplasty result (significant residual stenosis), an aggressive renarrowing process that occurs in response to the angioplasty, or combination of these two factors. It is evident from this discussion that the angiographic "risk factors" for "restenosis" are dependent on the definition used for restenosis. The most commonly utilized criterion, diameter stenosis ≥50% at follow up (and is the definition used in most of the studies relating lesion morphology/composition and restenosis), has been repeatedly shown to be related to the residual stenosis immediately following the procedure [reviewed in 27]. Therefore, it should be emphasized that this definition of restenosis is strongly influenced by the procedural result. "Risk factors" identified in many of these cases, reflect an inadequate result more than an aggressive renarrowing process. This should be stressed since the "angiographic risk factors" for the criterion DS > 50% at follow-up are really those factors that predispose to a less optimal post procedural angiographic result. This would explain the inclusion of several ACC/AHA Type B and C lesions as restenosis "risk factors". Other definitions, that focus more on the "renarrowing process" (ie. late loss) are closely related to the initial gain. "Angiographic risk factors" using this definition will actually reflect the angiographic parameters that are associated with large initial procedural gains and thus excellent angiographic results. There currently is no available definition that effectively combines these 2 criteria.

The commonly used restenosis definition, diameter stenosis >50%, is more likely to be associated with clinical events such as revascularization than definitions more reflective of the renarrowing process. From a functional and clinical point of view, the diameter stenosis and absolute minimal luminal diameter at follow-up are the most important quantitative angiographic measurements to correlate with late clinical events [30-32] (not withstanding errors inherent in determining reference diameters due to diffuseness of disease and involvement of the adjacent reference segments of the vessel in the renarrowing process). Based on follow-up minimal luminal diameter (MLD) values, QCA has been shown to effectively separate "clinical-event-positive" (ie. reintervention, bypass surgery, myocardial infarction or death) and "clinical-event-negative" patients [31]. In three drug studies, the difference in mean MLD between the two groups of patients was 0.37 mm for CARPORT, 0.42 mm for MERCATOR and 0.51 mm for PARK (all highly statistically significant). For patients who received a Palmaz-Schatz stent in the BENESTENT study, the difference in MLD between the two groups was even more impressive, 0.86 mm.

c. Restenosis Mechanisms Inadequately Evaluated by QCA

A second important issue to consider in analyzing angiographic restenosis studies is the mechanism(s) of restenosis. The formation of intimal hyperplasia has generally been regarded as the main process contributing to lumen loss (which is the measurement obtained from QCA), with variable contributions from vasospasm, thrombus formation and recoil. However, important observations from both experimental animal and human intravascular coronary artery studies have focused attention on "chronic remodelling", a poorly understood process by which the entire vessel actually constricts over time and as a consequence the lumen also becomes much smaller [33-35]. This appears to be a particularly important mechanism for restenosis in lesions treated by balloon angioplasty and directional atherectomy but relatively minor component of restenosis after stenting [36,37]. How do we incorporate these new perspectives into our understanding of how "angiographic variables and lesion composition" relate to restenosis, especially after the use of different devices? Can they explain the differences in outcome between atherectomy and stenting [38]? It should be quite apparent then that despite an extensive literature accumulation over the last 10 years, the data (often conflicting) remain incomplete. Angiographic studies have contributed important information to our knowledge of restenosis but needs to be assessed critically and supplemented by other imaging techniques which have contributed complementary (and at times contradictory) information.

4. Reviewing QCA Restenosis Studies: Caveats

Prior to discussing the relationship between lesion morphology and restenosis, a few general comments should be kept in mind while reviewing the results of angiographic studies.

a. Study design: Was angiographic follow-up consistently performed to limit bias (>85% of eligible patients)?

b. Angiographic analysis system: Has it been properly validated?

c. The Post Procedural Angiogram: The Achilles Heel of Quantitative Angiography: It should be noted that the post procedural angiographic result is the least reliable for quantitative measurements compared with the pre procedure and follow-up angiograms. This is related to the hazy appearance of the lesion with the presence of complex tears and dissections that further accentuate the non-circular geometry of the lesion that is assumed in comparisons of lesions by the criterion of minimal luminal diameter. Several studies have indicated that the post procedural diameter stenosis is probably the most important variable related to restenosis using the popular criterion, diameter stenosis > 50% [39]. Thus, problems in assessing the post procedural angiographic result could lead to erroneous conclusions in studies, including risk factor subanalyses. This possibility is suggested in a recent study relating intravascular ultrasound and QCA performed post angioplasty to QCA results at 6 months. Only post procedural residual area stenosis and minimal luminal diameter measured by IVUS, but not by angiography, were indicators of restenosis. Luminal areas obtained by intravascular ultrasound were significantly larger than both edge detection and videodensitometry with considerable deterioration of the agreement after balloon angioplasty and directional atherectomy [40,41].

Fewer problems have been encountered in the post procedural angiographic analysis of lesions treated by stenting and directional atherectomy [18,42,43]. The vessel luminal contours are typically smooth and much less ragged than after PTCA, facilitating the edge detection program. After stenting, the lesion also appears to assume a more circular geometry based on both IVUS studies and comparisons between angiographic edge detection and videodensitometric assessments [44]. This is important since vessel and lesion area measurements derived from angiographically determined diameters assume a circular configuration of the vessel. After coronary stenting, quantitative angiography appears to overestimate the minimal luminal diameter when compared to intravascular ultrasound [45]. However, the discrepancy between QCA and IVUS is significantly smaller after high pressure dilatation of the stent.

With directional atherectomy, it appears that there may be preferential expansions at the bases of the atherectomy cuts that results in relatively non-circular configuration post atherectomy [46], similar to balloon angioplasty [42]. This has been confirmed by angioscopy studies which have shown atherectomy bytes, outside the plaque area and non-confluent bytes in the plaque which resemble "vessel wall trenches" [47]. The initial atherectomy studies suggested that the major component of luminal improvement is actually "facilitated mechanical angioplasty" resulting from the high profile of the device and the low pressure balloon inflations rather than plaque removal, which accounted for only 28% of the effect (range 7-92%) [46]. The "Dottering" effect of the device was responsible for approximately 60% of the luminal improvement in one small study [48]. The same group found somewhat contradictory findings in a separate study that compared quantitative angiography, intravascular ultrasound and intracoronary angioscopy in 19 patients pre and post atherectomy [47]. They found that the achieved gain mainly resulted from plaque removal since plaque + media are decreased from 18.16 ± 4.47 mm^2 to 13.13 ± 3.1 mm^2 while vessel stretching only accounted for 15% of luminal area gain. Whether new approaches of more aggressive plaque removal will change the relationship of this device to restenosis remains to be shown in the BOAT (Balloon versus Optimal Atherectomy Trial). OARS (Optimal Atherectomy Restenosis Study) and EUROCARE (EUROpean Carvedilol Atherectomy REstenosis) trials).

d. Statistical Analysis:
Are adequate number of patients enroled in trial to test the number of potential risk factors. The majority of studies use a univariate analysis with multiple variables, which are probably not independent of each other eg. plaque size and reference diameter.

e. Restenosis definitions (see above)

5. Relationship of Lesion Morphology and Restenosis:

a.Vessel Size:
The measurement of the reference diameter will vary depending on the measurement system. In studies using calipers, the diameter of the "normal appearing" vessel proximal and distal to the lesion may be averaged. In quantitative systems such as the CAAS and Cardiac Measurement System, the reference segment can be defined by the user which is also quite subjective and variable, particularly in cases where the proximal part of the arterial segment shows a combination of stenotic and ectatic areas or in cases where a "normal" portion is just not clearly available. The preferable alternative is the determination of the reference segment by an automated process that is independent of the user. The CAAS system is able to incorporate an interpolated reference diameter that is derived solely from the information conveyed by the diameter function. This has previously been described in detail [49,50].

i) PTCA
Does the size of the vessel itself influence the late result after balloon angioplasty

or the newer devices? The most detailed study after PTCA was published in 1994 by David Foley and colleagues at the Thoraxcenter involving >3000 patients (3736 lesions) [51]. The lesions were divided into 9 equally sized groups according to vessel size. The main conclusion of the study was that increasing vessel size was independently predictive of decreasing late luminal loss and increasing follow-up minimal luminal diameter after successful balloon angioplasty.

To study the extremes of vessel size, the results of the two upper (n=731) and lower (n=734) noniles from this patient population have been reanalyzed for this book chapter. Several interesting observations emerged from this study. In larger vessels, significantly larger acute gains are achieved during angioplasty compared with smaller vessels (0.81 mm versus 0.54 mm). At follow-up, these larger vessels also demonstrate more late loss (0.24 versus 0.18 mm) but overall larger net gains (0.57 mm vs 0.36 mm) and larger minimal luminal diameters (1.84 mm vs 1.26 mm) and diameter stenoses (44% vs 40%). However, using two discrete restenosis criteria, DS% >50% at follow up and loss >0.4 mm, higher restenosis rates were seen in larger vessels (35% vs 26% Criterion 1; 35% vs 24% Criterion 2). This can be partly explained by the increasing severity of diameter stenosis of larger vessels at baseline (62% vs 53%). Unfortunately, the clinical importance (target vessel revascularization) of these "increased" restenosis rates in larger vessels is not provided but two important points should be emphasized. First, there may be discrepancies between the severity of stenosis and the need for vascularization in smaller versus larger vessels. In other words, >50% diameter stenosis may have a less propensity for provoking ischemia in a smaller artery than a larger artery. Increased diameter stenosis without consideration of vessel size may not necessarily indicate a requirement for more revascularization procedures. The absolute minimal luminal diameter at follow up also seems to be quite an important determinant in provoking ischemia [30]. The larger vessel group had overall a much larger minimal luminal diameter at follow-up (despite more severe % diameter stenosis). Secondly, as Foley et al have explained in their discussion, alternative devices could potentially have more impact in reducing the "restenosis rates" in larger vessels than in smaller vessels. This may explain some of the restenosis benefit of stents (which have been restricted to larger vessels) compared with devices used predominantly in smaller vessels (eg. excimer laser, rotational ablation).

Coronary stents have been limited essentially to larger vessels (ie. ≥3mm diameter) due to concern about subacute thrombosis in smaller arteries. This vessel size requirement was mandated in both the Stress and Benestent studies but was based on a visual analysis. The operators in some cases deployed stents in vessels smaller than 3.0 mm (based on QCA measurements). A meta-analysis on clinical and angiographic outcomes based on coronary vessel size in these two trials recently showed a relationship between vessel size and restenosis (DS≥50% at follow-up) in lesions treated either by stenting or PTCA [52]. In this study, both angioplasty and stent groups had lower restenosis rates and lower clinical event rates in vessels ≥3.0 mm than in vessels <3.0 mm. Restenosis rates were not different between the two devices in vessels <2.6 mm (approximately 40%). In larger (>3.4 mm) vessels, lower (but not statistically significant) restenosis rates were evident in stents (22% vs 30%) with equivalent (16%) event rates. However, in vessels 2.6-3.4 mm diameter, stents resulted in an impressive and significant reduction in angiographic restenosis and clinical events. Columbo's group also found an inverse relationship between restenosis and vessel size in stented coronary arteries [53]. The restenosis rates (DS>50%) in vessel diameter <3.0, 3.0-3.5 mm and >3.5 mm were 25% (n=129), 19% (n=156) and 6% (n=69), respectively.

b. Lesion length:
The measurement of lesion length in various studies has not been uniformly assessed and raises important methodologic issues. In some studies, lesion length is measured from the point at which the lumen is compromised by 50% diameter stenosis at the proximal or distal reference vessel site [53]. Since it can be quite difficult to know exactly where the "50% diameter stenosis" actually begins, this measurement is quite imprecise and subject to both intraobserver and interobserver variability. A full description of the methods used to determine lesions length using the computer based coronary angiographic analysis system (CAAS) is reviewed elsewhere [49]. Frame selection is important since lesion length can only be reliably measured in non-foreshortened views. In assessing the importance of lesion length as a risk factor, the cutoff that defines a "long lesion" should also be considered. In many studies (see below), the cutoff is at 8 mm. Few studies have utilized the AHA/ACC lesion classification which defines a "B" lesion as 10-20 mm in length and "C" lesion as >20 mm. This would provide much more meaningful data to the clinician but would also profoundly limit the number of lesions analyzed in these QCA studies as "long lesions".

An increased risk of restenosis (follow-up DS>50%) with incremental increases in lesion length (using the DS>50% criterion) has been a consistent finding in several stent [53,54], PTCA [55-57] and laser [28,58] studies. In the CARPORT study, Rensing et al found a significant difference in late loss (change in MLD at follow-up) in longer (>8.8 mm) lesions than in shorter lesions (0.38 mm vs 0.23 mm) but lesion length was not independently predictive in a multiple linear regression analysis [59]. Using a similar analysis with the MERCATOR study, Hermans found no relationship between lesion length (cutoff was 6.7 mm) and change in MLD at follow-up [60].

The relationship between increasing lesion length and increased risk of restenosis has led to considerable interest in using either different angioplasty strategy (eg.long balloons) or adjunctive techniques such as excimer laser, rotablator or coronary stenting. In stented arteries, the restenosis rates (DS≥50%) in lesions <9 mm, 9-15 mm and >15 mm were 11% (n=194), 21% (n=96) and 39% (n=62) [53]. The AMROE (Amsterdam-Miami-ROtterdam-Eindhoven) trial was a multicenter randomized trial comparing balloon angioplasty for long (≥10 mm by visual assessment) coronary lesions that has recently been published [29]. Lesion length and other quantitative variables were subsequently measured by the CAAS system. Discrepancies between the 2 methods of assessing lesion length were indicated by the CAAS derived mean lesion lengths of 9.41 and 8.91 mm in the laser and balloon angioplasty groups, respectively [28]. The median lesion length for the entire group was 8.93 mm (ie more than 50% of the patients deemed eligible for the trial actually had "short" lesions determined by the CAAS QCA system). In the group with long lesions (>8.98 mm by QCA), acute gains were similar in the two groups (laser 0.92 mm vs PTCA 0.83 mm) but the laser group had greater late loss (0.56 mm vs 0.32 mm, p=0.05), smaller net gain and higher restenosis rates using the DS>50% criterion (52% versus 32%). In a multiple linear regression analysis, laser was retained as an independent determinant of greater late loss and a smaller luminal diameter at follow-up, suggesting a device-specific effect. Of interest in this study, there was no difference in restenosis rates criteria (late loss, MLD or DS% at follow-up, DS>50%) in short versus long PTCA treated lesions although there were higher restenosis rates in long lesions versus short lesions treated by excimer laser. This is in contrast to an earlier study that did not show a relationship between restenosis rates and lesion length in excimer laser treated lesions [26].

Although multiple stents are usually implanted for long diffusely diseased lesions, they have also been used in specific situations such as incorrect placement of an initial stent or to cover dissections that extend beyond the length of the original lesion. Therefore, the limited data of late outcome of lesions treated with multiple stents lesions may not necessarily be restricted to long lesions. Strauss et al reported a 50% angiographic restenosis rate (DS≥50%) in 44 multiple Wallstent implanted lesions [61]. Recently two papers on multistent use were presented at the 1995 American Heart Association meeting. In 77 lesions (>20 mm in length) that were treated with 3 different stent types, Colombo's group reported restenosis rates ranging from 24-39% [54]. Follow up angiography was done in 70% of patients. Reimers and colleagures reported on late results in 48 patients that had multiple stents (4 different types) implanted in diffusely diseased arteries, predominantly for suboptimal results or as a bail-out [62]. All patients were treated with high pressure inflations and received oral anticoagulants. Restenosis (angiographic and "recurrence of angina") was observed in 25%. The angiographic follow-up rate was not stated. Therefore, insufficient data are currently available to assess the late effects of stenting on long lesions, either using multiple short stents or longer stents which will soon be readily available.

c. Eccentricity:
The major problem of assessing the importance of eccentricity as an angiographic risk factor for restenosis following balloon angioplasty is a consistent and reproducible definition. No other risk factor has been more evaluated yet less defined! The correlation between "eccentricity" determined by angiographic methods and pathologic examination has not been done and therefore the validity of angiographically-determined measurements is open to debate. The only quantitative systems that are programmed to measure eccentricity are the Reiber designed systems, CASS and CMS [49]. This is somewhat surprising since several of the new devices have been specifically targeted for eccentric lesions (eg. directional atherectomy, eccentric excimer laser catheters) despite our inability to reliably measure "eccentricity".

No consistent relationship between lesion eccentricity and restenosis after balloon angioplasty is apparent in the literature [59,60]. Recently, Schiele and colleagues presented data on the influence of angiographic "eccentricity" on restenosis after directional atherectomy [63]. Although the method of measuring eccentricity was not described, restenosis rates were significantly higher in moderately (51-75%) and highly (>75%) eccentric lesions compared with low (0-50%), despite "optimal early angiographic results". However, Kimball could find no relationship between an index of lesion symmetry and late luminal loss in lesions treated by either directional atherectomy or balloon angioplasty [64].

Intravascular ultrasound studies have also attempted to define lesion eccentricity. "Concentric" lesions are circumferential along the entire vessel wall as opposed to "eccentric" when a part of the vessel wall is disease-free. This has been quantified by an eccentricity index whereby the minimal luminal diameter/maximal luminal diameter is ≤ 0.5. However, data are not currently available relating IVUS determined eccentricity to late restenosis.

d. Ostial Location:

Lesions in the aorta-ostial position (native RCA, vein grafts) [65,66], and lesions within the first 3 mm of the left anterior descending and circumflex arteries or their major branches [67] are traditionally characterized as being "high risk" for standard balloon angioplasty. They are associated with poor immediate outcomes and higher restenosis rates. As a result these lesions are thought to represent a potential niche for new devices including directional atherectomy (DCA), rotational atherectomy, transluminal extraction catheter (TEC), excimer laser (ELCA) and endoluminal stents.

There are two potential reasons for increased restenosis rates with ostial lesions. First, due to technical challenges, acute gain in luminal diameter may be lower and residual diameter stenosis post procedure may be higher. This difficulty is significantly augmented at aorto-ostial sites where guider stability is a problem and calcium may be present. Intracoronary ultrasound studies demonstrate that significant residual plaque mass remains at these sites despite excellent angiographic result [68]. Second, the major contributor to increased rates of restenosis associated with ostial lesions is likely due to vessel wall elastic recoil. Elastic recoil is considered to be important for restenosis at other ostial sites, such as renal artery stenosis [69]. Pathological studies suggest that tissue composition is different and intimal proliferation is more eccentric at ostial sites [70], thus predisposing them to more aggressive restenosis. In addition, flow characteristics may vary at the ostial site with different shear stresses, predisposing them to increased platelet deposition and thrombus formation. Furthermore, determination of restenosis of ostial lesions by QCA poses a significant technical problem. Calculation of percent diameter stenosis depends on accurate measurement of the reference diameter of the vessel. At the ostial site, only the segment of vessel distal to the lesion can be used to measure the reference diameter, decreasing the accuracy and precision of calculations by QCA [49].

Recent data are challenging the traditional view that ostial lesions are associated with higher restenosis rates. The reasons for this discrepancy may arise from the fact that initial PTCA studies only included a small number of patients and had poor angiographic follow-up. In addition, the practice of PTCA in the 1980's may not have resulted in large luminal gains. Using the CAVEAT 1 database, Boehrer et al demonstrated that restenosis rates are comparable for lesions in the ostial and non-ostial locations of the LAD (non-ostial 57%, n=489; ostial 47%, n=74; p=0.16) [71]. The clinical outcomes were also not significantly different for ostial or non-ostial lesions whether patients had PTCA or atherectomy. In a comparative analysis of all patients undergoing PTCA or DCA for vein graft disease at the Cleveland Clinic between 1986 and 1992, the clinical, procedural and follow-up profile were not significantly different for patients who had ostial versus non-ostial disease [72]. Ostial location was not a predictor of higher restenosis rates in native vessels [73] or bypass grafts [74] undergoing ELCA therapy. Coronary stenting of ostial lesions, although technically challenging, has resulted in excellent longterm outcomes as it addresses both the issues of optimizing acute luminal gains and minimizing elastic recoil [75,76].

e. Proximal LAD:

Is there really an increased risk of restenosis in proximal LAD lesions? This is a particularly important question because of the large myocardial territory at risk in proximal LAD lesions and the long-term success of mammary artery conduits have often placed interventional cardiologists in a defensive posture. The issue of restenosis has been the subject of numerous conflicting studies, even within the same group. Review of studies with >100 patients from 1984-1991 (using a variety of angiographic analysis techniques and restenosis definitions (but mainly DS>50%), showed no difference in restenosis rates in 8 studies [9,54,77-82] and an increased incidence of restenosis in proximal LAD lesions in 4 trials [55,56,83,84]. In 1992, Hermans reported in 1234 patients (combined CARPORT and MERCATOR trials) that there were no statistical differences in restenosis rates between coronary segments using a DS>50% criterion (proximal LAD:LCX:RCA 33%:30%:28%) [85]. There were also no significant differences in late loss or relative loss, which normalized the changes for differences in reference diameters. However, in a later study (3072 patients) by the same group in which the results of the 4 restenosis trials were now pooled (CARPORT, MERCATOR, MARCATOR, PARK), lesion location in the LAD was significantly associated with greater late luminal loss and smaller minimal luminal diameter at follow-up as well as with greater percent stenosis at follow-up [51].

Do other devices have a beneficial effect on restenosis in proximal LAD lesions compared to balloon angioplasty? The results of directional atherectomy in proximal LAD lesions were studied as a post hoc subset in the CAVEAT trial and prospectively in Canadian Coronary Atherectomy Trial (CCAT). In the CAVEAT trial, patients with proximal LAD lesions had a significantly lower rate of restenosis (DS≥50% at follow-up) with atherectomy (51%) than with PTCA (63%), which was not associated with a better clinical outcome [23]. The CCAT study showed no differences in angiographic restenosis (DS>50%) in atherectomy treated lesions (46%) compared with PTCA (43%), despite a significantly lower residual % diameter stenosis post procedure (26% versus 33% post PTCA) [24]. No data are yet available for stenting or other alternative coronary devices.

6. Relationship of Lesion Composition and Restenosis:

a. Calcium and Thrombus:

Important issues in assessing the importance of calcium and thrombus as factors in restenosis are the ability of the imaging technique to detect the presence or absence of these factors and the investigators attempts to develop a reliable grading system of severity. At the present time, detection of calcium or thrombus by angiography remains quite subjective and there is little information of interobserver and intraobserver variability in the assessment of these factors in the published restenosis studies. An indication of interobserver variability can be found in comparing the incidence of angiographically visible calcium in two large restenosis studies analyzed at the same core laboratory. In the CARPORT study (697 patients), Rensing et al reported calcium in 233 of 666 lesions studied (35% overall) [59,86]. Meanwhile, Walter Hermans has reported in the MERCATOR trial (693 patients) that only 80 of 778 lesions contained calcium (10% overall) [60]. Since these study populations were otherwise comparable (and in fact results have been pooled for restenosis studies [51], it is doubtful that this level of discrepancy is based on real differences in the two study populations. However, it does emphasize the difficulty in evaluating calcification as a risk factor for restenosis. In Herman's study, calcified lesions were associated with less late loss in luminal diameter during follow-up (0.16 mm in calcified versus 0.28 mm in non calcified lesions). The authors suggested that this may be due to less acute gain in calcified lesions, which are more difficult to successfully dilate, although no supportive data were presented. In the CARPORT study, there were no differences in change in MLD at follow-up between calcified lesions (0.29 mm) and non calcified lesions (0.31 mm).

Other imaging techniques appear to be more reliable in detecting calcium and thrombus than angiography. Umans et al, identified calcium in 11 (1 diffusely calcified, 5 superficial focal and 5 deeply located calcification) of 26 atherectomy cases while angiography did not detect the presence of calcium in any of the cases [47]. Mintz et al detected lesion calcium in 73% of 1155 coronary lesions studies while only 38% were appreciated by angiography [87]. He also showed that calcium is more often subendothelial (72%), concordant in location with the maximal thickness of the plaque and involves the adjacent reference segment. A recent observation from Ozaki and colleagues is that the presence of calcium is an extremely important factor in discrepancies between quantitative angiography and intravascular ultrasound in measurements of luminal area [88]. By ultrasound, calcium is defined as bright echoes within a plaque with acoustic shadowing. This finding has had excellent correlation with histologic studies. These particular investigators devised a grading system for calcium as calcium free, focal deposit (<90° of the vessel circumference) and moderate or diffuse (>90°) and found that the correlation of IVUS and edge detection post angioplasty was 0.71 in calcium free lesions, 0.37 in the presence of focal calcium deposits and 0.15 in moderate to diffuse calcification. However, this correlation may not be due so much to the presence of calcium but rather its role in increasing shear stress within the plaque during coronary angioplasty [89], which could predispose calcified lesions to develop dissection or haziness. The presence and circumferential extension of calcium is also predictive of the development of dissection or fracture after PTCA, particularly when the arc of vessel calcium is >90° [90,91]. Ultrasound studies have also suggested that the prevalent mechanism of lumen enlargement in calcified plaques is a full thickness rupture of the plaque allowing a distention of the vessel adventitia, rather than plaque compression [92].

Calcium also appears to interfere with plaque removal during directional atherectomy. Umans et al showed that plaque reduction in cross-sectional area in ultrasonic non-calcified lesion was larger than calcified lesions (5.89 vs 4.13 mm^2). Subendothelial calcium appears to both limit tissue retrieval by DCA and increase the incidence of procedural complications [93]. Intracoronary ultrasound has shown though that rotational atherectomy achieves better results in diffusely calcified lesions, generating a regular smooth circular lumen [94]. IVUS studies by Kovach and colleagues have suggested that the excimer laser creates a "shattering effect", facilitating the use of adjunctive balloon angioplasty, rather than actually removing large areas of thick calcification [94]. Sufficient data are not yet available to assess the contribution of IVUS determined calcification and restenosis. In one small PTCA study (89 patients), Gorge and colleagues could not show an association between calcification and restenosis (DS>50% by QCA) [95].

Thrombus is poorly evaluated by angiography and intravascular ultrasound. Angioscopy appears to be the most reliable method of detection [96-99]. In a directional atherectomy study, thrombus was identified in 7 of 26 cases before the procedure by angioscopy but no cases were detected by the other two imaging techniques [47]. After atherectomy, angioscopy identified thrombus in 58% of cases compared to 0% and 4% by ultrasound and angiography, respectively. Angiographically determined thrombus at the dilatation site pre angioplasty does not seem to be a risk factor for restenosis but post angioplasty has been associated with more severe luminal narrowing at follow-up (risk ratio:2.6) [100]. However, due to the low sensitivity of angiography to detect thrombus, confirmation of this observation will need to await more rigorous studies with other technologies.

b) Plaque Composition

Several in-vitro studies have indicated that ultrasonic characteristics of the plaque are reasonably well correlated with the histologic composition of the lesion [101,102]. The presence and depth and circumferential extension of calcification can be appreciated (see above) and dense fibrous plaques of high reflectivity can be distinguished from less echogenic types of plaques. "Soft" plaques are defined by >80% of plaque area composed of tissue with an echogenicity lower than the adventitia, while fibrous plaques are as bright or brighter than the adventitia, but without acoustic shadowing characteristic of calcified plaques. "Mixed" plaques involve bright echoes with acoustic shadowing between 90^0 and 180^0 of vessel wall circumference or a mixture of soft and fibrous plaque with each component occupying <80% of the plaque area [90]. Thrombus and lipid deposits cannot be reliably detected with current technologies. Intravascular ultrasound studies have categorized coronary plaques according to "echogenic properties". It is premature to comment on long term lesion outcome related to these properties. Using a classification of soft, diffusely calcified and mixed, Gil and colleagues were unable to detect any influence on the acute procedural results (elastic recoil and relative gain) [90]. Additionally, these angiographic parameters were not influenced by lesion eccentricity (IVUS defined as minimal /maximal wall thickness <0.5) or plaque dissection (detected by IVUS in 65%). However, these studies suggested that plaque compression is the main mechanism of PTCA in soft plaques while vessel wall disruption and total vessel expansion is predominant in mixed and calcified plaques [90].

The PICTURE study (post intra-coronary treatment ultrasound restenosis evaluation) is a prospective study of 200 patients to identify ultrasonic markers of risk of late restenosis. Preliminary reports have suggested that there is no correlation between clinical and angiographic incidence of restenosis and lesion composition [103]. In 322 patients, Mintz et al found that the residual cross-sectional area stenosis measured with IVUS was an independent predictor of angiographic restenosis (DS>50%) in a multivariate analysis [104]. Restenosis occurred in >50% of the lesions with more than 70% residual area stenosis immediately after the procedure. This observation is compatible with the previously noted QCA association between less optimal procedural results and "restenosis" using a predetermined level or diameter stenosis at follow-up. An interim (135 patients) analysis of the GUIDE II trial (Guidance by ultrasound imaging for decision endpoints), a multicenter trial which will ultimately recruit 500 patients, has shown that residual plaque burden and luminal cross-sectional area after intervention were predictive of long term recurrence of symptoms [105].

Is there a relationship between lesion composition and dissections? A prospective pre and post interventional IVUS study recently reported the incidence of severe dissections (extension of the dissection channel ≥ 20° of the vessel circumference extending into the medial layer or a clearly identified second lumen) in 106 lesions classified according to tissue echolucency. There were no differences in the incidence of severe dissections (30-36%) between soft (hypo and isoechogenic), moderate (hyperechogenic) and heavily calcified (arc>90°) lesions [106].

c. Total Subacute/Chronic Occlusions

Registry data compiled from the National Heart Lung and Blood Institute (NHLBI) in 1985-1986 indicated that total occlusions represented 10% of all lesions attempted [107]. In the 50-75% of lesions that are actually successfully dilated by balloon angioplasty [108], restenosis is reported to occur in nearly 40% to 70% of lesions [109-112]. In general, interpretation of these restenosis rates are limited by poor rates of angiographic follow-up, which were driven predominantly by recurrent symptoms rather than a methodical approach. Restenosis has been related to postangioplasty lumen diameter [112-114], a shorter duration of occlusion [110] and occlusions in the left anterior descending and right coronary artery [114]. The mechanism(s) of restenosis may be somewhat different in total occlusions. While two studies have shown no significant deterioration in dilated lesions between the immediate post PTCA result and at 24 hours [115,116], Buller and colleagues recently demonstrated significant early recoil in 33 successfully treated subacute/chronic coronary occlusions [117]. More than 50% of patients met a ≥50% diameter stenosis criterion at 24 hours. Silent reocclusion occurred in 20% of patients, despite intravenous heparin and 60% of lesions had angiographically more severe dissections. Thus, combinations of "early recoil", "underappreciated dissections" and "thrombus burden" may be contributing to a marked early deterioration in these lesions that is quite different than the more delayed processes that occur after balloon angioplasty of stenotic, nonoccluded arteries.

Is there a role for the newer devices in total occlusions to decrease the high restenosis rates [118]? The laser guide wire (Prima Total Occlusion Device, Spectranetics) may improve acute procedural results (and thus subsequent later results) by permitting more successful crossings of the lesion (successful in 58% of cases) [119], which remains the major limitation. Excimer laser, directional atherectomy and high speed roational atherectomy have all been used to debulk plaque mass and optimize the procedural result [120-122] but no reliable angiographic follow-up data are available. Extremely encouraging results of chronic occlusions treated with the coronary Palmaz-Schatz stent have recently been reported. Goldberg et al found a restenosis rate (DS≥50%) of only 20% in 60 chronic occlusions, with only 1 reocclusion [123]. In a smaller study of 30 patients, a restenosis rate of 20% was described along with 2 cases of subacute thrombosis [124]. This apparent beneficial effect of stenting may be due to limiting dissection-induced reclosure since moderate to large dissections were noted in 37% of lesions. A randomized trial (TOSCA) is underway to determine whether heparin coated Palmaz-Schatz stents are superior to balloon angioplasty for restenosis in total occlusions.

d. Dissections:

Coronary angioplasty results in an angiographically visible dissection in 20-45% of the dilated lesions, depending on the study. A modified National Heart, Lung and Blood Institute classification has been developed to assess the severity of dissections (types A-F) [125]. How accurate and consistent are investigators in actually assessing the presence and severity of angiographic dissections? This is difficult to assess since the intraobserver and interobserver variations in defining angiographic dissections are rarely reported. In one study of successfully dilated coronary lesions, there was agreement between two observers on the presence or absence of dissections in 89% of lesions and 85% agreement on the severity [126]. The intraobserver variability for the presence or absence of dissection was 82% and 87%, and for the type of dissection was 80% and 76%. Major discrepancies in reporting of dissections also exist between the various imaging techniques. In the GUIDE 1 trial, dissections were identified in 40% by intravascular ultrasound compared to 19% by angiography [105].

Although there are conflicting reports in the literature, the bulk of evidence does not support a relationship between the presence of a dissection and restenosis. Early studies using visual estimation or hand held caliper measurements, suggested that a "therapeutic" dissection (ie. a dissection that did not compromise the lumen and preclude a "successful" angioplasty) may be protective against restenosis [8] or conversely, increase restenosis [54]. However, several large studies in the 1990's have consistently shown that the presence of an angiographically visible dissection has no effect on restenosis rates in a successfully dilated coronary lesion [56,126,127]. Hermans found no differences in restenosis rates between types A-C dissections (only 5 Types E-F were present). Similarly, the presence of a dissection had no significant effect on late loss after directional atherectomy [64].

e. Bypass Grafts:

The placement of saphenous veins as arterial conduits leads to a number of changes in the function and structure of the "arterialized" vein [128,129]. The mechanisms leading to restenosis in these conduits are not well understood and may not be the same as native arteries. In fact, the incidence of total occlusions at follow-up appears to be much higher in bypass grafts than in native coronary arteries, with reported rates of 10-25% after PTCA [130], directional atherectomy [130], transluminal extraction catheter (TEC) [131] and excimer lasers [74]. In general, venous bypass grafts, especially large, older vessels have diffuse, degenerative disease that respond poorly to PTCA with overall restenosis rates in the range of 50-70% [132-139]. Lesion location within the graft is also a determinant of restenosis rate. The aoto-ostial and proximal body lesions have higher restenosis rates compared to those at the distal anastamosis [132]. Newer devices such as directional atherectomy [130], excimer laser [74,140] and TEC [131] do not appear to have made significant improvements on the restenosis rates compared with conventional PTCA. In contrast, nonrandomized data in the form of single centre or multicentre angiographic follow-up studies have suggested a significant impact of stents on reducing restenosis rates, even before the era of high pressure balloon dilatation and intravascular ultrasound guidance [141]. In the European Multicenter experience with the Wallstent, 6 month stent restenosis rates using DS>50% was 34% [20]. Piana et al examined the results of stent placement in 200 consecutively treated graft lesions with either coronary (n=146) or biliary (n=54) stents and found an angiographic restenosis rate of 17% [142]. The multicenter US Palmaz-Schatz stent experience involved 589 patients (624 lesions) treated for focal vein graft lesions from 1990-1992 [143]. Follow up angiography, obtained in only 66% of patients, indicated an encouraging overall restenosis rate of 29.7%, and was associated with restenotic lesions and smaller vein grafts (<3mm). An ongiong randomized trial (SAVED trial - Stent versus balloon Angioplasty for aorto-coronary saphenous Vein bypass graft Disease) will more definitively assess the utility of stenting as primary prevention of restenosis [144].

7. Future:

It is expected that the technical advances in QCA systems will substantially improve the reliability of measurements. This includes the development of the gradient field transform algorithm for the tracking of dissections and complex lesions as well as dynamic algorithms with adaptive weighting of the first and second derivatives to overcome the present limitations of systems that overestimate small luminal diameters and underestimate large luminal diameters [145,146]. Important technical advances in intravascular ultrasound are also expected to occur. Imaging catheters will continue to reduce in size and it is anticipated that a guidewire type ultrasound probe would allow the opportunity for simultaneous imaging during a revascularization procedure. On-line three dimensional reconstruction of ultrasound images is another route for advancement. The role of angioscopy remains uncertain. Other than detection of thrombus, there seem little significant additional benefit conferred by this technology.

8. Final Thoughts:

Despite methodologic and technical limitations (definitions, angiographic analysis systems), a relationship clearly exists between restenosis and various lesion morphologies and compositions undergoing balloon angioplasty. It is also evident that of the newer technologies, coronary stenting will probably improve restenosis rates in specific lesion subtypes at high risk for restenosis. What message should the clinician and interventionalist take home from these "population based" studies in treating individual patients? Should specific lesion types or characteristics be contraindications to an interventional approach? In the CARPORT study, Rensing and colleagues developed a model to determine how accurately restenosis could

328

be predicted in individual patients, based on a number of angiographic morphologies and clinical characteristics [59]. Although several variables were identified to have an association with restenosis, the actual predictive value of the model (using a follow up 50% diameter stenosis criterion) for individual patients was poor. Their predictive accuracy was only 50% for patients with ≥ 0.4 mm late luminal loss. In the intermediate range of 0.1-0.4 mm of luminal loss, outcome was correctly predicted in only 10% of patients. Thus, morphology alone should not be an absolute contraindication to an interventional procedure, since many patients will still do well despite unfavorable lesion characteristics. Restenosis unfortunately remains an unpredictable event that can only be partially explained by lesion morphology and composition.

References:

1.   Ryan T, Faxon DP, Gunnar RM, et al. Guidelines for percutaneous transluminal coronary angioplasty: A report of the American College of Cardiology/American Heart Association Task Force on assessment of diagnostic and therapeutic cardiovascular procedures. J Am Coll Cardiol 1988;12:529-545

2.   Ellis SG, Vandormael MG, Cowley MJ, et al. Coronary morphologic and clinical determinants of procedural outcome with angioplasty for multivessel coronary disease. Implications for patient selection. Circulation 1990;82:1193-1202

3.   Gruentzig AR, Senning A, Siegenthaler We. Non-operative dilatation of coronary artery stenosis: Percutaneous transluminal coronary angioplasty. N Engl J Med 1979;301:61-68

4.   Mancini GBJ. Quantitative coronary arteriographic methods in the interventional catheterization laboratory: an update and perspective. J Am Coll Cardiol 1991;17:23B-33B

5.   Zir LM, Miller SW, Dinsmore RE, et al. Interobserver variability in coronary angiography. Circulation 1976;627-632

6.   Goldberg RK, Kleiman NS, Monor ST, Abukhalil J, Raizner AE. Comparison of quantitative coronary angiography to visual estimates of lesion severity pre and post PTCA. Am Heart J 1990;1:178-184

7.   Keane D, Haase J, Slager C, Montauban van Swijndregt E, Lehmann K, Ozaki Y, Di Mario C, Kirkeeide R, Serruys PW. Comparative validation of quantitative coronary angiography systems: results and implications from a multicenter study using a standarized approach. Circulation 1995;91:2174-2183

8.   Leimgruber PP, Roubin GS, Anderson HV, et al. Influence of intimal dissection on restenosis after successfrul coronary angioplasty. Circulation 1985;72:530-35

9.   Holmes DR, Vlietstra RE, Smith HC, et al. Restenosis after percutaneous transluminal coronary angioplasty (PTCA): a report from the angioplasty registry of the National Heart Lung and Blood Institute. Am J Cardiol 1984;53:77C-81C

10. Gould KL, Lipscomb K. Effects of coronary stenoses on coronary flow reserve and resistance. Am J Cardiol 1974;33:87-94

11. Gould KL, Kelley KO, Bolson EL. Experimental validation of quantitative coronary arteriography for determining pressure-flow characteristics of coronary stenosis. Circulation 1982;66:930-937

12. Rensing BJ, Hermans WRM, Deckers JW, de Feyter PJ, Tijssen JGP, Serruys PW. Luminal narrowing after percutaneous transluminal coronary balloon angioplasty follows a near Gaussian distribution. A quantitative angiographic study in 1445 successfully dilated lesions. J Am Coll Cardiol 1992;19:939-945

13. Kuntz RE, Safian RD, Levine MJ, Reis GJ, Diver DJ, Baim DS. Novel approach to the analysis of restenosis after the use of three new coronary devices. J Am Coll Cardiol 1992;19:1493-1500

14. Lehmann KG, Melkert R, Serruys PW. Contributions of frequence distribution analysis to the understanding of coronary restenosis. A reappraisal of the Gaussian Curve. Circulation 1996;93:1123-1132

330

15.   King SB III, Weintraub WS, Tao X, Hearn J, Couglas JS Jr. Bimodal distribution of diameter stenosis 4 to 12 months after angioplasty: implications for definitions and interpretation of restenosis. J Am Coll Cardiol 1991;17:345A (abstract)

16.   Beatt KJ, Serruys PW, Luijten HE, Rensing B, Suryapranata H, de Feyter P, van den Brand M, Laarman GJ, Roelandt J. Restenosis after coronary angioplasty: The paradox of increased lument diameter and restenosis. J Am Coll Cardiol 1992;19:258-266

17.   Kuntz RE, Safian RD, Carroza JP, Fischman RF, Mansour M, Baim Ds. The importance of acute luminal diameter in determining restenosis after coronary atherectomy or stenting. Circulation 1992;86:1827-35

18.   Serruys PW, Umans VAWM, Strauss BH, van Suylen RJ, de Feyter PJ. Quantitative angiography after directional coronary atherectomy. Br Heart J 1991;66:122-129

19.   Umans VAWM, Robert A, Foley D, Wijns W, Haine E, de Feyter P, Serruys PW. Clinical, histologic and quantitative angiographic predictors of restenosis following directional coronary atherectomy: a multivariate analysis of the renarrowing process and late outcome. J Am Coll Cardiol 1994;23:49-59

20.   Strauss BH, Serruys PW, Bertrand ME, et al. Quantitative angiographic follow-up of th ecoronary Wallstent in native vessels and bypass graft (European experience-March 1986-March 1990). Am J Cardiol 1992;69:475-81

21.   Serruys PW, de Jaegere P, Kiemeneij F, et al. A comparison of balloon-expandable -stent implantation with balloon angioplasty in patients with coronary artery disease. N Engl J Med 1994;331:489-495

22.   Fishman DL, Leon MB, Baim DS, et al. A randomized comparison of coronary stent placement and balloon angioplasty in the treatment of coronary artery disease. N Engl J Med 1994;331:496-501

23.   Topol EJ, Leya F, Pinkerton CA, et al. A comparison of directional atherectomy with coronary angioplasty in patients with coronary artery disease. N Engl J Med 1993;329:221-227

24.   Adelman AG, Cohen EA, Kimball BP, et al. A comparison of directional atherectomy with balloon angioplasty for lesions of the left anterior descending artery. N Engl J Med 1993;329:228-233

25.   Kuntz RE, Gibson CM, Nobuyoshi M, Baim Ds. Generalized model of restenosis after conventional balloon angioplasty, stenting and DCA. J Am Coll Cardiol 1993;21:15-25

26.   Bittl JA, Kuntz RE, Estella P, Sanborn TA, Baim DS. Analysis of late lumen narrowing after excimer laser-facilitated coronary angioplasty. J Am Coll Cardiol 1994;23:1314-20

27.   Kuntz RE, Baim DS. Defining coronary restenosis. Newer clinical and angiographic paradigms. Circulation 1993;88:1310-1323

331

28. Foley DP, Appelman YE, Strikwerda S, Piek JJ, Koolen JJ, Tijssen JP, de Feyter PJ, David GK, van Swijndregt EJ, Melkert R, Serruys PW. .A comparison of angiographic restenosis propensity of excimer laser coronary angioplasty and balloon angioplasty in longer coronary lesions.. In: *Short and long-term results of transluminal coronary interventions: an angiographic perspective.* Foley DP (PhD thesis). Erasmus University, Rotterdam 1995

29. Appelman YEA, Piek JJ, Strikwerda S, Tijssen JGP, de Feyter PJ, David GK, Serruys PW, Margolis JR, Koelemay MJ, Montauban van Swijndregt EWJ, Koolen JJ. Lancet 1996;347:79-84

30. Rensing BJ, Hermans WRM, Deckers JW, de Feyter PJ, Serruys PW. .Which angiographic parameter best describes functional status 6 months after successful single vessel coronary balloon angioplasty?.. In: *Restenosis after percutaneous transluminal coronary angioplasty. A Quantitative angiographic approach.* Rensing BJWM (PhD Thesis). Erasmus Univeristy, Rotterdam 1992.

31. Keane D, Melkert R, Herrman JP, Foley DP, Ozaki Y, Di Mario C, de Feyter PJ, Serruys PW. .Quantitative coronary angiography endpoints: a valid surrogacy for clinical events?. In: *de Feyter PJ, Di Mario C and Serruys PW (eds). Quantitative Coronary Imaging.* Barjesteh, Meeuwes & Co., Rotterdam 1995

32. Keane D, Serruys PW. .Quantitative coronary angiography: an integral component of interventional cardiology.. In: Topol EJ, Serruys PW (eds). *Current Review Of Interventional Cardiology, 2nd edition.* Current Medicine, Philadelphia, 1995:205-233

33. Post MJ, Borst C, Kuntz RE. The relative importance of arterial remodeling compared with intimal hyperplasia in lumen renarrowing after balloon angioplasty: a study in the normal rabbit and the hypercholesterolemic Yucatan micropig. Circulation 1994;89:2816-2821

34. Kakuta T, Currier JW, Haudenschild CC, Ryan TH, Faxon DP. Differences in compensatory vessel enlargement, not intimal formation, account for restenosis after angioplasty in the hypercholesterolemic rabbit model. Circulation 1994;89:2809-2815

35. Isner J. Vascular remodeling. Honey, I think I shrunk the artery . Circulation 1994;89;2937-2941

36. Kimura T, Kaburagi S, Tashima Y, Nobuyoshi M, Mintz GS, Popma JJ. Geometric remodeling and intimal regrowth as mechanisms of restenosis: observations from serial ultrasound analysis of restenosis (SURE) trial. Circulation 1995;92[suppl I]:I-76 (abstract)

37. Mintz GS, Kent KM, Satler LF, Wong SC, Hong MK, Griffin J, Pichard AD. Dimorphic mechanisms of restenosis after DCA and stents: A serial intravascular ultrasound study. Circulation 1995;92[suppl 1]:I-546 (abstract)

38. Umans VA, Robert A, Foley DP, Haine E, de Feyter PJ, Wijns W, Serruys PW. Clinical, angiographic and histologic predictors of restenosis after directional coronary atherectomy: a multivariate analysis of the renarrowing process and late outcome. J Am Coll Cardiol 1994;23:49-59

39.   Beatt KJ, Serruys PW, Hugenholtz PG. Restenosis after coronary angioplasty: new standards for clinical studies. J Am Coll Cardiol 1990;15:491-498

40.   Ozaki Y, Keane D, Di Mario C, Camenzid E, Baptista J, de Feyter P, Roelandt JRTC, Serruys PW. Comparison of coronary luminal quantification obtained from both geometric and videodensitometric quantitative angiography and from intracoronary ultrasound pre and post coronary intervention. Submitted

41.   Gorge G, Liu F, Ge J, Haude M, Baumgart D, Caspary G. Intravascular ultrasound variables predict restenosis after PTCA. Circulation 1995;92[suppl I]:I-148 (abstract)

42.   Umans VA, Strauss BH, de Feyter PJ, Serruys PW. Edge detection versus videodensitometry for quantitative angiographic assessment of directional coronary atherectomy. Am J Cardiol 1991;68:534-538

43.   Serruys PW, Strauss BH, Beatt KJ, Bertrand M, Puel J, Rickards AF, Kappenberger L, Meier B, Goy JJ, Vogt P, Sigwart U. Angiographic follow-up after placement of a self-expanding coronary stent. N Engl J Med 1991;324:13-17.

44.   Strauss BH, Juilliere Y, Rensing BJ, Reiber JHC, Serruys PW. Edge detection versus densitometry for assessing coronary stenting quantitatively. Am J Cardiol 1991;67:484-490

45.   Blasini R, Schuhlen H, Mudra H, et al. Angiographic overestimation of lumen size after coronary stent placement: Impact of high pressure dilatation. Circulation 1995;92[suppl I]:I-223 (abstract)

46.   Penny WF, Schmidt Da, Safian RD, Erny RE, Baim DS. Insights into the mechanism of luminal improvement after directional coronary atherectomyl Am J Cardiol 1991;67:435-437

47.   Umans VA, Baptista J, Di Mario C, von Birgelen C, de Jaegere P, de Feyter PJ, Serruys PW. Angiographic, ultrasonic and angioscopic assessment of the coronary artery wall and lumen area configuration after directional atherectomy: The mechanism revisited. Am Heart J 1995;130:217-27

48.   Umans VA, Haine E, Renkin J, De Feyter PJ, Wijns W, Serruys PW. The mechanism of directional coronary atherectomy. Eur Heart J 1993;14:505-510

49.   Strauss BH, Escaned J, Foley DP, Di Mario C, Haase J, Keane D, Hermans WRM, de Feyter PJ, Serruys PW. Technological considerations and practical limitations in the use of quantitative angiography during percutaneous coronary recanalization. Prog Cardiovasc Dis 1994;36:343-362

50.   Foley DP, Escaned J, Strauss BH, di Mario C, Haase J, Keane D, Umans VA, Hermans WR, Rensing BJ, de Feyter PJ, Serruys PW. Quantitative coronary angiography (QCA) in interventional cardiology: Application to scientific research and clinical practice. Prog Cardiovasc Dis 1994;36:363-384

51.   Foley DP, Melkert R, Serruys PW. Influence of coronary vessel size on renarrowing process and late angiographic outcome after successful balloon angioplasty. Circulation 1994;90:1239-1251

52.   Azar AJ, Ketre K, Goldberg S, Kiemeneij F, Leon MB, Serruys PW. A meta-analysis on the clinical and angiographic outcomes of stents vs PTCA in the different coronary vessel sizes in the Benestent-1 and Stress-1/2 Trials. Circulation 1995;suppl I:I-475 [abstract]

53. Hall P, Nakamura S, Maiello L, Almagor Y, Gaglione A, Goldberg SL, Tobis JM, Martini, Tucci G, Di Maggio M, Colombo A. .Clinical and angiographic outcome after Palmaz-Schatz stent implantation guided by intravascular ultrasound.. In: *de Feyter PJ, Di Mario C and Serruys PW (eds). Quantitative Coronary Imaging.* Barjesteh, Meeuwes & Co., Rotterdam 1995

54. Akira I, Hall P, Maiello L, Blengino S, Finci L, Ferraro M, Martini G, Colombo A. Coronary stenting of long lesions (greater than 20 mm)- A matched comparison of different stents. Circulation 1995;92[suppl 1]:1-688 (abstract)

55. Guiteras Val PG, Bourassa MG, David PR, et al. Restenosis after successful percutaneous transluminal coronary angioplasty: the Montreal Heart Institute experience. Am J Cardiol 1987;60:50B-55B

56. Vandormael MG, Deligonul U, Kern M, et al. Multilesion coronary angioplasty: clinical and angiographic follow-up. J Am Coll Cardiol 1987;10:246-252

57. Hirshfeld JW Jr, Schwartz JS, Jugo R, et al. Restenosis after coronary angioplasty: a multivariate statistical model to relate lesion and procedure variables to restenosis. J Am Coll Cardiol 1991;18:647-56

58. Foley DP, Melkert R, Serruys PW. Restenosis after percutaneous intervention: is there a device specificity? *Handbook of Interventional Cardiology.* Topol E and Serruys PW (eds). In press.

59. Rensing BJ, Hermans WR, Vos J, et al. Luminal narrowing after percutaneous transluminal coronary angioplasty. A study of clinical, procedural, and lesional factors related to long-term angiographic outcome. Coronary Artery Restenosis Prevention on Repeated Thromboxane Antagonism (CARPORT) Study Group. Circulation 1993; 88:975-985.

60. Hermans WRM, Rensing BJ, Foley D, Tijssen JGP, Rutsch W, Emanuelsson H, Danchin N, Wijns W, Chappuis F, Serruys PW. Patient, lesion and procedural variables as risk factors for luminal re-narrowing after successful coronary angioplasty. A quantitative analysis in 653 patients with 778 lesions. J Cardiovasc Pharm 1993;22:S45-S57

61. Strauss BH, Serruys PW, de Scheerder IK, Tijssen JGP, Bertrand M, Puel J, Meier B, Kaufmann U, Stauffer JC, Rickards AF, Sigwart U. Relative risk analysis of angiographic predictors of restenosis in the coronary Wallstent[R]. Circulation 1991;84:1636-1643

62. Reimers B, di Mario C, Nierop P, Pasquetto G, Camenzind E, Ruygrok P. Long-term restenosis after multiple stent implantation. A quantitative angiographic study. Circulation 1995;92[supplement 1]:1-327 (abstract)

63. Schiele TM, Marx R, Vogt M, Leschke M, Heintzen MP. Eccentricity of coronary arteries is a predictor of chronic restenosis after directional atherectomy. Circulation 1995;92[suppl I]:I-328 (abstract)

64. Kimball BP, Cohen EA, Adelman AG. Influence of stenotic lesion morphology on immediate and long-term (6 months) angiographic outcome: comparative analysis of directional coronary atherectomy versus standard balloon angioplasty. J Am Coll Cardiol 1996;27:543-551

65. Topol EJ, Ellis SG, Fishman J et al. Multicenter study of percutaneous transluminal angioplasty for right coronary ostial stenosis. J Am Coll Cardiol. 1987:9:1214-1218

334

66.   de Feyter PJ, van Suylen R-J, de Jaegere PPT, Topol EJ, Serruys PW. Balloon angioplasty for the treatment of lesions in saphenous vein bypass grafts. J Am Coll Cardiol 1993;21:1539-49

67.   Mathias DW, Mooney JF, Lange HW et al.Frequency of success and complications of coronary angioplasty of a stenosis at the ostium of a branch vessel. Am J Cardiol. 1991:67:491-495.

68.   Popma JJ, Leon MB, Mintz GS, Kent KM, Satler LF, Garrand TJ, Pichard AD. Results of coronary angioplasty using the TEC catheter. Am J Cardiol. 1992:70:1526-1532

69.   Sos TA, Saddekini S, Pickering TG, Laragh JH. Technical aspects of percutaneous transluminal angioplasty in renovascular disease. Nephron. 1986:suppll:45-50

70.   Stewart J, Ward D, Davies M, Pepper J. Isolated coronary ostial stenosis: observations on pathology. Eur Heart J. 1987:8:917-920.

71.   Boehrer JD et al. Directional atherectomy versus balloon angioplasty for coronary ostial and nonostial left anterior descending coronary artery lesions: results from a randomized multicenter trial. J Am Coll Cardiol. 1995:25:1380-1386

72.   Abdel-Meguid AE, Whitlow PL, Simpfebdorfer C, Sapp SK, Franco I, Ellis SG and Topol E. Percutaneous revascularization of ostial saphenous vein graft stenoses. J Am Coll Cardiol. 1995:26:955-960

73.   Ghazzal ZYB, Burton E, Weintraub WS, Litvack F, Rothbaum DA, Klein L, King SB. Predictors of restenosis after excimer laser coronary angioplasty. Am J Cardiol. 1995:75:1012-1014

74.   Strauss BH, Natarjan MK, Batchelor WB, Yardley DE, Sanborn TA, Power JA, Watson LE, Moothart R, Tcheng JE, Bittl JA, Chisholm RJ. Quantitative angiographic analysis of the vein graft lesions treated with excimer laser angioplasty: Immediate and follow-up results. Circulation 1995;92:348-356

75.   Colombo A, Itoh A, Maiello L. Coronary stent implantation in aorto-ostial lesions: immediate and follow-up results. J Am Coll Cardiol 1996;27[suppl A]:253A

76.   Zampieri P, Colombo A, Almagor Y, Marello L, Finci L. Results of coronary stenting of ostial lesions. Am J Cardiol 1994;73:901-903

77.   Kaltenbach M, Kober G, Scherer D, Vallbracht C. Recurrence rate after successful coronary angioplasty. Eur Heart J 1985;6:276-281

78.   DiSciascio G, Cowley MJ, Vetrovec GW. Angiographic patterns of restenosis after angioplasty of multiple coronary arteries. Am J Cardiol 1986;58:922-925

79.   Myler RK, Topol EJ, Shaw RE, et al. Multiple vessel coronary angioplasty in 494 consecutive patients. Cathet Cardiovasc Diagn 1987;13:1-15

80.   Black AJR, Anderson HV, Roubin GS, et al. Repeat coronary angioplasty: Correlates of a second restenosis. J Am Coll Cardiol 1988;11:714-718

81.   Renkin J, Melin J, Robert A, et al. Detection of restenosis after successful coronary angioplasty: improved clinical decision making with use of a logistic model combining procedural and follow-up variables. J Am Coll Cardiol 1990;16:1333-1340

82.   Rupprecht HJ, Brennecke R, Bernhard G, Erbel R, Pop T, Meyer J. Analysis of risk factors for restenosis after PTCA. Cathet Cardiovasc Diagn 1990;19:151-159

83.   Leimgruber PP, Roubin GS, Hollman J et al. Restenosis after successful coronary angioplasty in patients with single-vessel disease. Circulation 1986;73:710-717

84.   de Feyter PJ, Suryapranata H, Serruys PW, et al. Coronary angioplasty for unstable angina: immediate and late results in 200 consecutive patients with identification of risk factors for unfavourable early and late outcome. J Am Coll Cardiol 1988;12:324-333

85.   Hermans WRM, Rensing BJ, Kelder JC, de Feyter PJ, Seruys PW. Postangioplasty restenosis rate between segments of the major coronary arteries. Am J Cardiol 1992;69:194-200

86.   Rensing BJ, Hermans WRM, Vos J, Tijssen JGP, Rutsch W, Danchin N, Heyndrickx GR, Mast EG, Wijns W, Serruys PW. .Luminal narrowing after percutaneous transluminal coronary. A study of clinical, procedural and lesional factors related to long term angiographic outcome.. In: *Restenosis after percutaneous transluminal coronary angioplasty. A Quantitative angiographic approach.* Rensing BJWM (PhD Thesis). Erasmus Univeristy 1992, Rotterdam.

87.   Mintz GS, Popma JJ, Pichard AD, et al. Patterns of calcification in coronary artery disease.: A statistical analysis of intravascular ultrasound and coronary angiography in 1155 lesions. Circulation 1995;91:1959-1965

88.   Ozaki Y, Keane D, Di Mario C, Camenzid E, Baptista J, de Feyter P, Roelandt JRTC, Serruys PW. Comparison of coronary luminal quantification obtained from both geometric and videdensitometric quantitative angiography and from intracoronary ultrasound pre and post coronary intervention. Submitted

89.   Fitzgerald PJ, Ports TA, Yock PG. Contribution of localized calcium deposits to dissection after angioplasty in vivo assessed by intravascular ultrasound imaging. Circulation 1992; 86:64-70

90.   Gil R, Di Mario C, Prati F, von Birgelen C, Ruygrok P, Roelandt JRTC, Serruys PW. .Influence of plaque composition on mechanisms of percutaneous transluminal coronary balloon angioplasty assessed by ultrasound imaging.. In: *de Feyter PJ, Di Mario C and Serruys PW (eds). Quantitative Coronary Imaging.* Barjesteh, Meeuwes & Co., Rotterdam 1995

91.   Tenaglia AN, Buller C, Kisslo KB, et al. Mechanisms of balloon angioplasty and directional coronary atherectomy as assessed by intracoronary ultrasound. J Am Coll Cardiol 1992;20:685-691

92.   Botas J, Clark DA, Pinto F, et al. Balloon angioplasty results in increased segemental coronary distensibility: a likely mechanism of percutaneous transluminal coronary angioplasty. J Am Coll Cardiol 1994;23:1043-1052

93.   Matar FA, Mintz GS, Pinnow E, et al. Multivariate predictors of intravascular ultrasound endpoints after directional coronary atherectomy. J Am Coll Cardiol 1995;25:318-324

94.   Kovach J, Mintz GS, Javier S, et al. Mechanisms of lumen enlargement after excimer laser angioplasty and adjunct balloon angioplasty: a sequential intravascular ultrasound study. J Am Coll Cardiol 1994;23:449A (abstract)

95.   Gorge G, Liu F, Ge J, Haude M, Baumgart D, Caspary G. Intrvascular ultrasound variables predict restenosis after PTCA. Circulation 1995;92[suppl I]:I-148 (abstract)

96.   Ramee SR, White CJ, Collins TJ, Mesa JE, Murgo JP. Percutaneous angioscopy during coronary angioplasty using a steerable microangioscope. J Am Coll Cardiol 1991;17:100-5

97.   Mizuno K, Satomura K, Miyamoto A, et al. Angioscopic evaluation of coronary-artery thrombi in acute coronary syndromes. N Engl J Med 1992;326:287-91

98.   Den Heijer P, Foley D, Escaned J, et al. Angioscopic versus angiographic detection of intimal dissection and intracoronary thrombus. J Am Coll Cardiol 1994;24:649-654

99.   Mizuno K, Miyamoto A, Isojima K, et al. A serial observation of coronary thrombi in vivo by a new percutaneous transluminal coronary angioscope. Angiology 1992;43:91-99

100. Rensing BJ, Hermans WRM, Vos J et al Carport Group. Angiographic risk factors of luminal narrowing after coronary balloon angioplasty using balloon measurements to reflect stretch and elastic recoil at the dilatation site. Am J Cardiol 1992;69:584-91

101. Di Mario C, The SHK, Madrestma S, et al. Detection and characterization of vascular lesions by intravascular ultrasound: an in vitro study correlated with histology. J Am Soc Echocardiogr 1992;5:135-46

102. Gussenhoben EJ, Essed CE, Lancee CT, et al. Arterial wall characteristics determined by intravascular ultrasound imaging: an in vitro study. J Am Coll Cardiol 1989;14:947-52

103. Peters RJG, PICTURE study group. Prediction of the risk of angiographic restenosis by intracoronary ultrasound imaging after coronary balloon angioplasty. J Am Coll Cardiol 1995;25:35A (abstract)

109. Mintz GS, Chuang YC, Popma JJ, et al. The final % cross-sectional narrowing (residual plaque burden) is the strongest intravascular ultrasound predictor of angiographic restenosis. J Am Coll Cardiol 1995;25:35A (abstract)

105. GUIDE Trial Investigators. Discrepancies between angiographic and intravascular ultrasound appearance of coronary lesions undergoing interventions. J Am Coll Cardiol 1993;21:118A

106. Athanasiadis A, Schmid KM, Wullen B, Haase KK, Voelker W. Is the incidence of severe dissections predictable by pre-interventional intravascular ultrasound lesion morphology? Circulation 1995;92[suppl I]:I-148 (abstract)

107. Detre K, et al. Percutaneous transluminal coronary angioplasty in 1985-86 and 1977-81. N Engl J Med 1988;312:265

108. Plante S, Laarman G, de Feyter PJ, et al. Acute complications of percutaneous transluminal coronary angioplasty for totally occluded coronary arteries. Am Heart J 1991;121;417-426

109. Holmes DR Jr., Vlietstra RE, Reeder GS, et al. Angioplasty in total coronary artery occlusions. J Am Coll Cardiol 1984;3:845-9

109. Bell MR, Berger QB, Bresnahan JF, Reeder GS, Bailey KR, Holmes DR. Initial and long-term outcome of 354 patients after coronary balloon angioplasty of total coronary artery occlusions. Circulation 1992;85:1003-11

110. DiSciasco G, Vetrovec GW, Cowley MJ, Wolfgang TC. Early and late outcome of PTCA for subacute and chronic coronary occlusion. Am Heart J 1986;111:833-839

111. Serruys PW, Umans V, Heyndrickx GR, et al. Elective PTCA of totally occluded arteries not associated with acute myocardial infarction; short-term and long-term results. Eur Heart J 1985;6:2-12

112. Melchior JP, Meier B, Urban P, et al. PTCA for chronic total coronary arterial occlusion. Am J Cardiol 1987;59:535-8

113. Lange RA, Cigarroa RG, Hillis LD. Influence of residual antegrade coronary blood flow on survival after myocardial infarction in patients with multivessel coronary artery disease. Coronary Artery Dis 1990;1:59-63

114. Ellis SG, Shaw RE, Gershony G, et al. Risk factors, time course and treatment effect for restenosis after successful percutaneous transluminal coronary angioplasty of chronic total occlusion. Am J Cardiol 1989;63:897-901

115. Foley DP, Deckers J, van den Bos AA, Heyndrickx GR, Laarman GJ, Suryapranata H, Zijlstra F, Serruys PW. Usefulness of repeat coronary angiography 24 hours after successful balloon angioplasty to evaluate early luminal deterioration and facilitate quantitative analysis. Am J Cardiol 1993;72:1341-1347

116. Hanet C, Wijns W, Michel X, Schroeder E. Influence of balloon size and stenosis morphology on immediate and delayed elastic recoil after percutaneous transluminal coronary angioplasty. J Am Coll Cardiol 1991;18:506-511

117. Buller C, et al. Early recoil, dissection and reocclusion following PTCA of total coronary occlusions. Can J Cardiol 1994;10[suppl]:276A (abstract)

118. Puma JA, Sketch MH Jr, Tcheng JE, Harrington RA, Phillips HR, Stack RS, Califf RM. Percutaneous revascularization of chronic coronary occlusions: An overview. J Am Coll Cardiol 1995;26:1-11

119. Serruys PW, Leon M, Hamburger JN, et al. Recanalization of chronic total coronary occlusions using a laser guide wire: The Eu and US total experience. J Am Coll Cardiol 1996;27[suppl A]:152A

120. Holmes DR Jr, Forrester JS, Litvack F, et al. Chronic total obstruction and short-term outcome: The excimer laser coronary angioplasty registry experience. Mayo Clinic Proc 1993;68:5-10

121. Warth D, Cowley M. Percutaneous transluminal coronary rotational ablation of total coronary occlusions. Circulation 1992;86 Suppl I:I-781 (abstract)

122.   Hinohara T, Rowe MH, Roberstono GC, et al. Effect of lesion characteristics on outcome of directional coronary atherectomy. J Am Coll Cardiol 1991;17:1112-20

123.   Goldberg SL, Colombo A, Maiello L, Borrione M, Finci L, Almagor Y. Intracoronary stent insertion after balloon angioplasty of chronic total occlusions. J Am Coll Cardiol 1995;26:713-719

124.   Medina A, et al. Effectiveness of coronary stenting for the treatment of chronic total occlusions in angina pectoris. Am J Cardiol 1994;73:1222

125.   Dorros G, Cowley MJ, Simpson J, et al. Percutaneous transluminal coronary angioplasty: report of complications from the National Heart, Lung, and Blood Institute PTCA Registry. Circulation 1983;67:4:723-730

126.   Hermans WRM, Rensing BJ, Foley DP, Deckers JW, Rutsch W, Emanuelsson H, Danchin N, Wijns W, Chappuis F, Serruys PW. "Therapeutic dissection" and the occurrence of restenosis. A quantitative angiographic analysis in 778 lesions after successful angioplasty. J Am Coll Cardiol 1992;20:767-80

127.   Rupprect HJ, Brennecke R, Bernhard G, Erbel R, Pop T, Meyer J. Analysis of risk factors for restenosis after PTCA. Cathet Cardiovasc Diagn 1990;19:151-159

128.   Smith SH, Geer JC. Morphology of saphenous vein coronary artery bypass grafts. Arch Pathol Lab Med 1983;107:13-18

129.   Cox JL, Chiasson DA, Gotlieb AV. Stranger in a strange land: the pathogenesis of saphenous vein graft stenosis with emphasis on structural and functional differences between veins and arteries. Prog Cardiovasc Dis 1991;34;45-68

130.   Holmes DR JR, Topol EJ, Califf RM, et al. A multicenter, randomized trial of coronary angioplasty versus directional atherectomy for patients with saphenous vein bypass graft lesions. Circulation 1995;91:1966-1974

131.   Safian RD, Grines CL, May MA, Lichtenberg A, Juran N, Schreiber TL, Pavlides G, Meany TB, Savas V, O'Neill WW. Clinical and angiographic results of transluminal extraction coronary atherectomy in saphenous vein bypass grafts. Circulation 1994;89:302-312

132.   de Feyter PJ, van Suylen R-J, de Jaegere PPT, Topol EJ, Serruys PW. Balloon angioplasty for the treatment of lesions in saphenous vein bypass grafts. J Am Coll Cardiol 1993;21:1539-49

133.   Platko WP, Hollman J, Whitlow PL, Franco I. Percutaneous transluminal angioplasty of saphenous vein graft stenosis: long term follow-up. J Am Coll Cardiol 1989;14:1645-50

134.   Douglas JS, Gruentzig AR, King SB III, Hollman J, Ischinger T, Meier B, Craver JM, Jones EL, Waller EL, Bones DK, Guyton R. Percutaneous transluminal angioplasty in patients with prior coronary artery bypass surgery. J Am Coll Cardiol 1983;2:745-754

135.   Corbelli J, Franco I, Hollman J, Simpfendorfer C, Galan K. Percutaneous transluminal coronary angioplasty after previous coronary artery bypass surgery. Am J Cardiol 1985;56:398-403

136.   Reeder GS, Bresnahan JF, Holmes DR, Mock MB, Orszulak TA, Smith HC, Vlietstra RE. Angioplasty for aortocoronary bypass graft stenosis. Mayo Clin Proc 1986;61:14-19

137. Meester BH, Samson M, Suryapranata H, et al. Long-term follow-up after attempted angioplasty of saphenous vein grafts: the Thoraxcenter experience 1981-1988. Eur Heart J 1991;12:648-53

138. Webb JG, Myler RK, Shaw RE, et al. Coronary angioplasty after coronary bypass surgery: initial results and late utcome in 422 patients. J Am Coll Cardiol 1990;16:812-20

139. Plokker HWT, Meester BH, Serruys PW. The Dutch experience in percutaneous transluminal angioplasty of narrowed saphenous veins used for aortocoronary arterial bypass. Am J Cardiol 1991;67:361-6

140. Bittl JA, Sanborn TA, Yardley DE, Tcheng JE, Isner JM, Chokshi SK, Strauss BH, Abela GS, Schmidhofer M, Power JA. Percutaneous excimer laser coronary angioplasty of saphenous vein bypass graft lesions: Predictors of outcome. Am J Cardiol 1994;74:144-148

141. Eeckhout E, Kappenberger L, Goy JJ. Stents for intracoronary placement: current status and future directions. J Am Coll Cardiol. 1996:27:757-765

142. Piana RN, Moscucci M, Cohen DJ, Kugelmass AK, Senerchia C, Kuntz RE, Baim DS. Palmaz-Schatz stenting for treatment of focal venin graft stenosis: immediate results and long-term outcome. J Am Coll Cardiol 1994;23:1296-304

143. Wong SC, Baim DS, Schatz RA, Teirstein PS, King SB, Curry JR RC, Heuser RR, Ellis SG, Cleman MW, Overlie P, Hirshfeld JW, Walker CM, Litvack F, Fish D, Brinker JA, Buchbinder M, Goldberg S, Chuang YC, Leon MB. Immediate results and late outcomes after stent implantation in saphenous vein graft lesions: the multicenter US Palmaz-Schatz stent experience. J Am Coll Cardiol 1995;26:704-12

144. Savage M, Douglas J, Fischman D et al. Coronary stents versus balloon angioplasty for aorta-coronary saphenous vein bypass graft disease: interim results of a randomized trial. JACC. 1995:25:79A (abstract)

145. van der Zwet PMJ, Reiber JHC. A new approach for the quantification of complex lesion morphology: The gradient field transform (GFT): Basic principles and validation results. J Am Coll Cardiol 1994;24:216-224

146. Keane D, Gronenschild E, Slager C, Ozaki Y, Haase J, Serruys PW. In-vivo validation of an experimental adeaptive quantitative coronary angiography algorithm to circumvent overestimation of small luminal diameters. Cathet Cardiovasc Diagn 1995;36:17-24

Table 1. Combined American College of Cardiology/American Heart Association Lesion Classification

Type A Lesions (High success, >85%, Low Risk)
- discrete (<10 mm length)
- concentric
- readily accessible
- nonangulated segment, <45°
- smooth contour
- little or no calcification
- less than totally occlusive
- nonostial in location
- no major branch involvement
- absence of thrombus

Type B Lesions (Moderate success, 60-85%, Moderate Risk)
- tubular (10-20 mm length)
- eccentric
- moderate tortuosity of proximal segment
- moderately angulated segment, >45°, <90° double guide wires
- irregular contour
- moderate to heavy calcification
- total occlusions <3 months old
- ostial in location
- bifurcation lesions requiring
- some thrombus present

Type C Lesions (Low success, <60%, High Risk)
- diffuse (>2 cm length)
- excessive tortuosity of proximal segment
- extremely angulated segments >90° friable lesions
- total occlusions >3 months old
- inability to protect major side branches
- degenerated vein grafts with

Table 2. Binary Definitions of Restenosis

1) an increase in diameter stenosis (DS) of at least 30% at follow-up angiography (NHLBI I)
2) an immediate post-PTCA DS of <50% increasing to ≥70% at follow-up (NHLBI II)
3) an increase in stenosis severity to within 10% or less of the predilation DS at follow-up (NHLBI III)
4) a loss of at least 50% of the gain in luminal diameter achieved at PTCA (NHLBI IV)
5) an increase of the DS from <50% after angioplasty to ≥50% at follow-up (Emory)
6) a decrease in minimal luminal diameter of ≥0.72 mm with respect to post PTCA situation (Thoraxcenter)

14.

PITFALLS AND PRACTICAL APPROACH TO THE USE OF IMAGING TECHNIQUES IN DEVELOPING CLINICAL STRATEGIES

Terry R. Bowers MD, Barry M. Kaplan MD, and
William W. O'Neill MD, FACC

William Beaumont Hospital
Royal Oak, Michigan

INTRODUCTION

Coronary angiography remains the standard modality for determining the presence or absence of significant coronary artery disease in 1996. However, in the preceding chapters, angiography has been shown to be limited in predicting the functional significance of a stenosis on coronary blood flow. [1,2] Additionally, visual estimates of percent diameter stenosis are plagued with significant interobserver and intraobserver variability. [3,4] This variability has improved with the development of computer-based quantitative and digital techniques; [5,6] yet, QCA and the physiologic assessment of stenosis severity are weakly correlated, particularly in patients with multivessel disease [7] and intermediate lesions. [8,9] The clinical correlation between functional significance and the best quantitative angiographic techniques in "borderline" coronary artery lesions is poor, secondary to wide 95% confidence intervals. [10]

CLINICAL IMPERATIVES DRIVING ENDOVASCULAR IMAGING

The shortcomings of angiography, described in Table 1, have prompted technologic advances in endovascular imaging, which have created 3 frontiers for nonangiographic intravascular assessment; namely, Doppler ultrasound, 2-D ultrasound (IVUS), and angioscopy. Each of these modalities, including their foundations and technical aspects, have been discussed in detail in the preceding chapters.

TABLE 1.   The Limitations Of Digital Contrast Angiography

1.   Bias and lack of reproducibility of vessel dimensions.
2.   Difficulty in assessing "normal" reference vessel as opposed to diffuse disease.
3.   Difficulty in assessing "borderline" lesion significance.
4.   Underestimation of plaque burden (concentric vs. eccentric lesions).
5.   Inadequate assessment of lesion characteristics.
   • plaque composition (depth and extent of calcium and/or thrombus)
   • severity of eccentric lesions
6.   Lack of physiologic data.
7.   Post-intervention disparity in angiographic lumen dimensions compared with histologic and intravascular ultrasound measurements.
   • hazy result (erratic lumen borders)
   • suboptimal result (residual plaque with eccentric or concentric borders, clot, or dissection)
8.   Dissociation between clinical and angiographic findings.

The impetus to apply endovascular imaging techniques to clinical practice has intensified due to the apparent overwhelming discordance between angiographic lesion severity, the physiologic effects of the stenosis, and clinical outcome.[11] While technological advances have led to a plethora of tools to both assess and treat coronary lesions, the challenge will now be to apply these tools in a rational and cost-effective manner to improve clinical outcome. The intent of this chapter is to discuss the practical applications of each nonangiographic imaging modality in everyday clinical practice. In so doing, the clinical utility and pitfalls of each will be elucidated by way of examples and tables summarizing clinical investigations and our own experience. The clinically relevant situations and strategies, where these imaging devices are practically applied, are presented in Figure 1.

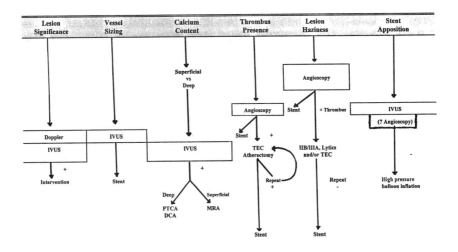

Figure 1. Schematic diagram representing the clinical algorithms guiding nonangiographic imaging applications.

A comparison of the utility of intracoronary Doppler, ultrasound and angioscopy with digital angiography is presented in Table 2. These techniques should not be viewed as competitive technologies. Each provides complimentary information, discussed throughout the chapter, which may be useful during angiography and percutaneous intervention.

TABLE 2   Comparison of Nonangiographic Imaging Modalities to Contrast Angiography

	DIGITAL ANGIO	ANGIOSCOPY	IVUS	DOPPLER
Vessel lumen detail	+	++++	++	-
Vessel wall detail		-	++++	-
Vessel dimensions	++	-	++++	-
Coronary flow	++	-	+	++++
Borderline lesions	+	++	+++	++++
Physiologic assessment	-	-	+	++++
Ostial lesions	+	-	+++	++
Detect diffuse disease	+	+++	++++	-
Assess Suboptimal results	+	+++	+++	+++
Differentiate Clot vs dissection	±	++++	+++	-
Continuous record	-	-	-	+++
Microvascular disease	-	-	-	++++
Ease of use	++++	+	++	+++
Predict complications	-	±	±	+
Predict restenosis	±	±	±	±
Device induced ischemia	-	+++	++	-

CHARACTERIZATION OF LESION SEVERITY

Intracoronary Doppler Blood flow Velocity

The most practical and well studied application for the nonangiographic imaging modalities is evaluation of the intermediate or borderline lesion. In our opinion, intracoronary Doppler blood flow velocity is the gold standard for assessment of lesion significance. However, in circumstances where Doppler velocimetry, translesional velocity gradient (TVG), and coronary flow reserve (CFR) are unreliable (Table 3), IVUS can also be used for assessment of lesion significance.[12,13] Rarely, angioscopy can be used to assess lesions of intermediate severity, particularly when associated with objective signs of ischemia; however, unless there is a concern regarding thrombus, we do not use it for this indication.

In the majority of intermediate lesions, invasive physiologic assessment utilizing distal CFR is a reliable means of determining the significance of such lesions.[14-23] In our catheterization laboratory, intracoronary adenosine is the preferred maximal vasodilator to assess hyperemic flow, because of its short duration of action, ease of use, and safety. In addition, cumulative doses of adenosine have no effect on resting blood flow velocity or cross-sectional area, as long as vessels are pretreated with intracoronary nitroglycerin to achieve maximal endothelial-independent vasodilatation. Therefore, repeated measurements can be performed during a single procedure.

Invasive physiologic assessment is particularly useful in patients with "unstable" chest pain syndromes without electrocardiographic changes; multiple lesions in the same or two different vessels; and lesions of intermediate severity (40-70% diameter stenosis) which may only be significant during periods of increased myocardial oxygen demand, but scintigraphic assessment is misleading or has not been performed (Figure 2).

Normal translesional velocity gradient and/or normal CFR support normal coronary blood flow; thus, intervention has been shown to be safely deferred in such lesions. [24,25] We currently view a distal CFR ≥ 2.0 utilizing the Flowire (Cardiometrics, Mountain View, CA) as normal, based on the scintigraphic support for this demarcation; [21-23] however, outcome data has not been obtained to support

348

this threshold. A distal reserve < 2.0 may be the threshold where ischemia is produced leading to an increase in adverse events; however, studies are ongoing.

Occasionally, there will be discordance between the Doppler derived parameters of TVG and CFR in relation to lesion significance. In suitable patients, without microvascular disease, there is preliminary support for CFR being a more reliable indicator of lesion significance; [26] however, an in-depth understanding of the limitations of the technique is paramount in interpreting conflicting data. (Table 3) Lastly, in intermediate lesion assessment, if microvascular abnormalities are suspected, CFR should be assessed in a reference vessel with minimal or no coronary lesions. Conditions leading to subclinical impairment of the microcirculation have little regional variability. A normal CFR in the reference vessel strengthens the reliability of the CFR assessed in the target vessel distribution.

Angio   # Doppler

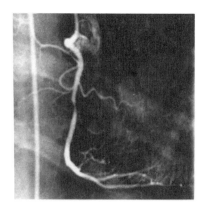
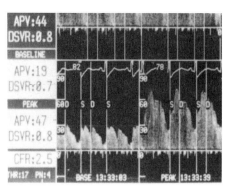

Figure 2. The angiographic and distal coronary blood flow velocity (resting and hyperemic) of a patient admitted to our institution with "unstable angina." Cardiac catheterization was performed which revealed single vessel disease with an intermediate (56% diameter stenosis) mid-RCA lesion found to be tightest in the RAO projection shown. Distal flow velocity assessment after intracoronary administration of 10 mcg Adenosine revealed a normal CFR of 2.5; therefore, intervention was deferred. The patient's symptoms returned 1 month later; however, a maximal stress cardiolyte scan was interpreted as normal, corroborating the physiologic interpretation of the Doppler assessment.

TABLE 3   Limitations in Interpretation of Intracoronary Doppler Velocity Assessment

Problem/Situation	Potential Effect
Doppler Wire Technical Considerations	
1. Inappropriate on-line IPV tracking	APV and DSVR may be falsely low; CFR and TVG calculated from APV may be erroneous
2. Inappropriate ECG gating from QRS	False diastolic and systolic time intervals; Erroneous DSVR
3. Unstable phasic Doppler signal	APV may be falsely low
4. Doppler probe not positioned to assess peak flow velocity	APV may be falsely low
Translesional Velocity Gradient (TVG, PDR)	
1. Ostial lesions	No proximal value to assess lesion
2. Single unbranched conduits	Continuity equation applies, TVG may be falsely low
3. Tortuous vessels	No distal value, unable to obtain reliable distal peak velocity
4. Diffuse distal disease	Falsely low TVG secondary to falsely elevated distal velocity
5. Tandem/sequential lesions	Falsely low TVG secondary to falsely elevated distal velocity because of distal lesional flow acceleration
6. Eccentric lesions	Falsely high TVG secondary to falsely elevated proximal velocity from acceleration at site of lesional flow convergence.
Coronary Flow Reserve (CFR)	
1. Abnormal microcirculation in downstream myocardium in patient with hypertrophy, diabetes, connective tissue disease, prior myocardial infarction, Syndrome X	May falsely lower CFR
2. Sequential lesions	Distal CFR is the result of the combined physiologic effect of all lesions in a single vessel at the time of assessment
3. Changes in vasomotor tone	May falsely lower CFR
4. Submaximal dose of vasodilator used	May falsely lower CFR
5. Transient increased in distal flow at time of assessment	May falsely lower CFR
6. Varying position of Doppler wire between baseline and hyperemic assessment	May falsely lower CFR
7. Varying hemodynamic conditions	May falsely lower CFR

Intravascular Ultrasound

Lesions may be angiographically indeterminate because of intermediate lesion stenosis or vessel tortuosity creating overlapping segments which cannot be definitively viewed. For the latter, IVUS provides precise quantitation of stenoses independent of the radiographic projection (Figure 3).[27] Ostial, bifurcation, and left main coronary lesions are particularly well suited for IVUS evaluation. Additionally, IVUS is useful for eccentric lesions, especially if the lesion appears angiographically severe in one projection but mild in a different projection. In these cases, as well as in patients with microvascular disease and other substrates for unreliable blood flow velocity assessment (Table 3), IVUS appears to be the modality of choice for quantitating luminal area and shape and thus lesion significance. As with Doppler assessment, preliminary data indicates that IVUS criteria can be used to defer intervention with a low frequency of target lesion revascularization at 1 year follow-up. [28] Larger, prospective studies will be required before this becomes an accepted application.

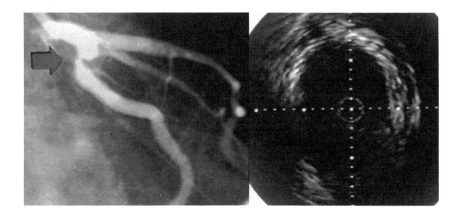

Figure 3. Ostial left circumflex artery lesion (left panel) appears angiographically significant despite IC nitroglycerin.. IVUS (right panel) reveals no lesion at the left main/left circumflex border where the angiogram is misleading due to overlapping vessel tortuosity. The distal coronary flow reserve by Doppler was normal.

The use of IVUS for quantitating luminal stenosis has improved assessment in the proximal coronary circulation.[29] The lack of physiologic data, however, necessitates an extrapolation of lesion significance from area stenosis. As discussed previously, velocity assessment, if possible, is superior for borderline lesion assessment, except in the case of left main coronary artery (LMCA) disease (Figure 4). The degree of LMCA stenosis is often the key deciding point on a referral for bypass surgery; yet, the prospective data supporting clinical decision making is based on angiographic diameter stenosis from the CASS database.[30] It is not uncommon for surgeons and cardiologists to disagree on the angiographic severity of LMCA stensoses, particularly if they are ostial in location. The prognostic importance of IVUS detected LMCA disease is unknown; but preliminary data suggest that IVUS may predict cardiovascular prognosis in patients with angiographically silent LMCA disease.[31] While awaiting larger more definitive studies, angiographically indeterminate LMCA lesions can be safely imaged with IVUS; [32] whereas, tight lesions should not be imaged.

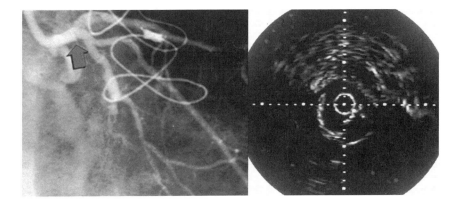

Figure 4. Angiogram reveals a discrete "slit" in the distal left main coronary artery of unclear significance (arrow in left panel). A stress thallium revealed anterior and lateral ischemia, yet the LAD and LCx vessels had no significant disease. IVUS (right panel) demonstrates a severe calcified plaque with acoustic shadowing of 200 degrees in the distal left main significantly decreasing luminal size.

Despite improvements in ultrasound equipment, IVUS devices remain ≥ 2.9 French (approximately 1 mm); therefore, assessment of borderline lesions in small, tortuous, or angulated vessels, and in eccentric lesions may be challenging. In our experience, the IVUS devices available today are reasonably flexible and successfully positioned in > 90% of the lesions assessed. Nevertheless, lesion inaccessibility remains a limitation of IVUS more commonly than Doppler flow assessment.

CHARACTERIZATION OF LESION MORPHOLOGY

Angioscopy

An equally important application of nonangiographic imaging has been the use of angioscopy and IVUS in the characterization of lesion morphology. Several studies confirm the superiority of angioscopy to contrast angiography (and probably intravascular ultrasound) in detecting and differentiating plaque, dissection, and thrombus. [33-35] Intracoronary thrombus is characterized by its red color against the white or yellow background of atherosclerotic plaque. Clearly, in saphenous vein bypass grafts, angioscopy is superior to angiography in detecting intraluminal thrombus and friable plaque. [36,37] We currently find angioscopy to be most useful in characterizing unstable lesions for the detection of thrombus (Figure 5) and other important intraluminal details, [38,39] and to guide therapy prior to and during percutaneous revascularization (Table 4).

The "culprit" lesions associated with unstable and post-infarct angina in saphenous vein grafts are frequently associated with thrombus. One study revealed that the incidence of thrombus in de novo unstable lesions ranged from 43-80%. [40] Other recent studies suggested that angioscopic identification of yellow, lipid rich plaque is typically associated with thrombus, whereas white, lipid poor plaque is infrequently associated with this entity. [41,42] In addition, diabetics with unstable angina may have a higher incidence of plaque ulceration and intracoronary thrombus than nondiabetics, which may partially explain the higher incidence of unstable ischemic syndromes in diabetics. [43] It is for these reasons that de novo lesions with a "hazy" appearance or an intraluminal defect on angiography are suspicious for thrombus and prompt us to perform angioscopy.   In several of these patients, angioscopy revealed white, or platelet rich, thrombus which has been recently described in the literature. [41] The presence of white or red thrombus may affect the risk of post intervention abrupt closure; the ideal treatment of this phenomenon is currently unknown, but may include IIb/IIIa inhibitors or extraction atherectomy (TEC). Angioscopy has recently been shown to be an effective clinical tool to detect subtle morphologic features which predict adverse outcomes after angioplasty [44]

Table 4. Clinical and Interventional Applications of the Nonangiographic Imaging Modalities

	Doppler Blood Flow Velocity Assessment	Intravascular Ultrasound	Angioscopy
CLINICAL	Intermediate lesions Syndrome X Transplant arteriopathy Bypass graft disease Functional recovery after MI *	Angiographically unrecognized disease Intermediate lesions Transplant vasculopathy	Intermediate lesions *
INTERVENTIONAL	Assess suboptimal results Predict complications 'trending' Assess no-reflow Monitor UK infusions * Dynamic turbulence *	Quantitative measurements Dissection assessment Guidance of directional atherectomy Coronary stent deployment Lesion calcification to guide rotational atherectomy	Characterize unstable lesions Saphenous vein bypass graft interventions Evaluate suboptimal results Post-interventional assessment of adequate results but unexplained defects ? Predict outcome of intervention

* postulated applications without strong evidence

354

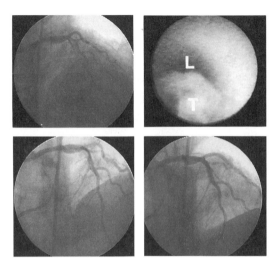

Figure 5. Angiography in a 33 year old female with an acute anterior wall myocardial infarction reveals a subtotal LAD occlusion with a filling defect (panel A). Angioscopy demonstrated a large thrombus (panel B) which was successfully removed by extraction atherectomy (panel C). Stent implantation was successfully performed (panel D) due to a residual dissection.

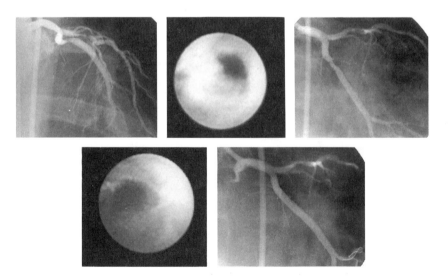

Figure 6. A 62 year old male presented with unstable angina and coronary angiography revealed a severe, hazy proximal lesion in the LCx (panel A). Angioscopy revealed a white thrombus at the lesion site (panel B). After extraction atherectomy, the stenosis improved (panel C) and angioscopy demonstrated complete thrombus removal (panel D). Stent implantation was performed with no residual stenosis and TIMI 3 flow (panel E).

Angioscopy is performed more frequently in saphenous vein grafts than in de novo lesions in our laboratory because of the high incidence of plaque friability and thrombus that has been detected in these conduits. Although there are no large scale clinical trials demonstrating a clear benefit of angioscopy in vein graft lesions, there is mounting evidence that angioscopy may improve outcome by guiding therapeutic strategies. We evaluated 27 lesions with a high clinical or angiographic suspicion for thrombus, including vein grafts (20 lesions) and native coronaries (7 lesions). We found that 17 of 27 lesions (63%) had thrombus by angioscopy. Extraction atherectomy, followed by repeat angioscopy, to document thrombus removal, was performed followed by stenting after the elimination of thrombus (Figure 7). In the absence of angioscopic thrombus, stents were implanted without extraction atherectomy (Figure 8). 93% of patients had a final residual stenosis < 10% without a major complication. Transient no-reflow, defined as no-reflow followed by recovery of TIMI 3 flow after intracoronary Verapamil occurred in 9 lesions (34%). Procedural failure occurred in 2 lesions (7%) due to sustained no-reflow despite intracoronary Verapamil. Following extraction atherectomy, all 17 lesions had angioscopic evidence of partial or complete thrombus removal. In addition, all 10 lesions without angioscopic thrombus underwent successful stent implantation without complications. No patients had Q-wave myocardial infarction, bypass surgery, stent thrombosis, or died in hospital. We concluded that stenting lesions with thrombus is feasible if thrombus removal can be achieved by extraction atherectomy. However, although angioscopy and extraction atherectomy may be useful adjuncts to stenting high risk lesions, the risk of no-reflow is not eliminated.

Therefore, our recommendations are: if thrombus is identified by angioscopy we utilize (TEC) atherectomy, usually without thrombolytic therapy. If repeat angioscopy confirms thrombus removal, then endoluminal stenting is typically employed; in contrast, stents are deployed without TEC if thrombus is not identified by angioscopy. [45] Stent deployment in the presence of thrombus is associated with an increased risk of subacute thrombosis and, therefore, is the driving force for prior evaluation. [46]

356

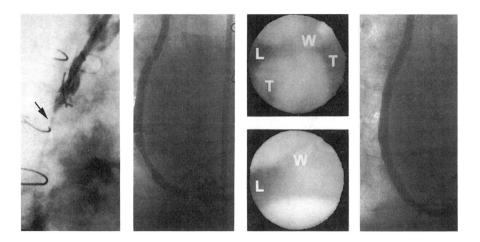

Figure 7. A total occlusion of a saphenous vein graft to the RCA was treated with intracoronary urokinase (panel A). After urokinase, two discrete 90% lesions are noted in the graft (panel B). Angioscopy demonstrated significant residual thrombus (panel C); therefore, extraction atherectomy was performed. After TEC, thrombus was completely removed (panel D) and stents were successfully deployed (panel E).

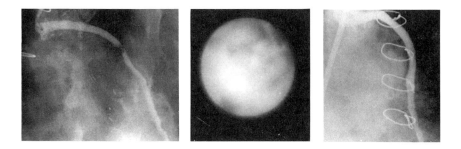

Figure 8. Angiogram of a vein graft to the LCx reveals a filling defect in the mid portion of the graft (left panel). Angioscopy demonstrates white plaque without any thrombus (middle panel); therefore, stent implantation was performed (right panel).

Recently we have reported that the identification of loose friable material in vein grafts identifies a high risk population for transient or sustained no-reflow. [47-48] Forty nine consecutive patients underwent prospective angioscopic evaluation prior to interventions on degenerated saphenous vein bypass grafts. Angioscopic plaque friability defined as loosely adherent and fragmented material protruding into the vascular lumen was visualized in 69% of lesions. Procedural complications included no reflow (47%) and distal embolization (16%). The presence of thrombus by angioscopy did not correlate with the occurrence of procedural complications; however, plaque friability was highly associated with no reflow and distal embolization. (Figure 9). Therefore, the presence of angioscopic plaque friability prior to percutaneous intervention is a potent predictor of procedural complications. These results may allow interventionalists to adjust procedural technique or device selection in vein graft interventions based on the baseline angioscopic findings. We recommend the use of extraction atherectomy to potentially remove friable debris before PTCA or stent implantation. Unfortunately, thrombolytics would be ineffective for friable debris removal despite their effect on thrombus. In the future, identification of plaque friability by angioscopy, will allow interventionalists to choose other devices such as the Angiojet (Possis, Boston, MA) or Hydrolyzer (Cordis, Miami, FL) which may be effective for removal of this debris.

The limitations of angioscopic evaluation in assessing lesion morphology include: difficulty in assessing aorto-ostial lesions because of difficulty ensuring a blood free imaging field, and the occasionally limited field of view due to the inability to steer currently available catheters. New flexible catheters with advanced fiberoptics will permit direct visualization of the luminal surface of virtually all native coronary arteries and bypass grafts. In addition, evaluation of the proximal left anterior descending or circumflex lesions are not advised because of the need for transient occlusion of the left main coronary artery. Additionally, in lesions with significant friability or thrombus, angioscopy can cause the no-reflow phenomenon. In our experience, transient but reversible no-reflow occurs after angioscopy in 30-40% of cases. As is usually the case, the risks and benefits of an adjunctive imaging device need to be weighed on a case by case basis.

358

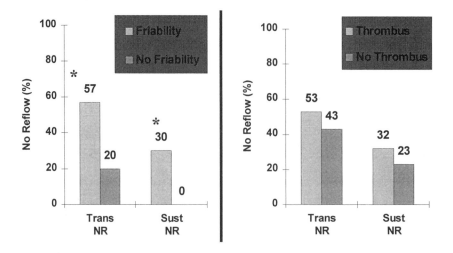

Figure 9. Vein graft friability was a significant predictor of procedural complications including no-reflow and distal embolization. Thrombus visualized by angioscopy; however, did not predict procedural complications.

Intravascular Ultrasound

Unlike angioscopy, IVUS generates a cross-sectional tomographic image which depicts both the lumen and the structure of the vessel wall. The utility of IVUS lies in its ability to differentiate the various plaque components in the vessel wall. The most important from the standpoint of performing a therapeutic intervention, and typically the easiest to identify, is calcium. IVUS, in our opinion, is useful in three realms prior to intervention: 1) Calcium presence and distribution; 2) Vessel sizing; and 3) Plaque composition and distribution.

Calcium

Several studies have reported that ultrasound is more sensitive than fluoroscopy in the detection and localization of calcification. [49-50] Calcium is identified by its bright reflectance and the acoustic shadowing which it creates. In previous studies, calcium has been detected by ultrasound at a rate of 60-70%

compared with flouroscopically identified calcium seen in 20-40%. With currently available atherectomy devices the depth and extent of calcification can dramatically affect the efficiency of plaque removal. The presence of superficial calcification, which may not be detectable by fluoroscopy, precludes successful tissue removal by DCA [51] and may also preclude adequate expansion of intracoronary stents. In addition, although fluoroscopic calcification has been considered a contraindication to directional atherectomy, IVUS studies suggest that lesions with deep calcification can undergo successful atherectomy. [52] Importantly, Rotablator atherectomy can effectively ablate superficial calcified portions of plaque (Figures 10,11); additionally, calcium removal and luminal enlargement is increased when large burrs are utilized (burr/artery ratio > 0.7) [53]

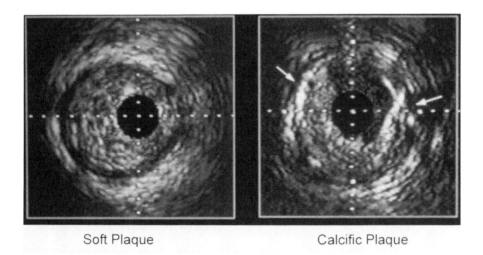

Soft Plaque   Calcific Plaque

Figure 10. The differentiation between soft plaque and calcific plaque by IVUS. The arrows indicate the increased echogenicity and shadowing seen with calcification.

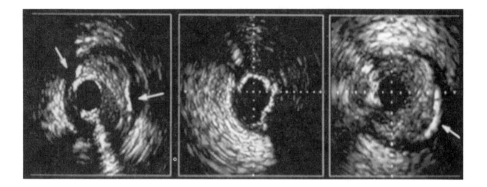

Figure 11. The differentiation of calcium location by IVUS: deep (left panel), superficial (middle panel), and mixed (right panel).

The potential advantages of a lesion specific interventional strategy are self-evident. Emerging data from the GUIDE study [54] (Guidance by Ultrasound Imaging for Decision Endpoints) revealed that preinterventional assessment with IVUS resulted in a change in strategy in over half the cases studied. This was predominately secondary to the finding of lesion calcification. If significant superficial calcification is not visualized angiographically, and attempts made to angioplasty the lesion fail secondary to incomplete balloon expansion despite high pressures, the opportunity to perform rotational atherectomy during that intervention can be lost; secondary to the fear of dissection propagation with the atherectomy device. If IVUS is performed prior to intervening, lesion calcification can be treated properly before attempting PTCA or stent implantation. It remains to be seen if these changes in strategy will lead to improvements in outcome.

Vessel Sizing

Intraluminal dimensions, including diameter and area stenosis, and wall thickness measurements by IVUS have correlated highly with both histologic and quantitative angiographic methods. [55-59] However, correlations were found to be weaker when eccentric atherosclerotic lesions were evaluated, particularly when IVUS is compared to quantitative angiography. [60-61] Clearly, before intervention, IVUS is a more reliable indicator of intraluminal shape and area than angiography. Vessel sizing is an important application of IVUS, especially when assessing the normal reference segment and the maximal device size which can be used.

In the era of intracoronary stenting, IVUS has proven to be useful in guiding the stent and post-dilatation balloon size. Incomplete apposition of the stent may correlate with a worse long-term outcome (Figure 12), while incomplete expansion amy be a factor leading to restenosis [62] Furthermore, IVUS has demonstrated that angiographically normal reference segments frequently have occult atherosclerosis and/or unexpected ectasia resulting in a systematic undersizing of the stents deployed. [63-64] In and of itself, however, reference segment disease has not been shown to be an independent predictor of clinical events, [64] but quantitation of atherosclerotic plaque burden may aid in prediction of restenosis. [65] To date, prospective data have not documented a clear advantage for device sizing by IVUS; the AVID trial is currently prospectively assessing angiographic vs. IVUS- directed stent placement [66].

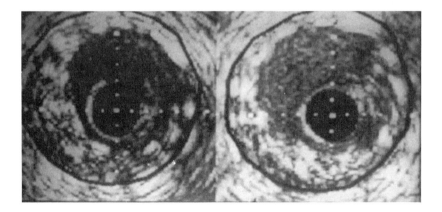

Figure 12. Incomplete stent apposition to the vessel wall with a gap between the stent struts and the vessel wall on the left lateral aspect of this image (left), treated with a larger high pressure balloon resulting in a fully deployed stent by IVUS (right).

Despite its reliable measurements, IVUS is vulnerable to geometric distortion particularly when the ultrasound beam is not orthogonal to the vessel wall. Fortunately, in the small coronary arteries this is rare because of the limited degree of obliquity, minimizing the image distortion; however, this limitation is most pronounced in vessels which are highly eccentric and post-intervention. In addition, the degree of calcification, both superficial and deep, and how it impacts on stent sizing, currently remains unknown. We feel that if the stent struts clearly appose the calcified wall despite submaximal expansion, adverse outcomes will be minimized. However, there is no currently available data to address this issue.

Plaque Composition and Distribution

Intravascular ultrasound allows detailed high quality cross-sectional imaging of the coronary artery wall, the major components of the atherosclerotic plaque, and the changes that occur in coronary artery anatomy during the atherosclerotic disease process. [67-68] Clearly, IVUS has an increased sensitivity for detecting minimal atherosclerosis, making it ideal for quantitating atherosclerosis in trials of regression with lipid-lowering therapy. However, this is not practical and does not translate into clinical utility. Along these lines, a promising application of IVUS is that of plaque-risk stratification. Histologic correlates of lesions at high risk for rupture are those which are highly lipid-laden plaque with a thin fibrous cap, [69] referred to as "soft plaque." The propensity of plaques to become unstable and undergo fissuring and thrombosis is directly related to the amount of extra-cellular lipid. [70-71] IVUS has the potential to characterize the plaque contents and stratify atherosclerotic lesions into those at high risk. [72] Echolucent "soft" plaques have a high lipid content, are less echogenic than surrounding adventitia, and have been shown to occur more frequently in unstable angina than "fibrous" plaques.

Although the lipid-rich reference segment plaque may be the precursor of the clinically unstable lesion, it remains to be seen if ultrasound tissue characterization can translate into an effect on outcome. The current gray scale image analysis is sometimes inadequate for accurate tissue characterization. Future developments in signal analysis may lead to more reliable methods of separating atherosclerotic plaque into its component elements. Lastly, it is important to realize that although ultrasound reveals detailed views of the vessel wall, image reconstruction is based upon acoustic reflections and not actual histology. For instance, IVUS may be unreliable in distinguishing plaque from media, particularly in diseased arteries.

POST INTERVENTION ASSESSMENT

Intravascular ultrasound, coronary blood flow velocity assessment, and angioscopy may all be used to assess the results of percutaneous intervention. A broad spectrum of therapeutic decisions hinge upon assessment of coronary lumen dimensions and characteristics for which we have historically relied on coronary angiography. Angiography, however, has been quite limited in several realms (Table 1) which will be delineated in the following sections.

Intravascular Ultrasound

Intravascular ultrasound has proven useful in determining the mechanism of successful balloon angioplasty. [73-77] Ultrasound studies have shown that the primary mechanism of balloon angioplasty is plaque rupture or dissection, although stretching of the vessel wall and plaque compression remain other potential mechanisms. Although angiography frequently can detect intimal dissections, it is inadequate at providing an accurate assessment of the severity and extent of dissection. [80-81] Pathologic studies after balloon angioplasty have shown a poor correlation with the angiogram, with the high degree of intimal disruption and residual plaque often going undetected angiographically. IVUS is accurate in measuring luminal area after balloon angioplasty and providing accurate measurements of angioplasty-induced dissection. Limited intimal disruption may be necessary to reduce elastic recoil and restenosis after balloon angioplasty, however, we do not routinely use IVUS to ensure such "cracks" are present; nevertheless, further studies may prove this is necessary.

Mechanistic considerations aside, IVUS can be clinically applied to catheter-based treatment strategies. IVUS can determine the depth and extent of dissection, guide the use of directional atherectomy, assess vessel calcification to guide rotational atherectomy, and aid in coronary stent deployment. There is emerging data that IVUS imaging after angioplasty can identify morphologic patterns at high risk for abrupt closure; extensive dissections that encompass an arch of more than 180° or are > 1 cm in length may be inherently unstable. [82] In addition, the more accurate measure of lumen dimensions following angioplasty by ultrasound may reveal that lumen cross-sectional area or residual plaque burden are important predictors of long term outcome. Specifically, a greater acute gain after angioplasty may result in less restenosis; although further studies are necessary to confirm prior preliminary reports using quantitative angiography [83]. Again, post-angioplasty assessment with ultrasound has been shown to provide surprising and unknown information in a high percentage of cases, as shown by the GUIDE study. [54] However, prospective outcome data utilizing this information is still not available.

DCA

Clinical experience with directional atherectomy has shown excellent initial angiographic results, however, this technique continues to be plagued with higher than expected rates of restenosis. Restenosis may be the result of either inadequate removal of atheroma or deep medial and adventitial trauma induced by aggressive cutting. [84] IVUS supports that the major mechanism of luminal improvement after DCA is plaque removal. [85] A larger lumen after atherectomy could result in lower restenosis rates based on the acute gain hypothesis; and aggressive plaque removal may be more safely accomplished with ultrasound guidance. Although this technique is feasible, it is challenging and still unproven. Technically, careful positioning of the intravascular ultrasound image relative to the fluoroscopic view to determine accurate localization of plaque is tedious. Sequential ultrasound examinations between DCA passes to determine the extent of plaque removal and assess the need for additional cuts then need to be performed. We believe that the development of the combined atherectomy/ultrasound devices to directly visualize the residual atheroma will bring this technique to the forefront. When more aggressive and targeted plaque removal can be reliably performed and assessed it will then be necessary to determine the impact of this strategy on long term recurrence rates before it becomes an accepted technique.

MRA

In contrast, the presence of superficial calcification which may not be detected by fluoroscopy precludes successful tissue removal by DCA. [85-86] Effective cutting is inhibited by the rim-like distribution of calcium at the luminal border significantly reducing yields of tissue. Because of these reduced yields, fluoroscopic calcification has been considered a contraindication to directional atherectomy; however, preliminary data suggests that lesions with deep calcification can undergo successful directional atherectomy. [87] With the advent of rotational atherectomy (Rotablator), lesions with superficial calcification or dense fibrotic plaque can be effectively treated. [88] We currently utilize Rotablator atherectomy for lesions which are fluoroscopically calcific, reserving IVUS for lesions which fail to yield to angioplasty or are aorto-ostial or bifurcation in location. In these latter circumstances, IVUS may provide important information about calcium location, prompting use of directional atherectomy or stents in cases where the calcification is deep. Anecdotally, ultrasound has been useful in conjunction with Rotablator atherectomy to guide upsizing to a larger burr and in performing definitive adjunction balloon angioplasty to improve acute gain. [89] Calcified vessels typically are unreliably sized by angiography. Since burr and balloon sizing has been shown to potentially impact on post MRA restenosis rates, more exact decisions regarding burr and balloon sizes may be critical to long term success and can be achieved with IVUS. There are ongoing ultrasound studies to assess the efficacy of post-ablation angioplasty to achieve better lumen enlargement and determine its ultimate effect on outcome. [90] However, we do not yet understand enough about the long term implications of these findings, particularly regarding calcium localization, to rationally influence the decision to utilize specific devices.

Stents

Intracoronary ultrasound imaging has proved to be useful in conjunction with coronary stent deployment. In addition to accurate vessel sizing, the extent of the lesion or dissection can be assessed to assist with stent placement and ensure complete coverage of the dissection flap. Ultrasound in our laboratory is currently utilized for this indication, as well as to assess for complete stent expansion and wall contact in complex cases (Figure 12). Emerging data suggests that "incomplete apposition" results in a higher rate of early stent thrombosis; [91] however, incomplete or irregular stent expansion in areas of calcification are not well understood. Intuitively, it seems that optimizing stent expansion will ultimately lead to decreased acute clinical events. IVUS studies have demonstrated a high rate of incomplete apposition despite "successful" deployment by angiography. This has prompted the routine use of high pressure balloon post-dilatation after stent deployment. It remains to be seen if IVUS will be useful or necessary after stenting when high pressure balloon inflations are utilized. Although optimization of stent deployment with IVUS would appear to be ideal, the need to use higher pressures or larger balloons to fully deploy all stent struts, can also lead to other complications such as dissections proximal or distal to the stent. Lastly, neointimal proliferation that is responsible for the restenosis phenomenon in stents can be delineated with IVUS and differentiated from thrombus formation. Anecdotally, we have utilized excimer laser in this circumstance to eradicate the neointimal proliferation and hopefully impact recurrent restenosis.

Intracoronary Doppler Velocity Assessment

Coronary blood flow velocity may be used to assess the results of percutaneous intervention. Normalization of average peak velocity (APV) and the diastolic to systolic velocity ratio (DSVR), restoring a diastolic predominance to coronary flow has been reported after successful PTCA, [92] directional atherectomy, [93] excimer laser atherectomy, [93] Rotablator atherectomy, [94] and stent implantation. [95-97] In contrast, normalization of coronary flow reserve (CFR) after successful PTCA is inconsistent. We hypothesized that the etiology of this inconsistent normalization of CFR may be due to angiographically inapparent disturbances in flow that remain after angioplasty. To test this hypothesis we studied 17 patients who underwent successful angioplasty by performing intracoronary Doppler flow velocity assessment at baseline, after angioplasty, and then ultimately after successful de novo stent implantation. Utilizing a CFR ≥ 2.0 as a normal range, all 17 patients had normalization of CFR after successful stent implantation. (Figure 13) This same observation has been supported by other recent studies all suggesting that successful implantation of Palmaz-Schatz stents immediately after angiographically successful, but physiologically inadequate, PTCA may normalize CFR. [97-99]

These data support that an abnormal CFR after intervention, specifically balloon angioplasty or stenting, is due to epicardial factors and not transient microvascular dysfunction. IVUS observations reveal that a high volume of residual atheroma persists after PTCA, [100] giving further support to Doppler-derived findings after this intervention. Preliminary data reveal that elimination of the residual lumen narrowing after angioplasty, characterized by IVUS, correlates with improvement and ultimate normalization of CFR by Doppler assessment. [97] Thus, PTCA may be associated with angiographically inapparent flow disturbances despite what appears to be successful lumen enlargement by angiographic criteria. Stents clearly improve lesion geometry and laminar flow, probably by eliminating residual lumen narrowing and tacking up dissections. In contrast, rotablator atherectomy induces significant increases in basal flow velocity, unlike stenting, and therefore abnormal post-procedure CFR may be secondary to microparticulate debris causing "acquired microvascular dysfunction." [101] (Figure 14)

"Suboptimal" results after intervention characterized by intraluminal haziness, moderate residual stenosis, or nonflow limiting dissection may be ideal indications for Doppler flow assessment. Preliminary data from the DEBATE study group suggests that distal flow velocity measurements after PTCA can predict recurrent ischemia and restenosis. [102] There are ongoing studies evaluating whether Doppler evaluation after intervention will impact on PTCA outcome and/or guide further intervention, i.e. stenting.

In our laboratory, patients at risk for "no-reflow" are monitored during intervention to assess the utility of intracoronary Verapamil for restoring flow, since Doppler flow velocity is a sensitive means of monitoring flow. Furthermore, patients with acute myocardial infarction who are undergoing primary PTCA are a group who may benefit from Doppler assessment after intervention to distinguish inapparent residual stenosis from microvascular dysfunction. [103] Additionally, doppler assessment immediately after primary PTCA may provide useful information regarding myocardial viability; however, the preliminary nature of the evidence precludes routine Doppler studies in these groups.

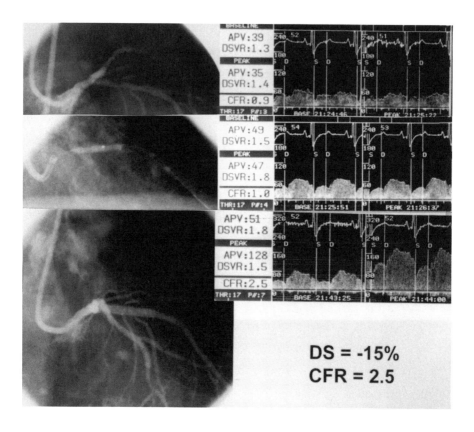

Figure 13. Sequential angiograms with the accompanying Doppler derived flow reserves before and after balloon angioplasty and stent implantation. Despite an adequate angiographic result after PTCA, the CFR remained severely impaired . After stent implanatation there was normalization of CFR to > 2.0 in this case as in all 17 patients assessed after stenting.

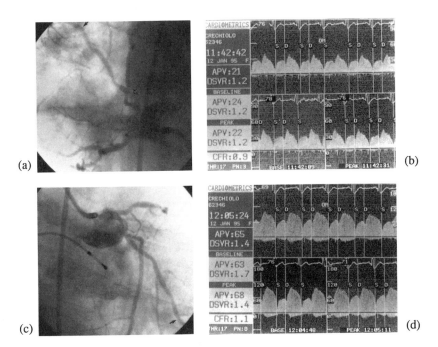

(a)   (b)

(c)   (d)

Figure 14. Baseline angiogram (panel A) with a proximal LCx lesion (open arrow) and the corresponding distal basal and hyperemic blood flow velocity (APV) (panel B) revealing an abnormal coronary flow reserve (CFR=0.9). After Rotablator atherectomy and adjunctive balloon angioplasty, the luminal stenosis decreased to 15% (panel C); however the CFR remained abnormally low (1.1) due to a parallel increase in basal and hyperemic APV (panel D). In 19 of 22 patients studied, similar increases in basal flow of approximately 150% above preintervention levels were observed after Rotablator therapy.

Intracoronary Doppler assessment provides the unique opportunity to record continuous blood flow velocity over time. Post-intervention "trending," as it is called, is used following coronary intervention to identify angiographically inapparent flow disturbances due to dissection, vasospasm, platelet aggregation, or changes in vasomotor tone. [104-106] Cyclic flow variations, which are evident by dramatic swings in coronary blood flow velocity presumably due to accumulation and dislodgement of platelet aggregates and microthrombi, have been associated with abrupt closure following PTCA. [107] Whether Doppler assessment is instantaneous or continuous, it provides physiologic data which is not available by any other method at the time of coronary intervention. Further work is necessary; however, we are hopeful that post-intervention "trending" will identify patients with unstable flow patterns who may benefit from stents or new anti-platelet agents. [108] The duration of continuous flow velocity monitoring after intervention that is necessary to exclude an acute adverse event currently remains unknown.

Angioscopy

Evaluation of the hazy or suboptimal result after percutaneous intervention may be the most valuable role for percutaneous coronary angioscopy. [109] Angioscopy can reliably differentiate thrombus, dissection, and plaque. [109-110] It is providing an ever expanding role in clinical practice because it provides a full-color 3-dimensional perspective of the coronary surface morphology. The ability to discriminate among colors in angioscopy makes it relatively easy to distinguish between thrombus and plaque, even if the clot burden is very small. The high resolution of angioscopic images can disclose minute luminal changes that are useful in monitoring post-intervention results. [44] These distinctions are clinically important because their treatment and outcome are different: if thrombus is identified, treatment strategies might include systemic or intracoronary thrombolytic therapy; local delivery of heparin, urokinase, or glycoprotein receptor inhibitors; or TEC atherectomy. In contrast, stenting would be highly effective for treating obstructive dissection flaps, circumstances in which thrombolytic drugs would have no role and would subject the patient to unnecessary risks. In our opinion, angioscopy is the gold standard for evaluation of thrombus presence and removal.

The angioscope may have clinical utility in stratifying the risk of complications after angioplasty in vessels that have a hazy appearance by angiography. Preliminary data revealed that angioscopic findings (but not IVUS findings) were important predictors of outcome one year after percutaneous intervention of native vessels and vein grafts treated with a variety of devices. [44,111] In addition, angioscopic thrombus may also be associated with a higher incidence of restenosis after percutaneous intervention. [112] Furthermore, restenosis may be impacted by angioscopy where intimal splits are not observed, and thus, further intervention with atherectomy or stent implantation may be indicated. Lastly as mentioned previously, in saphenous vein grafts, plaque friability by angioscopy prior to intervention is a predictor of procedural complications. Angioscopy can also be used to monitor these interventions and ensure complete friability and thrombus removal after extraction atherectomy (TEC). Studies have demonstrated that staging degenerated vein graft interventions with initial extraction atherectomy followed by one month of anticoagulation prior to PTCA/stenting may decrease untoward events. The appearance of residual friability after TEC by angioscopy may be an indication to stage the procedure and proceed with PTCA/stent at a later date.

Angioscopic evaluation after stent placement may be valuable for determining the adequacy of circumferential stent expansion, [113] although IVUS seems more practical for this application. IVUS, however, is very insensitive for thrombus detection and, therefore, angioscopy would be the nonangiographic imaging modality of choice to identify the nature of residual defects inside stents. White et al [114] have shown that the angioscope can reliably differentiate thrombotic occlusion from intimal dissection in patients with abrupt closure following angioplasty. The future of coronary angioscopy as an everyday tool relies upon the impact of the information provided on improving clinical outcomes. Specifically, if plaque color, lesion ulceration, thrombus and friability are predictive of procedural success or complications, then angioscopy will become an accepted imaging modality which warrants the additional cost and time necessary to perform the procedure.

COMPLICATIONS AND PROCEDURE SAFETY

Doppler Guidewire

In general, each of the non-angiographic imaging modalities can be performed safely as an adjunct to other percutaneous interventions or as a stand alone procedure. Although complications are unusual they appear to be based upon operator experience and procedural complexity. The hierarchy of complexity of the nonangiographic imaging devices is Doppler guidewire, IVUS, followed by angioscopy which is the most demanding. Doppler guidewire instrumentation of severe lesions is rarely associated with lesion injury, specifically, coronary dissection or vessel closure. [114] In our experience, no complication has resulted as a direct result of Doppler guidewire insertion; however, if the guidewire does not advance into the distal vessel easily, a transport device is placed into the distal vessel over a softer, finer guidewire, and an exchange for the Doppler guidewire is made.

Intravascular Ultrasound

Intravascular ultrasound is performed with a $\geq$ 2.9 French device and, therefore, the risk of causing transient ischemia when imaging severe stenoses or small vessels is higher than with that of the Doppler guidewire; ECG changes occurred in as many as 3.5% of patients. [115] It appears that the small risk of untoward effects comes in the form of transient coronary spasm which occurs in up to 5% of patients, but responds rapidly to intracoronary nitroglycerin In our experience, coronary thrombosis occurred in 1 patient during catheter manipulation across an unstable lesion. The ultrasound device was exchanged out for an angioplasty balloon and vessel patency was restored. The patient ultimately did well, however, despite the relative safety of coronary ultrasound, any intracoronary instrumentation carries the risk of vessel injury and the necessary personnel and equipment should be immediately available to treat any untoward complications. We feel that the adverse effects are very limited with this device and it can be safely performed in all patients.

Angioscopy

Coronary angioscopy can also be safely performed, however, this too is a $\geq$ 3.0 device in size. Like ultrasound, it requires distal wire position and transient ischemia may occur when the imaging device is placed beyond severe stenoses. In a large multicenter registry of 1,746 procedures, angiographic complications included dissection (due to the guidewire, balloon occlusion, or imaging bundle) in 2.8% and abrupt closure in 1.0%. [116] Rupture of the occlusion cuff leading to coronary artery perforation has been reported in 1 patient. [117] Improper technique can also lead to air emboli from the flush solution during angioscopic visualization. Although severe angiographic complications are unusual, 9% of lesions treated with PTCA may require a touch-up balloon inflation after angioscopy to improve lumen smoothness. [118] Angioscopy in degenerated vein grafts may be associated with transient or sustained no-reflow in nearly half the lesions, and in our experience identified a high risk subgroup for sustained no-reflow after further percutaneous intervention. [119] Although cuff inflation >60 seconds can lead to transient ischemia, and should not be performed, the incidence of major ischemic complications remains < 1%. [120] As with IVUS, lesion assessment should only be performed with the ability to restore vessel patency if one of the rare complications does occur.

UNUSUAL USES OF IMAGING DEVICES

Adjunctive imaging devices are also useful to guide new or unusual coronary interventions. In 1996, new devices or interventional procedures are available which require vessel imaging to avoid complications. We will describe three cases where use of Doppler, IVUS and angioscopy were imperative for the successful completion of unconventional procedures.

1. The use of venous allografts mounted on stents to treat coronary pseudoaneurysms has been recently reported in the literature (Figure 15). IVUS added critical information regarding vessel size and the adequacy of stent apposition to the vessel wall. The visualization of the allograft/vessel border by angioscopy and IVUS assured us of complete pseudoaneurysm coverage.

2. The issue of competitive flow in a bypass graft or a "steal" syndrome caused by anomalous vascular conduits and fistulas can be easily resolved with Doppler flow measurements. We recently used Doppler to demonstrate an increase in flow in the left internal mammary artery after coil embolization of a large unclipped LIMA to pulmonary artery fistula.

3. Traditionally, performance of rotational atherectomy within coronary stents has not been performed because of the risk of stent strut disruption with the Rotablator device. Nevertheless, since stent restenosis is largely secondary to neointimal proliferation, rotational atherectomy would

potentially be a useful device to treat this phenomenon. We recently performed angioscopy on a patient who developed in-stent restenosis 5 months after the primary procedure, demonstrating complete coverage of the stent struts with white plaque. Rotational atherectomy was safely performed yielding an excellent angiographic result.

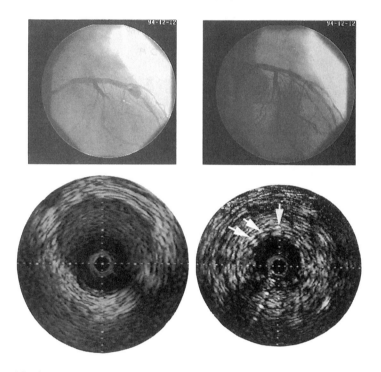

Figure 15. A coronary pseudoaneurysm three months after rotational atherectomy is treated with a stent-saphenous vein allograft. IVUS demonstrates the pseudoaneurysm before and after allograft placement.

FUTURE DIRECTIONS

A unified theme for each of the nonangiographic imaging devices propelling them into the future is going to be the ability of these modalities to predict and influence outcome. With future technical advances in device technology, leading to lower profile designs in both intravascular ultrasound and angioscopy, these modalities will become user friendly and permit large prospective, multicenter trials testing their ability to predict outcome. In addition, combination devices will improve our understanding of coronary artery pathophysiology and will likely improve our therapeutic capability. Current investigation with a combined imaging catheter providing on-line intravascular ultrasound with a tip-mounted Doppler flow probe will further improve our understanding of coronary vasomotion and the functional responses of the stenosis to current interventions. Directional atherectomy devices with ultrasound probes mounted on their tip are currently available and are being utilized to assess whether selective and aggressive plaque removal may be more safely accomplished, and reduce the risk of restenosis.

Three dimensional reconstruction of the coronary artery utilizing serial intravascular ultrasound images is also being developed, [121-122] and may add to our ability to impact on individual lesion assessment and therapy. Furthermore, added visualization in 3-dimensions with refinement in signal processing to allow more definitive tissue characterization, may ultimately give us control over the heterogeneous disease processes that involve the coronary artery. Lastly, nonangiographic imaging modalities will be paramount in cardiology when they can be performed non-invasively, and yet give reliable information regarding lesion characteristics which affect clinical decision making. Magnetic resonance imaging with radiotracer angiography, in our opinion, is the most promising and exciting modality presently emerging. However, the desire to achieve positive clinical endpoints and improve outcome must be the primary focus for the use and application of all new modalities.

CONCLUSION

The ability to visualize the internal anatomy of a coronary artery with IVUS and angioscopy, or translate visual assessments into physiology with Doppler flow, represent a significant advance in interventional cardiology. As we have mentioned throughout the chapter, the clinical applicability of these techniques are only now being discovered. Doppler will likely impact outcome of patients with intermediate lesions. IVUS will continue to be useful for preintervention assessment and treatment of dissections, while angioscopy will become an integral part of treating thrombotic lesions. Impacting clinical outcome is our prime motivation; however, should this not be the case, these devices will continue to have numerous research applications. Use of Doppler, IVUS and angioscopy, has led to an increased understanding of the atherosclerotic process and the effects of interventional devices on the coronary artery. This increased understanding of coronary anatomy and physiology may eventually lead to an ability to cure or inhibit progression of atherosclerotic heart disease.

References

1. White CW, Wright CB, Doty DB, Hiratza LF, Eastham CL, Harrison DG, Maras ML. Does visual interpretation of the coronary arteriogram predict the physiologic importance of a coronary stenosis? NEJM 1984;310:819-824.

2. Marcus ML, Skorton DJ, Johnson MR, Collins SM, Harrison DG, Kerber RE. Visual estimates of percent diameter coronary stenosis: "a battered gold standard." J Am Coll Cardiol 1988;11:882-885.

3. DeRouen TA, Murphy JA, Owen W. Variability in the analysis of coronary arteriograms. Circulation 1977;55:324-328.

4. Beauman GJ, Vogel RA. Accuracy of individual and panel interpretations of coronary arteriograms: Implications for clinical decisions. J Am Coll Cardiol 1990;16:108-113.

5. Gould KL, Kelley KO, Bolson EL. Experimental validation of quantitative coronary arteriography for determining pressure-flow characteristics of coronary stenosis. Circulation 1982;66:930-937.

6. Reiber JHC, Van der Zwet PMJ, Koning G, et al. Accuracy and precision of quantitative digital coronary arteriography: observer, short -, and medium-term variabilities. CCD 1993;28:187-19?.

7. Harrison DG, White CW, Hiratzka LF, Doty DB, Barnes DH, Eastham CL, Marcus ML. The value of lesion cross-sectional area determined by quantitative coronary angiography in assessing the physiologic significance of proximal LAD coronary arterial stenoses. Circulation 1984;69:1111-1119.

8. Donohue TJ, Kern MJ, Aguirre FV, Bach RG, Wolford T, Bell C, Segal J. Assessing the hemodynamic significance of coronary artery stenosis. Analysis of translesional pressure-flow velocity relations in patents. J Am Coll Cardiol 1993;22:449-458.

9. Tron C, Kern MJ, Donohue TJ, Bach RG, Aguirre FV, Caracciola EA, Moore JA. Comparison of quantitative angiographically derived and measured translesion pressure and flow velocity in coronary artery disease. Am J Cardiol 1995;75:111-1217.

10. Zijlstra F, Fioretti P, Reiber JHC, Serruys PW. Which cineangiographically assessed anatomic variable correlates best with functional measurements of stenosis severity? A comparison of quantitative analysis of the coronary cineangiogram with measured coronary flow reserve and exercise/redistribution thallium-201 scintigraphy. J Am Coll Cardiol 1988;12:686-691.

11. Topol EJ, Nissen SE. Our preoccupation with coronary luminology. The dissociation between clinical and angiographic findings in ischemic heart disease. Circulation 1995;92:2333-2342.

12. Doucette JW, Corl PD, Payne HM, Flynn AE, Goto M, Nassi M, Segal J. Validation of a doppler guidewire for intravascular measurement of coronary artery flow velocity. Circulation 1992;85:1899-1911.

13. McGinn AL, White CW, Wilson RF. Interstudy variability of coronary flow reserve. Influence of heart rate, arterial pressure and ventricular preload. Circulation 1990:81:1319-1330.

14. Gould KL, Lipscomb K, Hamilton GW. Physiologic basis for assessing critical coronary stenosis. Am J Cardiol 1974;33:87-94.

15. Gould KL, Lipscomb K, Hamilton GW. Compensatory changes of the distal coronary vascular bed during progressive coronary constriction. Circulation 1975;51:1085-1094.

16. Kirkeeide R, Gould KL, Parsel L. Assessment of coronary stenoses by myocardial imaging during coronary vasodilation. VII. Validation of coronary flow reserve as a single integrated measure to stenosis severity accounting for all its geometric dimensions. J Am Coll Cardiol 1986;7:103-113.

17. Gould KL, Kirkeeide R, Buchi M. Coronary flow reserve as a physiologic measure of stenosis severity. Part I. Relative and absolute coronary flow reserve during changing aortic pressure. Part II. Determination from arterographic stenosis dimensions under standardized conditions. J Am Coll Cardiol 1990;15:459-474.

18. Demer L, Gould KL, Kirkeeide RL. Assessing stenosis severity: Coronary flow reserve, collateral function, quantitative coronary arteriography, position imaging, and digital subtraction angiography: a review and analysis. Prog Cardiovasc Dis. 1988:30:307-322.

19. Wilson RF, Marcus ML, White CW. Prediction of the physiologic significance of coronary arterial lesions by quantitative lesion geometry in patients with limited coronary artery disease. Circulation 1987;75:723-732.

378

20.	Donohue TJ, Kern MJ, Aguirre FV, Bach RG, Wolford T, Bell C, Segal J. Assessing the hemodynamic significance of coronary artery stenosis. Analysis of translesional pressure-flow velocity relations in patients. J Am Coll Cardiol 1993;22:449-458.

21.	Kern MJ, Deligonul, Tatineni S, Serota H, Aguirre FV, Hilton TC. IV adenosine continuous infusion and low dose bolus administration for determination of coronary vascular reserve in patients with and without coronary artery disease. J Am Coll Cardiol 1991;18:718-729.

22.	Miller DD, Donohue TJ, Younis LT, Bach RG, Aguirre FV, Wity MD, Goodgold HM, Chaitman BR, Kern MJ. Correlation of pharmacologic technesium 99m-sestamibi myocardial perfusion imaging with post-stenotic coronary flow reserve in patients with angiographically intermediate coronary artery stenosis. Circulation 1994;89:2150-2160.

23.	Joye JD, Schulman DS, Lesorde D, Farah T, Donohue BC, Reichek N. Intracoronary doppler guide wire versus stress single-photon emission computer tomographic thallium 201 imaging in assessment of intermediate coronary stenoses. J Am Coll Cardiol 1994;24:940-947.

24.	Kern MJ, Donohue TJ, Aguirre FV, Bach RG, Caracole EA, Wolford T, Mechem CT, Flynn MS, Chaitman B. Clinical outcome of deferring angioplasty in patients with normal tranlesional pressure-flow velocity measurements. J Am Coll Cardiol 1995;25:178-187.

25.	Lesser JT, Wilson RF, White CW. Physiologic assessment of coronary stenosis of intermediate severity can facilitate patient selection for coronary angioplasty. Coronary Art Dis. 1990;1:697-705.

26.	Joye JD; Lasorda D; Farah T; Donahue BC; Schulman DS. CFR vs. translesional velocity gradient by Doppler guidewire in assessing intermediate coronary stenoses. J Am Coll Cardiol 1995;25:336A.

27.	White CJ, Ramee SR, Collin TJ, Jain A, Mesa JE. Ambiguous coronary angiography: clinical utility of intravascular ultrasound. Cathet Cardiovasc Diagn 26(3):200-203, 1992.

28.	Mintz GS, Bjoher TA, Kent KM, Pichard AD, Satler LF, Popma JJ, Morgan K, Leon MB. Clinical outcomes of patients not undergoing coronary artery revascularization as a result of intravascular ultrasound imaging. J Am Coll Cardiol 1995:25:61A.

29.	Nishimura RA, Higano ST, Holmes DR Jr. Use of intracoronary ultrasound imaging for assessing left main coronary artery disease. Mayo Clin Proc 1993;68:134-140.

30.	Alderman EL, Bourass MF, Cohen LS, et al. Ten-year follow-up of survival and myocardial infarction in the randomized coronary artery surgery study. Circulation 1990;82:1629.

31.	Burns WB, Hermiller JB, Kisslo KB, Culp SC, Davidson CJ. Prognostic significance of left main coronary artery disease detected by intravascular ultrasound. J Am Coll Cardiol 1995;25:143A

32.	Harris WO, Itigano ST, Reeder GS, Lerman A. Assessment of indeterminate left main coronary artery lesions with intravascular ultrasound. Circulation 1994;90:I-157.

33.	Litvack F, Grundfest WS, Lee ME, et al. Angioscopic visualization of blood vessel interior in animals and humans. Clin Cardiol 1985;8:65-70.

34.	Grundfest WS, Litvack F, Sherman T, et al. Delineation of peripheral and coronary detail by intraoperative angioscopy. Ann Surg 1985;202:394-400.

35.	Sanborn TA, Rygaard JA, Westbrook BM, et al. Intraoperative angioscopy of saphenous vein and coronary arteries. J Thorac Cardiovasc Surg 1986;91:339-343.

36.	White CJ, Ramee SR, Collins TJ, et al. Percutaneous angioscopy of saphenous vein coronary bypass grafts. J Am Coll Cardiol 1993;21:1181-1185.

37.	Annex BH, Larkin TJ, O'Neill WW, et al. Evaluation of thrombus removal by transluminal extraction coronary atherectomy by percutaneous coronary angioscopy. Am J Cardiol 1994;74:606-609.

38.	King SB III: Role on new technologies in balloon angioplasty. Circulation 1991;84:2574-2579.

39.	Forrester JS, Eigler N, Litvack F: Interventional Cardiology: the decade ahead. Circulation 1991;84:942-944.

40.	Waxman S, Mittleman MA, Manxo K, Saaower M, et al. Culprit lesion morphology in subtypes of unstable angina as assessed by angioscopy. Circulation 1995;92:I-79.

41.	Waxman S, Saaower M, Mittleman MA, Nesto RW, et al. Characterization of the culprit lesion underlying thrombus: insights from angioscopy. Circulation 1995;92:I-353.

42.	Uchida Y, Nakamura F, Tomaru T, Mortia T, et al. Prediction of acute coronary syndromes by percutaneous coronary angioscopy in patient with stable angina. Am Heart J 1995;130:195-203.

43.	Silva JA, Escobar A, Collins TJ, Ramee SR, White CJ. Unstable angina. A comparison of angioscopic findings between diabetic and nondiabetic patients. Circulation 1995;92:1731.

44. White CJ, Ramee SR, Collins TJ, et al. Coronary thrombi increase PTCA risk, angioscopy as a clinical tool. Circulation 1996;93:253-258.

45. Annex BH, Ajluni SC, Larkin TJ, et al. Angioscopic guided interventions in a saphenous vein bypass graft. Cathet Cardiovasc Diagn 1994;31:330-333.

46. Nath FC, Muller DWM, Ellis SG, et al. Thrombosis of a flexible coil coronary stent: frequency, predictors and clinical outcome. J Am Coll Cardiol 1993;21:622-627.

47. Kaplan BM, Safian RD, Grines CL, et al. Usefulness of adjunctive and extraction atherectomy before stent implantation in high-risk aorto-coronary saphenous vein grafts. Am J Cardiol 1995;76:822-824.

48. Tilli FV, Kaplan BM, Safian RD, Grines CL, O'Neill WW. Angioscopic plaque friability: a new risk factor for procedural complications following saphenous vein graft interventions. J Am Coll Cardiol (in-press)

49. Mintz GS, Douek P, Pichard AD, et al. Target lesion calcification in coronary artery disease: an intravascular ultrasound study. J Am Coll Cardiol 1992;20:1149-1155.

50. Pichard AD, Mintz GS, Satler LF, Lent KM, Popma JJ, Kovach JA, Leon MA. The influence of pre-intervention intravascular ultrasound imaging on subsequent transcatheter treatment strategies. J Am Coll Cardiol 1993;21:133A.

51. Tuzcu EM, Berkalp B, DeFranco AC, Ellis SG, Whitlow PW, Franco I, Raymond RE, Nissen SE. The dilemma of diagnosing coronary calcification: angiography vs. intravascular ultrasound. J Am Coll Cardiol 1995 (in-press).

52. Fitzgerald PJ, Muhlberger VA, Moes NY, et al. Calcium location within plaque as a predictor of atherectomy tissue retrieval: an intravascular ultrasound study. Circulation 1992;86:I-516.

53. Kaplan BM, Stewart RE, Reddy VM, O'Neill WW, Safian RD. A prospective study of large vs. small burrs: Intravascular ultrasound substudy in the coronary angioplasty and rotablator atherectomy trial (CARAT). J Am Coll Cardiol 1996 (in press).

54. Fitzgerald PJ, Mullen WL, Yock PG, and the GUIDE Trial Investigators. Discrepancies between angiographic and intravascular ultrasound appearance of coronary lesions undergoing intervention. A report of phase I of the GUIDE Trial. J Am Coll Cardiol 1993;21:118A.

55. Potkin BN, Bartorelli AL, Gessert JM, et al. Coronary artery imaging with intravascular high-frequency ultrasound. Circulation 1990;81:1575-1585.

56. Pandian NG, Kreis A, O'Donnell T. Intravascular ultrasound estimation of arterial stenosis. J Am Soc Echocardiogr 1989;2:390-397.

57. Nissen SE, Gurley JC, Grines CL, et al. Intravascular ultrasound assessment of lumen size and wall morphology in normal subjects and patients with coronary artery disease. Circulation 1991;84:1087-1099.

58. St Goar FG, Pinto FJ, Stadius ML, et al. In vivo coronary intravascular ultrasound imaging: Correlation with angiography. J Am Coll Cardiol 1991;18:952-958.

59. Willard JE, Netto D, Demian SE, et al. Intravascular ultrasound imaging of saphenous vein grafts in vitro: comparison with histologic and quantitative angiographic findings. J Am Coll Cardiol 1992;19:759-764.

60. Hogdson JM, Graham SP, Sheehan H, et al. Percutaneous intravascular ultrasound imaging: Validation of a real time synthetic aperture array catheter. Am J Card Imaging 1991;5:65-71.

61. Tobis JM, Mahon DJ, Moriuchi M, et al. Intravascular ultrasound imaging following balloon angioplasty. Int J Card Imaging 1991;6:191-205.

62. Wong SC, Chuang Y, Schatz R, etal. Predictors for adverse clinical events are different in stents and PTCA: Results from the Stent Restenosis Study. J Am Coll Cardiol 1995;25:125

63. Nissen SE, DeFranco AC, Raymond RD, Franco I, Eaton G, Tuzcu EM. Angiographically unrecognized disease at "normal" reference sites: a risk factor for sub-optimal results after coronary intervention. Circulation 1993;88(4):41.

64. Mintz GS, Painter JA, Pichard AD, Kent KM, Satler LF, Popma JJ, Chuang YC, Bucher TA, Sokolowicz LE, Leon MB. Atherosclerosis in angiographically "normal" coronary artery reference segments: an intravascular ultrasound study with clinical correlations. J Am Coll Cardiol 1995;25(7):1479-1485.

65. Nissen SE, Tuzcy EM, DeFranco AC, et al. Intravascular ultrasound evidence of atherosclerosis at "normal" reference sites predicts adverse clinical outcomes following percutaneous coronary interventions. J Am Coll Cardiol 1994;23:271A.

66. Russo R, Teirstein P for the AVID investigators. Angiography vs. intravascular ultrasound-directed stent placement. Circulation 1995;92:I-546.

67.   Hodgson JMCB, Reddy KG, Suneja R, Nair RN, Lesnefsky EJ, Sheehan HM. Intracoronary ultrasound imaging: Correlation of plaque morphology with angiography, clinical syndrome and procedural results in patients undergoing coronary angioplasty. J Am Coll Cardiol 1993;21:35.

68.   Tobis JM, Mallery J, Mahon D, et al. Intravascular ultrasound imaging of human coronary arteries in vivo. Analysis of tissue characterizations with comparison to in vitro histologic specimens. Circulation 1991;83:913-926.

69.   Richardson PD, Davies JM, Born GVR. Influence of plaque configuration and stress distribution on fissuring of coronary atherosclerotic plaques. Lancet 1989;2:941-944.

70.   Ambrose JA, Tannenbaum MA, Alexopoulos D, et al. Angiographic progression of coronary artery disease and the development of myocardial infarction. J Am Coll Cardiol 1988;12:56-62.

71.   Davies M. A macroscopic and microscopic view of coronary thrombi. Circulation 1990;82 Suppl III:III-1138-1146.

72.   Keren G, Leon MB. Characterization of atherosclerotic lesions by intravascular ultrasound: possible role in unstable coronary syndromes and in interventional therapeutic procedures. Am J Cardiol 1991;68:85B-91B.

73.   Castaneda-Zuniga WR, Formanek A, Tadavarthy M, et al. The mechanism of balloon angioplasty. Radiology 1980;135:565-571.

74.   Block PC, Myler RK, Stertzer S, et al. Morphology after transluminal angioplasty in human beings. N Engl J Med 1981;305:382-385.

75.   Farb A, Virmani R, Atkinson JB, et al. Plaque morphology and pathologic changes in arteries from patients dying after coronary balloon angioplasty. J Am Coll Cardiol 1990;16:1421-1429.

76.   The SHK, Gussenhoven EJ, Zhong Y, et al. Effect of balloon angioplasty on femoral artery evaluated with intravascular ultrasound imagining. Circulation 1992;86:483-493.

77.   Losordo DW, Rosenfeld K, Pieczek A, et al. How does angioplasty work? Serial analysis of human iliac arteries using intravascular ultrasound. Circulation 1992;86:1845-1848.

78.   Waller BF. "Crackers, breakers, stretchers, drillers, scrapers, shavers, burners, welders, and melters": the future treatment of atherosclerotic coronary artery disease? A clinical-morphologic assessment. J Am Coll Cardiol 1989;13:969-987.

79.   Leimgruber PP, Roubin GS, Anderson HV, et al. Influence of intimal dissection on restenosis after successful coronary angioplasty. Circulation 1985;72:530-535.

80.   Holmes DR Jr, Vlietstra RE, Mock MB, et al. Angiographic changes produced by percutaneous transluminal coronary angioplasty. Am J Cardiol 1983;51:676-683.

81.   Waller BF. Morphologic correlates of coronary angiographic patterns at the site of percutaneous transluminal coronary angioplasty. Clin Cardiol 1988;11:817-822.

82.   Waller BF, Orr CM, Pinkerton CA, et al. Coronary balloon angioplasty dissections: "the good, the bad and the ugly." J Am Coll Cardiol 1992;20:701-706.

83.   Kuntz RE, Safian RD, Carozza JP, Fischman RF, Mansour M, Baim DS. The importance of acute luminal diameter in determining restenosis rates after coronary atherectomy and stenting. Circulation 1992;86:1827-1835.

84.   Garratt KN, Holmes DR JR, Bell Mr, et al. Restenosis after directional coronary atherectomy: differences between primary atheromatous and restenosis lesions and influence of subintimal tissue resection. J Am Coll Cardiol 1990;16:1665-1671.

85.   Tenaglia AN, Buller CE, Kisslo KB, et al. Mechanisms of balloon angioplasty and directional coronary atherectomy as assessed by intracoronary ultrasound. J Am Coll Cardiol 1992;20:685-691.

86.   Hinohara T, Rowe MH, Robertson GC, et al. Effect of lesion characteristics on outcome of directional coronary atherectomy. J Am Coll Cardiol 1991;17:1112-1120.

87.   Fitzgerald PJ, Muhlberger VA, Moes NY, et al. Calcium location within plaque as a predictor of atherectomy tissue retrieval: an intravascular ultrasound study. Circulation 1992;86(Suppl I):1-516.

88.   Mintz GS, Potkin BN, Keren G, et al. Intravascular ultrasound evaluation of the effect of rotational atherectomy in obstructive atherosclerotic coronary artery disease. Circulation 1992;86:1383-1393.

89.   Safian RD; Niazi K; Strzelecki M; et al. Detailed angiographic analysis of high-speed rotational atherectomy in human coronary arteries. Circulation 1993;88:961-968.

90. Yock PG, Fitzgerald PJ, Mullen WL. Intravascular ultrasound in strategic approaches in coronary intervention. Editors Stephen G Ellis, David R Holmes, Jr. Williams and Wilkens Company, 1996;121-130.

91. Goldberg S, Columbo A, Almager Y, et al. Has the introduction of intravascular ultrasound guidance led to different clinical results in the deployment of intracoronary stents? Circulation 1994;90:I-612.

92. Segal J, Kern MJ, Scott NA, King III SB, Doucette JW, Heuser RR, Ofili E, Siegel R. Alterations of phasic coronary artery flow velocity in humans during percutaneous coronary angioplasty. J Am Coll Cardiol 1992;20:276-286.

93. Segal J. Applications of coronary flow velocity during angioplasty and other coronary interventional procedures. Am J Cardiol 1993;71:17D-25D.

94. Bowers TR, Stewart RE, O'Neill WW, Reddy VM, Khurana S, Safian RD. Plaque pulverization during Rotablator atherectomy: does it impair coronary flow dynamics? J Am Coll Cardiol 1995;25:96A.

95. Bach R, Kern MJ, Bell C, et al. Clinical application of coronary flow velocity for stent placement during coronary angioplasty. Am J Heart 1993;125:873-880.

96. Bowers TR, Safian RD, Stewart RE, Benzuly KH, Shoukfeh MM, O'Neill WW. Normalization of CFR after stenting, but not after PTCA. J Am Coll Cardiol 1996 (in press).

97. Kern MJ, Aguirre FV, Donohue TJ, Bach RG, Caracole EA, Wolford TL, Khoury A, Mechem C. Impact of residual lumen narrowing on coronary flow after angioplasty and stent: intravascular ultrasound Doppler and imaging data in support of physiologically-guided coronary angioplasty. Circulation 1995;92:I-263.

98. Verna E, Gil R, DiMario C, Sunamura M, Gurne O, Porenta G. Does coronary stenting flowing balloon angioplasty improve distal coronary flow reserve? Circulation 1995;92:I-536.

99. Haude M, Baungart DM Casoaru G, Erbel R. Does adjunct coronary stenting in comparison to balloon angioplasty has an impact on Doppler flow velocity parameters? Circulation 1995;92:I-547.

100. Tobis JM, Mallery J, Mahon D, et al. Intravascular ultrasound imaging of human coronary arteries in vivo: analysis of tissue characterizations with comparison to in vitro histological specimens. Circulation 1991;83:913-926.

101. Bowers TR, Stewart RE, O'Neill WW, Reddy VM, Safian RS. The effect of Rotablator atherectomy and adjunctive balloon angioplasty on coronary blood flow. Circulation (in submission)

102. The D.E.B.A.T.E. Study Group. Are flow velocity measurements after PTCA predictive of recurrence of angina or of a positive exercise stress early after balloon angioplasty? Circulation 1995;92:I-264.

103. Nemoto T, Kimure K, Shimizu T, Mochida Y, et al. Coronary artery flow velocity waveform in acute myocardial infarction with angiographic no-reflow. Circulation 1995;92:I-325.

104. Eichhorn E, Grayburn PA, Willard JE, Anderson HV, Bedotto JB, Carry M, Kahn JK, Willerson JT. Spontaneous alterations in coronary blood flow velocity before and after coronary angioplasty in patient with severe angina. J Am Coll Cardiol 1991;17:43-52.

105. Anderson HV, Kirkeeide RL, Stuart Y, Smalling RW, Heibig J, Willerson JT. Coronary artery flow monitoring following coronary interventions. Am J Cardiol 1993;71:62D-69D.

106. Kern MJ, Aguirre FV, Donohue TJ, Bach RG, Caracole EA, Flynn MS, Wolford T, Moore JA. Continuous coronary flow velocity monitoring during coronary interventions: velocity trend patterns associated with adverse events. Am Heart J 1994;128:426-434.

107. The D.E.B.A.T.E. Study Group. Cyclic flow variations after PTCA are predictive of immediate complications. Circulation 1995;92:I-725.

108. Anderson HV, Revana M, Rosales O, Brannigan L, Stuart YH, Weisman H, Willerson JT. Intravenous administration of monoclonal antibody to the platelet GP IIb/IIIa receptor to treat abrupt closure during coronary angioplasty. Am J Cardiol 1992;69:1373-1376.

109. White CJ, Ramee SR, Collins TJ, et al. Percutaneous coronary angioscopy: applications in interventional cardiology. J Interven Cardiol 1993;6:61-67.

110. Sassower MA, Abela GS, Koch JM, et al. Angioscopic evaluation of periprocedural and postprocedural abrupt closure after percutaneous coronary angioplasty. Am Heart J 1993;126:444-450.

111. Feld S, Ganim M, Vaughn WK, Kelly R, et al. Utility of angioscopy and intravascular ultrasound in predicting outcome following coronary intervention. Circulation 1995;92:I-785.

382

112. Bauters C, Lablanche JM, McFadden E, Hamon M, Bertrand ME. Angioscopic thrombus is associated with a high risk of angiographic restenosis. Circulation 1995;92:I-401.
113. Teirstein PS, Schatz RA, Rocha-Singh KJ, et al. Coronary stenting with angioscopic guidance. J Am Coll Cardiol 1992;19:223A.
114. Kern MJ, Donohue TJ. Stenosis severity assessment with intracoronary Doppler in Coronary Revascularization and Imaging. Williams and Wilkens 1996;159-170.
115. Erbel RM, Ge J, Gerber T, et al. Safety and limitations of intravascular ultrasounds experience with 325 consecutive procedures. Circulation 1992;86:I-779.
116. Waxman S, Mittleman MA, Manxo K, Saaower M, et al. Culprit lesion morphology in subtypes of unstable angina as assessed by angioscopy. Circulation 1995;92:I-353.
117. Wolff MR, Resar JR, Stuart RS, et al. Coronary artery rupture and pseudoaneurysm formation resulting from percutaneous coronary angioscopy. Cathet Cardiovasc Diagn 1993;28:47-50.
118. Alfonso F, Hernandez R, Goicolea J, et al. Angiographic deterioration of the previously dilated coronary segment induced by angioscopic examination. Am J Cardiol 1994;74:604-606.
119. Kaplan BM, Safian RD, Grines CL, et al. Usefulness of adjunctive angioscopy and extraction atherectomy before stent implantation in high-risk aorto-coronary saphenous vein grafts. Am J Cardiol 1995;76:822-824.
120. Lablanche JM, Gerschwind H, Cribier A, et al. Coronary angioscopy safety survey: European multicenter experience. J Am Coll Cardiol 1995;25:154A.
121. Rosenfield K, Losordo DW, Ramaswamy K, et al. Three dimensional reconstruction of human coronary and peripheral arteries from images recorded during two dimensional intravascular ultrasound examination. Circulation 1991;84:1938-1956.
122. Coy KM, Park JC, Fishbein MC, et al. In vitro validation of three dimensional intravascular ultrasound for the evaluation of arterial injury after balloon angioplasty. J Am Coll Cardiol 1992;20:692-700.

Index

acute coronary syndromes, 216–217
adenosine, 137, 141, 146, 347
ambiguous coronary lesions, 39–40
Ambrose classification system, 54, 62–63, 67, 72, *see also* type I lesions; type II lesions; type III lesions
American College of Cardiology/American Heart Association (ACC/AHH) classification, 21, 22–23, 251, 252, 253, 262, 265, 267, 268, 269, 311, 319, *see also* type A lesions; type B lesions; type C lesions
  description of, 340
  relevance of, 266
Amsterdam-Miami-Rotterdam-Eindhoven (AMROE) trial, 319
aneurysms, 305
angina, *see* stable angina; unstable angina
angiography, 1–23, 31, 161–170, 346
  of ambiguous coronary lesions, 39–40
  angioscopy compared with, 11–12, 95, 214–216
  atherosclerosis not detected by, 161–162, 169–170, 241, 245, 281
  autopsy and natural history studies compared with, 164–166
  of calcified lesions, 18–19, 42, 285, 304
  of complex lesions, 2–4
  contrast streaming and, 13
  of coronary arterial flow, 19–20
  coronary flow reserve and, 141–143
  of eccentric lesions, 4–7, 285
  of filling defects, 9–12
  intravascular ultrasound compared with, 12, 38–40, 42, 43–44, 245, 246, 284–288
  of irregular lesions, 14–15
  lesion length and, 16–17, 319
  lesion physiology predicted from, 137–140
  limitations of, 32–33, 161–162, 169–170, 230, 241, 281, 343–344

  morphology of, 168–169
  of ostial lesions, 321
  percutaneous transluminal coronary angioplasty and, 286
  postmortem, 71
  post-procedural, 316
  prior to myocardial infarction, 162–164, 168–169
  prior to Q-wave myocardial infarction, 179
  progression of disease and, 167–168
  quantitative luminal measurements and, 40
  of restenosis, 311–312, 313–317, 318, 319, 321, 325
  of rough lesions, 14–15
  silent disease on, 38–39
  stent deployment and, 43–44, 296–297
  of ulcerations, 7–8
  vessel size and, 318
Angiojet, 357
angioplasty, *see* percutaneous transluminal coronary angioplasty
angioscopy, 83–98, 211–238, 344, 375–376
  acute coronary syndromes defined with, 216–217
  angiography compared with, 11–12, 95, 214–216
  characterization of lesion morphology with, 352–357
  choice of vessel, 88
  classification of images, 213–214
  clinical applications of, 353
  clinical presentation in, 89–91
  comparative utility of, 346
  complications of, 372–373
  during coronary and peripheral vascular surgery, 220–221
  during coronary interventions, 91, 217–219, 353
  description of equipment, 85–87
  description of procedure, 89

historical development of, 83–85
limitations of, 230
new technology in, 212–213
post-intervention assessment with,
    370–371
preparation in, 88–89
restenosis and, 90, 95, 218–219, 312
safety of, 87–88, 372–373
stent placement and, 219
unstable angina and, 196, 216, 217, 354
unusual uses of, 373–374
angulated stenosis, 259–260
animal studies, *see* experimental studies
aorto-ostial lesions, 263, 321
application-specific ultrasound processing
    software (ASUP), 104
aspirin, 195, 299
atherectomy, 2
angioscopy and, 218, 220–221
computerized 3-D intravascular
    reconstruction and, 112
directional, *see* directional coronary
    atherectomy
proximal LAD and, 322
restenosis and, 322
atherectomy index, 292
atherosclerosis, 239–247, *see also* plaque
angiography limitations in detection of,
    161–162, 169–170, 241, 245, 281
autopsy and natural history studies of,
    165–166
contribution to coronary artery disease
    and mortality, 240
intravascular ultrasound detection of,
    245–246
risk stratification of, 40
transplant, 39–40
automatic pull-back devices, 41
autopsy studies, 164–166, 287
average peak velocity (APV), 366, 369
AVID trial, 361

Balloon versus Optimal Atherectomy Trial
    (BOAT), 317
BENESTENT, 315
bifurcation lesions
intravascular ultrasound of, 39, 350
percutaneous transluminal coronary
    angioplasty and, 253, 256–257
protected, 257
unprotected, 257
biliary Palmaz-Schatz stents, 297
biplane analysis, 64, 67
blood speckle, 36
branched artery system, 148–149

bridging collaterals, 253, 254

calcified lesions, 48, 260–261, 282
angiography of, 18–19, 42, 285, 304
characteristics of, 18–19
directional coronary atherectomy and,
    294
intravascular ultrasound of, 37–38, 40,
    244, 287, 288, 294, 304–305,
    323–324, 358–360
restenosis and, 322–324, 325
rotational atherectomy and, 302, 303–304
Canadian Coronary Atherectomy Trial
    (CCAT), 294, 296, 322
Cardiac Measurement System (CMS), 317,
    320
cardiac transplantation, 39–40, 148,
    245–246
cardioscopes, 84
CARPORT study, 315, 318, 322, 323,
    327–328
catheters, angioscopy, 85–87
catheters, intravascular ultrasound, 242,
    246, 305
design of, 33–34
improvements in, 283
laboratory techniques for, 34–35
c7E3, 259
Cleveland Clinic, 259, 269, 321
closure, 216, 219, 258, 261, 262, 369
CLOUT, 291
collagen, 181, 293
collage type 1, 199
collage type 3, 199
complex lesions, 189, 190–192
angiography of, 2–4
angioscopy of, 90
characteristics of, 54
computerized techniques and, 71–72
histologic and biochemical correlates of,
    2–4
restenosis and, 68, 75
complications, 371–373
of angioscopy, 372–373
of Doppler guidewires, 371–372
of intravascular ultrasound, 372
of percutaneous transluminal coronary
    angioplasty, 268
computerized techniques, 53–77
background on, 53–54
clinical applications of, 61–69
method in, 55–57
morphometric parameters in, *see*
    integrated error/cm; number of
    major features/cm; peaks/cm;

scaled edge length ratio; summed
maximum errors/cm
reproducibility in, 61
computerized three-dimensional
intravascular reconstruction, 103–118,
282–284, 375
archival storage in, 106
concept of, 104–105
current and future applications of,
112–118
image processing algorithms
requirements in, 105
utility of, 106–107
computerized tomography (CT), 18–19,
103, 104, 105
contrast streaming, 13
cornary surgery, 220–221
coronary angiographic analysis system
(CAAS), 313, 317, 319
coronary angiography, see angiography
Coronary Angioplasty versus Excisional
Atherectomy Trial (CAVEAT), 264,
265, 294, 296, 321, 322
coronary arterial flow, see coronary blood
flow
coronary artery bypass surgery (CABG),
179–180, 196
emergent, 254, 258, 263, 264
myocardial infarction after, 163–164, 169
percutaneous transluminal coronary
angioplasty and, 254, 258,
263–265, 326–327
restenosis in grafts, 326–327
coronary artery disease, 240
Coronary Artery Surgery Study (CASS),
166, 167, 169, 320, 351
coronary blood flow
angiography of, 19–20
in branched artery system, 148–149
changing stenosis morphology and, 130
grading system for, 19–20, 253
inlet geometry and shear stress in, 136
length and diameter of stenosis in,
133–136
lesion severity and, 137
variable lesion geometry and, 131–133
velocity, see velocity flow
volume, see volume flow
coronary flow reserve (CFR), 139,
347–348, 366–367, 368, 369
angiography and, 141–143
distal bed vasodilation and, 123–126
coronary Palmaz-Schatz stents, 297
crescendo angina, 198
culprit lesions, 168–169, 185, 189, 216, 352

curvature analysis, 15, 55–56, 72–73
curvature peaks, 56, 57
curvature signature, 15, 56–57, 58, 60, 64,
66
cytokines, 199

DEBATE study, 367
diabetes, 126, 149, 352
diastolic to systolic velocity ratio (DSVR),
148, 150, 151, 152, 154, 366
diffuse disease, 162, 286
dipyridamole, 141
directional coronary atherectomy (DCA),
3, 366
calcified lesions and, 323, 359
coronary artery bypass grafts and,
326–326
eccentric lesions and, 292–293, 305, 320
future implications for, 295–296
guided, 295, 296
intravascular ultrasound and, 41–42,
291–296, 304
luminal gain and, 314
morphologic features of, 291–292
ostial lesions and, 321, 350
post-intervention assessment and,
364–365
restenosis and, 317, 320, 325, 326–327,
364
total occlusion and, 325
trial data on, 293–294
dissections, 363
angiography of, 214–215, 288
angioscopy of, 214–215, 352, 370
directional coronary atherectomy and,
292
percutaneous transluminal coronary
angioplasty and, 149–152, 291
restenosis and, 326
rotational atherectomy and, 303
stents and, 297, 305
distal bed vasodilation, 123–126
distal embolization, 256, 258, 264–265
Doppler guidewires, 138, 148, 371–372
Doppler ultrasound, 121, 126, 140, 141,
142, 344, 375–376
characterization of lesion severity and,
347–349
clinical applications of, 353
comparative utility of, 346
dissections and, 149
interventional applications of, 353
intravascular ultrasound compared with,
350, 352

386

post-intervention assessment by, 366–370
unusual uses of, 373
Dottering effect, 317

eccentric lesions, 152, 189, 190
  angiography of, 4–7, 285
  characteristics of, 4–7
  directional coronary atherectomy and, 292–293, 305, 320
  intravascular ultrasound of, 38, 39, 292–293, 321, 350
  percutaneous transluminal coronary angioplasty and, 261–262, 320
  restenosis and, 320–321
echogenic plaque, 293–294, 324
echolucent plaque, 293–294
elastic recoil, 321, 322
endoluminal grafts (ELG), 118
endoluminal stents, 321
Ermenonville classification system, 12
EUROpean Carvedilol Atherectomy REstenosis (EUROCARE) trials, 317
European Multicenter study, 327
European Working Group on Coronary Angioscopy, 12, 213
Evaluation of c7E3 in the Prevention of Ischemic Complications (EPIC), 91, 259
excimer lasers, 366
  angioscopy and, 218
  calcified lesions and, 305, 324
  coronary artery bypass grafts and, 326–326
  intravascular ultrasound and, 305
  ostial lesions and, 321, 322
  restenosis and, 319, 320, 322, 325, 326–327
  total occlusion and, 325
exercise, 131
experimental studies
  of angioscopy during coronary interventions, 217
  of lesion severity, 137
  of shear stress, 136
  of variable lesion geometry, 131–133

fibrin, 183, 194–195, 197, 200, 293
fibrinogen, 200
fibrinopeptide A (FPA), 3
fibrous plaque
  intravascular ultrasound of, 37–38, 40, 47, 244, 362
  restenosis and, 324
  rupture of, 198–200

filling defects, 9–12, 188, 257
Flowire, 347
foam cells, 198, 264
fractal analysis, 56, 57
friable plaque, 352, 357, 371

Gaussian distribution model, 313
geometric remodeling, 281, 286
Gianturco-Rubin stents, 44, 107, 297
Global Utilization of Streptokinase and t-PA for Occluded Coronary Arteries (GUSTO) Study, 74
glycoprotein IIb/IIIa receptor inhibition, 200, 353, 370
grade 0 flow, 19–20
grade 1 flow, 19–20, 253
grade 2 flow, 19–20
grade 3 flow, 19–20
grade 0 thrombi, 10
grade 1 thrombi, 10
grade 2 thrombi, 10
grade 3 thrombi, 10
grade 0 ulcerations, 7
grade 1 ulcerations, 7
grade 2 ulcerations, 7
gray scale analysis, 244
Guidance by Ultrasound Imaging for Decision Endpoints (GUIDE) trial, 289, 290, 325, 326, 360, 364
guided directional coronary atherectomy (GDCA), 295, 296

heparin, 35, 152, 195, 258, 370
holmium lasers, 218
Hydrolyzer, 357
hyperemia, 126, 127, 134, 140, 145
hypertension, 149

ImageCath®, 85–87
inlet geometry, 136
integrated error/cm, 58, 61
  description of, 56
  restenosis and, 68, 69, 70
  unstable angina and, 62, 63, 65, 72
Interferon-gamma, 199
International Atherosclerosis Project, 240
intimal disruption, 216, 217, 233, 236
intimal thickening, 245–246
intravascular ultrasound (IVUS), 31–50, 239–247, 281–306, 344, 375–376
  abnormal morphology in, 37
  ambiguous coronary lesions and, 39–40
  angiographically silent disease and, 38–39

angiography compared with, 12, 38–40, 42, 43–44, 245, 246, 284–288
angioscopy and, 91, 95
artifacts of, 35–36
atherosclerosis detected with, 245–246
of calcified lesions, 37–38, 40, 244, 287, 288, 294, 304–305, 323–324, 358–360
catheters in, *see* catheters, intravascular ultrasound
characterization of lesion morphology with, 352, 358–363
characterization of lesion severity with, 347, 349–352
clinical applications of, 353
comparative utility of, 346
complications of, 372
device selection and, 304–305
diagnostic applications of, 38–39
directional coronary atherectomy and, 41–42, 291–296, 304
of eccentric lesions, 38, 39, 292–293, 321, 350
future directions of, 44
interventional applications of, 40–44, 353
limitations of, 35–36, 246
normal anatomy and, 36–37
percutaneous transluminal coronary angioplasty and, 41, 49, 284–291, 305, 363
plaque composition determined by, 244, 362–363
plaque distribution determined by, 362–363
plaque quantification by, 243–244
post intervention assessment by, 363–366
quantitative luminal measurements, 40
rationale for use of, 242
restenosis and, 29, 41, 289, 312, 316, 323–324, 325
risk stratification of atherosclerotic lestions and, 40
rotational atherectomy and, 43, 302–304, 305
safety of, 35, 372
stent placement and, 43–44, 296–302, 305
systems in, 242–243
theoretical advantages of, 33
three-dimensional, *see* computerized three-dimensional intravascular reconstruction
unusual uses of, 373
INtravascular ultraSound PredIctors REstenosis (INSPIRE), 290

irregular lesions, 54, 166
angiography of, 14–15
characteristics of, 14–15
myocardial infarction and, 169
scaled edge length ratio and, 57
ischemia, 88, 126, 131
ischemic preconditioning, 181, 194
isoproterenol, 133

Johnson and Johnson stents, 298

laser balloons, 314
laser guide wires, 325
left anterior descending (LAD) lesions, 152, 322, 354
left main coronary artery (LMCA) lesions, 350, 351
left ventricular ejection fraction, 166
left ventricular hypertrophy, 126, 149
lesion diameter, 133–136
lesion geometry, 131–133
lesion length
angiography and, 16–17, 319
coronary blood flow and, 133–136
determination of, 16
percutaneous transluminal coronary angioplasty and, 253, 254, 262–263
restenosis and, 74–75, 319–320
lesion physiology, 137–140
lesion severity
coronary blood flow and, 137
intravascular ultrasound and, 347, 349–352
non-Q wave myocardial infarction and, 184–188
low density lipoprotein (LDL) cholesterol, 198
luminal diameter, 285–286, 325
minimal, 314–315, 316, 319, 320, 323
luminal gain, 314
luminal narrowing, 240

macrophages, 183, 199
magnetic resonance imaging (MRI), 103, 104, 105
MAPS Study Group, 259, 260, 265
Mayo Clinic, 163
mechanical transducers, 34, 36, 282
MERCATOR study, 315, 318, 322, 323
methoxamine, 133
Microvision® system, 85
minimal luminal diameter, 314–315, 316, 319, 320, 323
minimal residual stenosis, 296–297
mixed plaque, 324

Monckeberg medial sclerosis, 18
mortality rates
    atherosclerosis as major contributor to,
        240
    for percutaneous transluminal coronary
        angioplasty, 263, 264
MRA, 365
multi-element electronic designs, 34
myocardial infarction, 161–170, *see also*
        non-Q wave myocardial infarction;
        Q-wave myocardial infarction
    angiography prior to, 162–164, 168–169
    angioscopy and, 216, 217
    autopsy and natural history studies of,
        164–166
    irregular lesions and, 15
    from non-stenotic lesions, 162–164
    percutaneous transluminal coronary
        angioplasty and, 164, 169, 264
    rough lesions and, 14, 54, 169
    shear stress and, 136
    thrombi characterisitics in, 194–195
    ulcerations and, 7–8, 198
myocardial perfusion imaging, 141–143

napkin-ring lesions, 38
National Heart Lung and Blood Institute
        Registry of Coronary Angioplasty, 21,
        251, 262, 325, 326
natural history studies, 164–166
neolumen: balloon ratio (NLBR), 288
nicardipine, 167
nitroglycerin, 130, 133, 134, 347, 372
non-Q wave myocardial infarction,
        177–201
    moderate coronary stenosis and, 179–181
    stenosis severity, thrombus burden and
        time course in, 184–188
    thrombosis and vasospasm in, 181–183
    unstable angina distinguished from, 186,
        197
non-stenotic lesions, 162–164
non-uniform rotational distortion (NURD),
        36, 282–283
no-reflow phenomenon, 355, 357, 367, 373
nuclear echocardiography, 31
number of major features/cm, 58, 61
    description of, 56–57
    restenosis and, 68, 69, 70, 72
    unstable angina and, 62, 63, 65

onionskin pattern, 37
Optimal Atherectomy Restenosis Study
        (OARS), 294, 296, 317

Optimal Stent Implantation (OSTI) study,
        298
Oracle-Micro™, 34
Oracle™, 44
ostial lesions, 321–322, 350

Palmaz-Schatz stents, 50, 107, 109, 297,
        314, 315, 326, 327, 367
    biliary, 297
    coronary, 297
Palmaz 204 stents, 112
PARK, 315, 322
passive collapse, 132
peaks/cm, 58
    description of, 56
    restenosis and, 68, 69, 70
    unstable angina and, 61–62, 63, 64, 65,
        72
percent diameter stenosis, 285–286,
        343–344
percutaneous transluminal coronary
        angioplasty (PTCA), 2, 20–23, 161,
        251–269, 357
    angioscopy and, 12, 88, 217–218
    angulated stenosis and, 259–260
    aorto-ostial lesions and, 263
    balloon size and, 263, 290–291
    bifurcation lesions and, 253, 256–257
    calcified lesions and, 260–261, 323, 324,
        360
    closure and, *see* closure
    computerized 3–D intravascular
        reconstruction and, 112
    coronary artery bypass grafts and, 254,
        258, 263–265, 326–327
    degree of stenosis and, 256
    directional coronary atherectomy
        compared with, 42, 291
    dissections and, 149–152
    Doppler ultrasound and, 366–369, 371
    eccentric lesions and, 261–262, 320
    future implications for, 290–291
    improvements in, 253
    interobserver variability in lesion
        assessment, 265–266
    intravascular ultrasound and, 41, 49,
        284–291, 305, 363
    lesion length and, 253, 254, 262–263
    luminal gain and, 314
    morphologic features of, 284–290
    myocardial infarction and, 164, 169, 264
    ostial lesions and, 321
    plaque composition and, 324
    proximal left anterior descending lesions
        and, 322

proximal tortuosity and, 259–260
restenosis following, 90, 289, 290,
    311–312, 316, 317–319, 320, 321,
    322, 324, 325
success rates for, 253, 254, 257–258,
    260, 266, 267
thrombi and, 10–11, 257–259
total occlusion and, 253–256, 265
trial data on, 289–290
unstable angina and, 195–196, 258, 259
percutaneous transluminal coronary
    rotational atherectomy (PTCRA), see
    rotational atherectomy
peripheral vascular surgery, 220–221
pincushion distortion, 216
plaque, see also atherosclerosis; specific
    techniques for removing
angioscopy of, 90–91, 352, 370
calcified, see calcified lesions
color of, see white plaque; yellow plaque
echogenic, 293–294, 324
echolucent, 293–294
fibrous, see fibrous plaque
friable, 352, 357, 371
intravascular ultrasound determination
    of composition, 244, 362–363
intravascular ultrasound determination
    of distribution, 362–363
intravascular ultrasound quantification
    of, 243–244
restenosis and composition of, 324–325
rotational atherectomy for, see rotational
    atherectomy
soft, see soft plaque
stable, see stable plaque
ulcerated, see ulcerations
unstable, see unstable plaque
plaque burden, 240, 246–247, 285, 286
plaque compression, 287
plaque disruption
angioscopy and, 235, 237
classification of, 229
in complex lesions, 3
percutaneous transluminal coronary
    angioplasty and, 284, 287, 288, 289
plaque fracture, 287, 289
plaque plus media, 282
plaque rupture, 169, 363
angioscopy of, 90
conditions favoring, 198–200
disease progression and, 189
lesion location and, 192
non-Q wave myocardial infarction and,
    197–198
platelet aggregation, 181, 182–183, 216

platelet derived growth factor (PDGF), 199
Post IntraCoronary Treatment Ultrasound
    Result (PICTURE), 290, 324–325
postmortem angiography, 71
post-stenotic flow velocity, 145–148
pressure-flow relationships, 121–123, 126
length and diameter of stenosis in,
    133–134
variable lesion geometry and, 133
Prima Total Occlusion Device, 325
Program on the Surgical Control of
    Hyperlipidemias (POSCH), 167, 180
protected bifurcation lesions, 257
proximal left anterior descending (LAD)
    lesions, 322
proximal to distal flow velocity ratio (P/D),
    144–145, 146, 148, 151
proximal tortuosity, 259–260
P-selectin, 3

quantitative luminal measurements, 40
Q-wave myocardial infarction, 177, 190,
    197, 355
angiography prior to, 179
intravascular ultrasound and, 290
non-Q wave myocardial infarction vs.,
    168
percutaneous transluminal coronary
    angioplasty and, 254
stenosis severity, thrombus burden and
    time course in, 184–188

red thrombi, 194, 213, 229, 352, 353
remodeling, 38, 41, 281, 286, 315
reocclusion, see restenosis
residual stenosis, 314–315, 316
minimal, 296–297
restenosis, 311–340
angiography of, 311–312, 313–317, 318,
    319, 321, 325
angioscopy and, 90, 95, 218–219, 312
binary definitions of, 341
computerized techniques and, 64–69,
    73–77
definitions and evaluation of, 312–314
directional coronary atherectomy and,
    317, 320, 325, 326–327, 364
eccentric lesions and, 320–321
echogenic plaque and, 294
inadequate evaluation of, 315–316
intravascular ultrasound of, 41, 289, 290,
    312, 316, 323–324, 325
lesion composition and, 322–324
lesion length and, 74–75, 319–320
lesion morphology and, 317–322

luminal gain and, 314
ostial lesions and, 321–322
plaque color and, 90
plaque composition and, 324–325
review of studies, 316–317
risk factros for, 315
stent, 297
vessel size and, 317–319
right coronary artery stenosis, 87–88
ring-down artifact, 283
Rotablator™, 43
rotational atherectomy, 365, 366, 367
calcified lesions and, 305, 359
high speed, 325
intravascular ultrasound and, 43,
302–304, 305
morphologic features of, 302–303
ostial lesions and, 321
restenosis and, 325
stents and, 373–374
total occlusion and, 325
rough lesions, 54
angiography of, 14–15
characteristics of, 14–15
myocardial infarction and, 14, 54, 169
scaled edge length ratio and, 57

safety, 371–373
of angioscopy, 87–88, 372–373
of Doppler guidewires, 371–372
of intravascular ultrasound, 35, 372
saphenous vein grafts, 355, 356, 371
scaled edge length ratio, 59, 61
description of, 57
restenosis and, 68, 69, 70, 75
unstable angina and, 63
Serial Ultrasound REstenosis (SURE), 290
shear stress, 136
shoulder to shoulder definition, 262
silent disease, 38–39
single pass technique, 293
single photon emission computed
tomographic (SPECT) thallium
imaging, 142
single plane analysis, 64, 67
slotted tube stents, 297
snow-plow effect, 256–257
soft plaque
calcified lesions differentiated from, 359
intravascular ultrasound of, 37, 47, 244,
287, 362
restenosis and, 324, 325
solid-state transducers, 282
stable angina, 166, 190, 196
angiography and, 12

angioscopy and, 216, 218
computerized techniques and, 61–64, 65,
72–73
eccentric lesions and, 6
lesion length and, 17
percutaneous transluminal coronary
angioplasty and, 257–258
reocclusion and, 68, 75
soft plaque and, 287
ulceration and, 7–8
white plaque and, 95, 218
stable plaque
angioscopy of, 213–214, 232, 235
classifiction of, 229
steal syndrome, 373
stent restenosis, 297
stents, 2, 366
angioscopy during placement of, 219
calcified lesions and, 359, 360
endoluminal, 321
future implications for, 301–302
Gianturco-Rubin, 44, 107, 297
intravascular ultrasound and, 43–44,
296–302, 305
Johnson and Johnson, 298
luminal gain and, 314
morphologic features of, 296–297
ostial lesions and, 321
Palmaz-Schatz, see Palmaz-Schatz stents
Palmaz 204, 112
post-intervention assessment and,
365–366
rotational atherectomy and, 373–374
slotted tube, 297
trial data on, 297–301
Wallstent, 320, 327
Wiktor, 297
wire, 297
stent thrombosis, 298–299
Stent versus balloon Angioplasty for
aorto-coronary saphenous Vein
bypass graft (SAVED) trial, 327
streptokinase, 64, 76, 179, 185
stress echocardiography, 31
STRUT registry, 302
summed maximum error/cm, 58, 61
description of, 56
restenosis and, 68, 69, 70
unstable angina and, 62, 63, 65, 72
syndrome X, 126

Thorax Center, 253, 318
thrombi
angiography of, 215

angioscopy of, 213–214, 215, 216, 217,
    234, 235, 352–355, 370
classifiction of, 229
color of, *see* red thrombi; white thrombi
complex lesions and, 3
coronary symptoms and, 194–198
filling defects and, 9–12
grading system for, 10
percutaneous transluminal coronary
    angioplasty and, 257–259
in rapid disease progression, 181–183
restenosis and, 75–76, 322–324
stent, 298–299
unstable angina and, 181–183, 190, 195
Thrombolysis and Angioplasty in Unstable
    Angina (TAUSA) trial, 195, 258–259
Thrombolysis in Myocardial Infarction
    (TIMI) studies, 7, 10, 19–20, 185,
    195, 253, 265, 355
thromboxane A2, 183
thromboxane B2, 183
thrombus burden, 184–188
ticlopidine, 299
t-lymphocytes, 199
TOSCA, 326
total occlusion
    percutaneous transluminal coronary
        angioplasty and, 253–256, 265
    Q-wave myocardial infarction and, 197
    restenosis and, 325–326
tPA, 195
transducer ring-down, 36
transforming growth factor-β (TGF-β), 199
translesional flow velocity, 143–145
translesional velocity gradient (TVG), 347,
    348
transluminal extraction catheter (TEC),
    353, 355, 370, 371
    coronary artery bypass grafts and,
        326–327
    ostial lesions and, 321
transplant atherosclerosis, 39–40
type I lesions, 6–7, 67
type II lesions, 3, 6–7
type IIa lesions, 67
type IIb lesions, 67
type III lesions, 67
type A lesions, 251
    characteristics of, 21–22, 252, 340
    percutaneous transluminal coronary
        angioplasty and, 21–22, 265, 266
type B lesions, 311
    characteristics of, 21–22, 252, 340
    percutaneous transluminal coronary
        angioplasty and, 21–22

restenosis and, 315, 319
type B1 lesions, 21, 251, 311
type B2 lesions, 21, 251, 266, 311
type C lesions, 251, 311
    characteristics of, 21–22, 252, 340
    percutaneous transluminal coronary
        angioplasty and, 21–22, 265, 266
    restenosis and, 315, 319

ulcerations, 71, 181
    angiography of, 7–8
    angioscopy of, 90, 352
    characteristics of, 7–8
    grading system for, 7
    myocardial infarction and, 7–8, 198
    restenosis and, 76–77
unprotected bifurcation lesions, 257
unstable angina, 177–201
    angiography and, 12, 168
    angioscopy and, 196, 216, 217, 354
    computerized techniques and, 60, 61–64,
        65, 72–73
    curvature and, 60, 72–73
    dissections and, 149
    Doppler ultrasound assessment of, 347,
        348
    eccentric lesions and, 6
    lesion length and, 17
    moderate coronary stenosis and, 179–181
    non-Q wave myocardial infarction
        distinguished from, 186, 197
    percutaneous transluminal coronary
        angioplasty and, 195–196, 258, 259
    reocclusion and, 68, 75, 77
    shear stress and, 136
    soft plaque and, 287
    stenosis severity, thrombus burden and
        time course in, 184–188
    thrombi in, 181–183, 190, 195
    ulcerations and, 7–8, 352
    vasospasm in, 181–183
    yellow plaque and, 95
unstable plaque, 177–201
    moderate coronary stenosis and, 179–181
    stabilization to prevent, 200–201
    stenosis severity, thrombus burden and
        time course in, 184–188
    thrombosis and vasospasm in, 181–183
urokinase, 195, 217, 259, 370

vasopressin, 133
vasospasm, *see* vessel spasm
velocity flow, 121–123, 140, 160
    in branched artery system, 148
    changing stenosis morphology and, 130

dissections and, 150
post-stenotic, 145–148
translesional, 143–145
variable lesion geometry and, 131
volume flow data vs., 126–127
volume flow vs. in stenosis severity,
127–130
Verapamil, 355, 367
vessel size
intravascular ultrasound determination
of, 360–362
percutaneous transluminal coronary
angioplasty and, 253
restenosis and, 317–319
vessel spasm
in rapid disease progression, 181–183
rotational atherectomy and, 302
volume flow, 121–123, *see also*
pressure-flow relationships
in branched artery system, 148
changing stenosis morphology and, 130
variable lesion geometry and, 131

velocity flow data vs., 126–127
velocity flow vs. in stenosis severity,
127–130

Wallstent, 320, 327
water melon-seed effect, 263
Western Washington Studies, 19
white plaque, 192
angioscopy and, 90–91, 95, 98, 218
in classification system, 229
restenosis and, 218
stable angina and, 95, 218
white thrombi, 194, 353
Wiktor stents, 297
wire stents, 297

yellow plaque, 192
angioscopy and, 90, 93, 95, 98, 218
in classification system, 229
restenosis and, 218
unstable angina and, 95